EQUINE CARDIOLOGY

MARK W. PATTESON
MA, VetMB, PhD, DVC, Cert VR, MRCVS

b

Blackwell
Science

© 1996 by
Blackwell Science Ltd
Editorial Offices:
Osney Mead, Oxford OX2 0EL
25 John Street, London WC1N 2BL
23 Ainslie Place, Edinburgh EH3 6AJ
238 Main Street, Cambridge
  Massachusetts 02142, USA
54 University Street, Carlton
  Victoria 3053, Australia

Other Editorial Offices:
Arnette Blackwell SA
  1, rue de Lille, 75007 Paris
  France

Blackwell Wissenschafts-Verlag GmbH
  Kurfürstendamm 57
  10707 Berlin, Germany

  Feldgasse 13, A-1238 Wien
  Austria

First published 1996

Set in 10/12 pt Souvenir
by DP Photosetting, Aylesbury, Bucks
Printed and bound in Great Britain
at the Alden Press Limited, Oxford
and Northampton

DISTRIBUTORS

Marston Book Services Ltd
PO Box 87
Oxford OX2 0DT
(*Orders:* Tel: 01865 791155
          Fax: 01865 791927
          Telex: 837515)

North America
  Blackwell Science, Inc.
  238 Main Street
  Cambridge, MA 02142
  (*Orders:* Tel: 800 215-1000
            617 876-7000
            Fax: 617 492-5263)

Australia
  Blackwell Science Pty Ltd
  54 University Street
  Carlton, Victoria 3053
  (*Orders:* Tel: 03 347-0300
            Fax: 03 349-3016)

A catalogue record for this title
is available from the British Library

ISBN 0–632–03299–5

Library of Congress
Cataloging-in-Publication Data

Patteson, Mark.
    Equine cardiology/Mark Patteson.
      p. cm.
    Includes bibliographical references
and index.
      ISBN 0–632–03299–5
    (pk. : alk. paper)
      1. Horses–Diseases. 2. Veterinary
    cardiology. I. Title.
SF959.C37P38 1995
636.1'089612–dc20   95-661
                              CIP

Contents

List of Tables

Preface

To state that veterinary medicine is a balance between art and science is a cliché; however, it can be seldom more applicable than to equine cardiology. Judgements are usually based on a subjective assessment, often with a very limited amount of objective information. Equine cardiology often involves giving a prognosis for the future exercise capacity, or safety, of a horse with cardiac disease. There are seldom clear right or wrong answers in these situations. Each case requires judgement based on scientific facts, practical application of the principles derived from them and common sense. However, recent developments, particularly echocardiography, have led to a much greater understanding of cardiac disease, and objective information is now more easily obtained. A thorough understanding of disease, diagnostic techniques and treatment makes it much easier to give a reasoned judgement, upon which a professional opinion is based. The aim of this book is to help to provide a basis for these judgements, and to enable practising vets and students feel that cardiology can be an interesting subject for them and not just for specialists.

In this book there is some overlap between chapters in order to allow easy access to all relevant information at a glance. Quick reference to important information has been made as easy as possible by including salient points in tables within the text. More detailed discussions are also provided and, for those with the time and interest for further study, there is an extensive list of further reading.

There are very few long-term follow-up studies of horses with heart disease and many questions remain unanswered. Much of this book is based therefore on the opinion of the author. For some rare conditions, the text is based on a compilation of published information. Opinions will always be based on a blend of personal experience and information derived from publications and outside influence. If this book helps vets to understand cardiology from both viewpoints then it will have achieved its objectives.

Mark Patteson

Acknowledgements

This book would not have been written without the encouragement and help which others have given me in developing an interest in equine cardiology. This interest evolved during my years in practice and at the University of Bristol School of Veterinary Science. The opportunity to indulge my special interest came through a Horserace Betting Levy Board research training scholarship and was encouraged by referrals from vets in practice and from the stimulation of teaching students. Many colleagues have contributed to my learning, but I owe particular thanks to Dr Christine Gibbs and Dr Paul Wotton. I would also like to pay tribute to Dr Jim Holmes, who was influential in the development of equine cardiology. I was fortunate enough to work with Dr Holmes during the first year of my PhD. I would also like to acknowledge the contribution to the subject made in recent years by Dr Virginia Reef, who has been a guiding light to many cardiologists with an interest in horses, as evident from the number of her publications in the reading list. I am extremely grateful to Paul Wotton and Jill Richardson who read the text and made valuable comments. I would never have completed the book without the encouragement and understanding of my wife Jo.

MWP

List of Abbreviations

2DE	two-dimensional echocardiography
1°AVB	first degree atrioventricular block
2°AVB	second degree atrioventricular block
3°AVB	third degree atrioventricular block
AF	atrial fibrillation
AML	anterior mitral leaflet
ANS	autonomic nervous system
AoV	aortic valve
APC	atrial premature complex
AR	aortic regurgitation
ASD	atrial septal defect
AV	atrioventricular
CHD	congenital heart disease
CHF	congestive heart failure
CT	chordae tendineae
CW	continuous wave
DE	Doppler echocardiography
ECG	electrocardiogram
IVS	interventricular septum
LA	left atrium
LAD	left atrial diameter
LRT	lower respiratory tract
LRTD	lower respiratory tract disease
LV	left ventricle
LVD	left ventricle diameter
LVFW	left ventricular free-wall
LVOT	left ventricular outflow-tract
MR	mitral regurgitation
MV	mitral valve
PA	pulmonary artery
PAVB	partial atrioventricular block
PDA	patent ductus arteriosus
PMI	point of maximal intensity
PRF	pulse repetition frequency
PV	pulmonary valve
PWD	pulsed-wave Doppler echocardiography

RA	right atrium
RCC	right coronary cusp (aortic valve)
RV	right ventricle
RVFW	right ventricular free-wall
SA	sinoatrial
TR	tricuspid regurgitation
TV	tricuspid valve
URT	upper respiratory tract
VF	ventricular fibrillation
VPC	ventricular premature complex
VSD	ventricular septal defect
VTI	velocity/time integral

Chapter 1

Cardiac Anatomy and Physiology

A knowledge of normal anatomy is fundamental to an understanding of both the normal function of the cardiovascular system and the disease processes affecting it. Familiarity with anatomical detail is essential for accurate auscultation and further studies such as echocardiography. A sound knowledge of the physiology of the circulation is required so that the effects of drugs and disease on the heart can be understood. A knowledge of the electrophysiology of the equine heart is essential for the application and interpretation of electrocardiography in this species, in which there are important differences from other species. The response of the cardiovascular system to exercise is an especially important consideration in an athletic species such as the horse.

In this chapter, the normal anatomy and physiology of the equine cardiovascular system are described, with reference to considerations which are of particular importance in this species.

1.1 The circulation

The circulatory system is required to perfuse the tissues of the body with a medium suitable to maintain cell life. It delivers oxygen and nutrients and removes waste products for elimination by the kidneys, liver and lungs. Effective circulation depends on normal electrical activation and mechanical function of the heart, normal cardiac structure and appropriate regulation. The important components of the circulatory system are the heart, great arteries (aorta and pulmonary artery), arterioles, capillaries, venules, great veins and lymphatics. The system is divided into two circuits in series, one supplying systemic requirements and the other serving the pulmonary tissues.

Control of the cardiovascular system is mediated by regulatory centres in the brain via the autonomic nervous system (ANS). The ANS has a neural and a humoral component. Regulation takes place at the level of the heart, vessels and local tissues. In addition, mechanisms regulating renal function and respiration have a profound effect on the cardiovascular system.

1.2 The structure of the heart

The heart is made up of three principal structures, the myocardium, endocardium and pericardium.

1.2.1 The myocardium

The myocardium actively contracts to pump blood into the great arteries and actively relaxes in early diastole to ensure emptying of the veins and filling of the ventricles. It is surrounded by the epicardium and lined by endocardium.

Myocardial cells

The bulk of the myocardium is made up of muscular fibres which contract when they are depolarised. They have the important property that, unlike skeletal muscle, they have a refractory period which prevents tetanic contraction. As a result, electrical stimulation is required for each contraction. Some myocardial cells are specialised for transmission of electrical signals through the heart, forming a specialised conduction system. The electrophysiology of these tissues is different from that of the contractile part of the myocardium and is discussed in more detail below.

Each myocyte is made up of many myofibrils which are aligned along the long axis of the cell. In turn, each myofibril is made up of sarcomeres which are joined in series. The sarcomeres contain interdigitating myofilaments made up of contractile proteins. The cell surface is covered with sarcoplasmic reticulum, which forms invaginations between each of the sarcomeres. This is the source of calcium, which is released when the membrane is depolarised. The contractile fibres contain four proteins. Two proteins form filaments which overlap; the thicker filament is myosin, the thinner, actin. Two regulatory proteins, troponin and tropomyosin, are involved in the formation of cross-bridges between the two filaments. When the cell is stimulated by an excitatory impulse, a complex movement of ions, particularly the release of calcium stored in the sarcoplasmic reticulum, results in an increase in the overlap of the myofilaments and a consequent reduction in the length of the filament and cell, i.e. contraction. Together, the cells form two functional syncytia, divided at the atrioventricular junction, which allow the spread of depolarisation wavefronts throughout the atrial and ventricular myocardium.

Cardiac chambers

The heart is divided into four chambers: two atria which act as priming chambers, and two ventricles, which are the main pumps. In the horse, the heart is positioned almost vertically on the sternum, with the long-axis in a dorso-ventral direction.

The cardiac chambers are adapted for maximum efficiency for the requirement of pumping blood through a high pressure and a low pressure circuit connected in series. The left ventricle (LV) drives blood through the high pressure, high resistant systemic circulation. It is constructed like a piston, forming a cylindrical chamber suited to high pressure pumping. The inflow tract is formed by the mitral valve and the caudal wall of the ventricle, the outflow tract by the cranial wall (interventricular septum) and the centrally positioned aortic valve. These tracts are arranged in a 'V' shape (Figure 1.1). The right ventricle (RV) has a large surface area in comparison to its volume and is more suited to low pressure pumping. The inflow tract is on the right cranial side of the heart, the

Cranial   Caudal

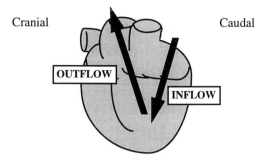

Fig. 1.1 V shape inflow/outflow of LV.
The LV has a 'V' shape relationship between the inflow and outflow tract resembling a piston.

outflow tract is on the left cranial side of the heart (Figure 1.2). Together they form a 'U' shape (Figure 1.3). The RV wraps around the cranial aspect of the LV and its contraction is intimately related to that of the LV. Under normal circumstances, the interventricular septum, which divides the ventricles, contracts as part of the LV.

The atria are situated dorsal to the ventricles and act as receiving chambers, storing returning venous blood until it can empty into the ventricles in early diastole. Blood returns to the right atrium from the caudal vena cava, cranial vena cava and the sinus venosus. Pulmonary veins feed the left atrium with blood returning from the lungs. The lining of the atria is trabeculated, suiting them to their task of storing blood prior to ventricular filling. The atria are relatively thin walled because they pump against low pressure in the normal heart. The right atrium is larger than the left atrium, and at post-mortem examination is usually less tightly contracted.

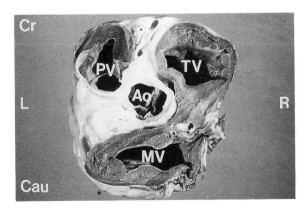

Fig. 1.2 Valve positions.
A cross-section through the heart at the level of the atrioventricular ring shows the position of the valves. The aorta (**Ao**) is centrally positioned, with the tricuspid valve (**TV**) right and cranial, the pulmonary valve (**PV**) left and cranial, and the mitral valve (**MV**) left and caudal.

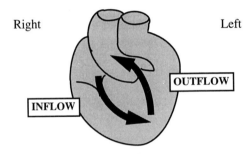

Fig. 1.3 U shape inflow/outflow of RV.
The RV has a 'U' shaped structure and wraps round the cranial aspect of the LV making it suitable for pumping into a low pressure circuit.

Coronary arteries

The coronary arteries are divided into two main trunks. The right coronary artery usually takes more blood flow than the left. The arteries leave the aorta from the sinuses of Valsalva, where their openings are guarded by the valves. Their position in the sinuses ensures that coronary blood flow is not obstructed by the valve leaflets. The majority of coronary blood flow occurs during diastole.

1.2.2 The endocardium

The chambers of the heart are lined with endocardium which is responsible for maintaining a smooth surface, free from thrombi which would have a deleterious effect on the circulation. The endocardium may also have a number of local biochemical regulatory roles, but these are poorly understood. In addition, the endocardium is developed to form the cardiac valves, which maintain movement of blood through the cardiac chambers in series, and prevent back-flow. Abnormalities of the valves may result in regurgitation of blood, which reduces the efficiency of the heart. Valvular regurgitation is a very common abnormality in the horse. Valves can also be stenosed, restricting outflow and increasing the work load on the chambers. However, valvular stenosis is a very rare abnormality in the horse (see section 6.1).

Two types of valve are present in the heart. The atrioventricular (AV) valves divide the atria from the ventricles. They are supported by connective tissue fibres called the chordae tendineae and by the papillary muscles. The tricuspid valve (right AV valve) divides the right side of the heart, has three principal leaflets and is supported by three or more papillary muscles. The mitral valve (left AV valve) divides the left side of the heart and consists of two main leaflets and a number of smaller leaflets. The septal (anterior) mitral leaflet is the largest and divides the inflow and the outflow tracts. The other main leaflet is the caudal (posterior) mitral leaflet. The left and right commissural leaflets are situated between the main leaflets and are variable in number and configuration. The mitral valve is supported by chordae tendineae which branch from two large papillary muscles. Both the right and left papillary muscles support chordae tendineae to the septal and caudal valve leaflets. The chordae tendineae consist of major and minor chordae, with the larger structures supporting the tips of the valves, and chordae of gradually decreasing thicknesses inserting nearer the valve base. The valves normally have a thicker edge than body, but nodule formation on these valves is a common disease process of variable significance (see section 2.4.3). Together, the papillary muscles, chordae and valve leaflets make up a functional unit – the valve apparatus.

The semi-lunar valves are three leaflet structures which are positioned between the ventricles and the great arteries. The aortic valve divides the LV from the aorta. Each valve leaflet has a small nodule in the middle of its leading edge (the corpora Aranti). Slit-like fenestrations are often found along the leading edge of the leaflets, but these are a normal finding. The leaflets are termed the right coronary, left coronary and non-coronary cusps, to reflect their position relative to the coronary arteries. The pulmonary valve divides the RV from the pulmonary artery and is similar in structure to the aortic valve. Similar nodules (corpora Morgoni) and fenestrations may be seen. The pulmonary valve leaflets are much thinner structures than the aortic valve leaflets.

1.2.3 The pericardium

The pericardium is a fibrous sac which surrounds the heart, separating it from the lungs, and its function is mechanical. The heart can function normally in the absence of the pericardium, but operates more efficiently if it is present. It acts as a barrier to infection and allows free movement of the heart within the thoracic cavity. It limits the expansion of the ventricles during diastole, preventing expansion beyond their elastic limits. Disease of the pericardium limits cardiac output by causing diastolic failure, because it prevents normal filling of the atria and ventricles, particularly on the right side (see section 2.2.10).

1.3 The peripheral cardiovascular system

The peripheral cardiovascular system has an essential role in the distribution of blood to supply the requirements of tissues and to remove waste products. It is not just a simple conduit, but controls the relative distribution of blood to different tissues in the body according to demands.

The *aorta* has a highly elastic wall, which stores the force of ventricular contraction so that blood continues to be pumped around the circulation even in diastole. The stiffness of the aorta is controlled by autonomic stimulation and affects impedance to flow. If the aorta becomes abnormally stiff, the load on the LV is increased, and circulation is less efficient.

The *arterioles* are also elastic, but in addition they contain smooth muscle. Their diameter, and therefore the resistance which they offer to blood flow, is controlled by direct innervation, by systemic humoral factors, and by local vasoactive compounds. The relative size of arterioles in different tissues controls the relative distribution of blood within the body. A co-ordinated response is required so that blood pressure is maintained.

The *capillaries* are the site of exchange of nutrients and waste products. The permeability of the capillary wall can alter under some circumstances. The balance of osmotic and hydrostatic pressures across the capillary wall controls the net flow of fluid and electrolytes into the extracellular space. Selective permeability of the capillary walls is required to prevent too much protein crossing the wall and altering the osmotic pressure of the intestinal fluid.

The *venules* collect blood from the capillaries and return it to the great veins. The majority of circulating blood volume is contained within the venules; control of the tone of their walls plays an important role in maintaining blood pressure. When there is a demand for increased cardiac output, constriction of the venules maintains an adequate preload to allow cardiac output to respond to demands.

The *great veins* play a similar role to venules in control of blood pressure and circulating blood volume. The *spleen* also acts as a reservoir for blood, and can release a large number of red cells into the circulation during exercise to increase the oxygen carrying capacity of blood.

The *lymphatic system* is responsible for returning excess interstitial fluid into the venous circulation. This ensures that the interstitial fluid maintains a suitable osmolarity and concentration of electrolytes and proteins.

1.4   Cardiac physiology

In order to interpret auscultatory findings and to appreciate the pathophysiological changes in normal and diseased animals, it is particularly important to understand the mechanical and electrical events which occur during the cardiac cycle. The movement of blood is dependent on pressure gradients between the chambers and the great vessels. The pressure gradients are affected by significant disease processes and changes in these pressure gradients are responsible for signs of congestive heart failure (see section 2.2.1). The acceleration and deceleration of blood during the cardiac cycle is responsible for the normal transient sounds heard during auscultation. The pressure gradients and the rate of change of the gradients are responsible for the characteristics of cardiac murmurs which may occur with normal and abnormal blood flow. The pressures within the atria, ventricles and aorta at different points during the cardiac cycle are shown in Figure 1.4.

1.4.1   The cardiac cycle

The cardiac cycle can be divided into distinct periods determined by electrical and mechanical events.

Systolic events
Systole is the period during which the ventricles develop pressure to drive blood into the great arteries. It can be divided into three intervals.

(1) Electromechanical delay   Electromechanical delay is the time taken for the electrical stimulus to result in activation of the ventricular muscle.

(2) Isovolumetric contraction   The period of isovolumetric contraction is the time when the ventricles have begun to contract, but the volume of the chambers has not yet changed. It occurs immediately after the period of electromechanical delay, following electrical stimulation of the ventricles. During

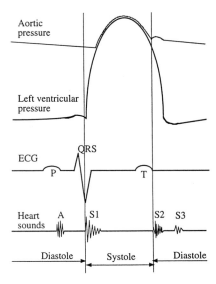

Aortic
pressure

Left ventricular
pressure

ECG

QRS

P

T

Heart
sounds

A

S1

S2 S3

Diastole

Systole

Diastole

Fig. 1.4 **Pressure changes in chambers and vessels.**

this period, intraventricular pressure increases until it is sufficient to open the semi-lunar valves and eject blood into the great arteries. The AV valves have already closed at the onset of isovolumetric contraction, although at slow heart rates they may have slightly re-opened and the increasing ventricular pressure forces them closed.

The *pre-ejection period* includes both electromechanical delay and isovolumetric contraction.

(3) The ejection period Once the semi-lunar valves have opened, the ventricles can eject the forward stroke volume into the systemic circulation. There is a short period during which the velocity of blood flow accelerates to a peak, after which there is a gradual decline until the point at which the aortic and pulmonary artery pressures are sufficiently high to prevent further ejection of blood. In the aorta, the majority of blood flow occurs during the first third of the ejection period. In the pulmonary artery the peak velocity of outflow occurs slightly later in systole.

The duration of *electromechanical systole* is the sum of the pre-ejection period and the ejection period. The length of this period depends on loading conditions and contractility, and is often greater for pulmonary flow.

The force of contraction largely develops from a reduction in the diameter of the ventricles, rather than a shortening of their length. However, the AV ring is drawn towards the ventricles, resulting in a fall in pressure in the atria which draws in blood from the great veins.

Diastolic events
Diastole is the period during which the filling of the ventricles occurs. It can be divided into four intervals. Blood flow principally occurs during two of these periods.

(1) Isovolumetric relaxation At the end of systole, the semi-lunar valves shut and the ventricles relax, resulting in a fall in the intraventricular pressure, initially with no change in the chamber volume. This is an active process, known as the period of isovolumetric relaxation. It ends when the pressure in the ventricles falls to below that in the atria and the AV valves open.

(2) Early diastolic filling At resting heart rates, the majority of the filling of the ventricles occurs during this 'passive' period, when the blood stored in the atrial 'priming' chambers flows rapidly into the ventricles. The period ends when the elastic properties of the ventricle prevent further filling and the intraventricular pressure rises above that in the atria. In fact, relaxation of myocardial cells is an energy consuming process and normal myocardial function is required for normal relaxation and filling.

(3) Diastasis In the horse, at resting heart rates, diastasis is the longest period in diastole. During this phase only a small amount of blood flows from the atria, but this makes a negligible contribution to ventricular filling, the atria acting as conduits for venous return.

(4) Atrial contraction The second period of diastole during which there is significant blood flow is when the ventricles are actively filled by blood from atrial contraction. Atrial contraction has a 'pump-priming' action by increasing the ventricular pressure immediately prior to systole. This increases the strength of ventricular contraction. In the horse, atrial contraction provides only a small proportion of diastolic filling at resting heart rates. However, at higher heart rates, or in animals with abnormal diastolic filling, it is a much more significant component of filling and is essential to maintain preload.

The events of the cardiac cycle are summarised in Figure 1.5.

1.4.2 Autonomic control of the cardiovascular system

The cardiovascular system is under control of both neuronal and humoral components of the ANS. The system acts both on the heart itself and on the peripheral vasculature. The principal aim of the autonomic control of the cardiovascular system is to maintain blood supply to vital organs, particularly the brain. This requires adequate blood pressure, which can be maintained in the short term by altering systemic resistance and cardiac output. In the longer term, blood pressure is controlled by adjusting blood volume via a complex homeostatic mechanism involving the hypothalamus, pituitary gland, adrenal gland and kidney.

The heart is innervated by the sympathetic and the parasympathetic nervous system. Parasympathetic fibres are carried in the vagus nerve and their discharge results in a decreased heart rate and, to a lesser extent, reduced contractility. The sympathetic nervous system acts on the heart via direct neuronal control and also via the release of adrenaline and noradrenaline, mediated by beta receptors. This results in an increased heart rate and increased myocardial contractility. The cardiac centre in the medulla controls both the central and peripheral circulatory system via the ANS. Information on blood pressure is fed to the brain from

A: isovolumetric contraction

D: early diastolic filling

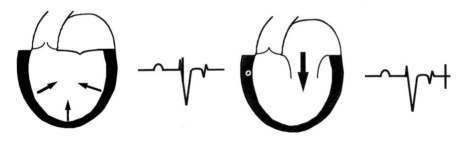

B: ejection period

E: diastasis

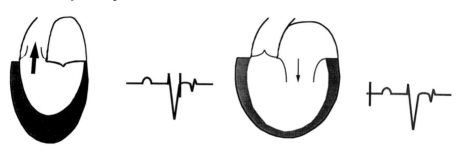

C: isovolumetric relaxation

F: atrial contraction

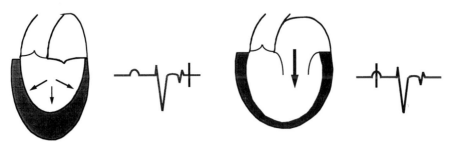

Fig. 1.5 The phases of the cardiac cycle, A–F (see text).

baroreceptors in the ventricles, aortic arch and carotid bodies. The pattern of autonomic control of the heart is shown in Figure 1.6.

1.4.3 Control of cardiac output

Cardiac output depends on stroke volume and heart rate. Stroke volume is dependent on three important factors: preload, afterload and contractility. All of

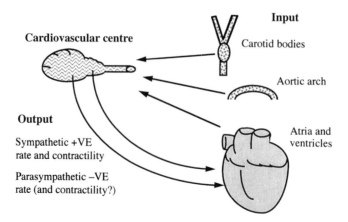

Fig. 1.6 Autonomic control.
Autonomic tone is controlled by the cardiovascular centre in the medulla of the brain. Heart rate and contractility are dependent on the balance between sympathetic and parasympathetic output. Input comes from a number of sources: changes in blood pressure are detected in the aortic arch, carotid bodies and ventricles, and volume changes are detected in the atria. Additional information comes from other centres in the brain.

these factors are inextricably linked (Figure 1.7). It is important that each of these is understood because they are important concepts in cardiology. However, any discussion of these factors invariably includes a substantial amount of over-simplification.

Preload
Preload is the force distending the ventricles. It can be assessed by measuring end-diastolic pressure, or estimated from measurement of end-diastolic dimensions of the ventricles. An intrinsic property of myocardial cells, within normal limits, is that the force of their contraction depends on the length to which they are stretched. The greater the stretch (within certain limits), the greater the force

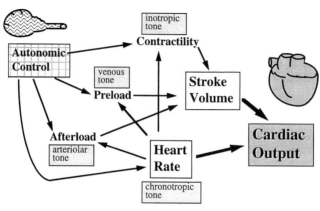

Fig. 1.7 Factors affecting cardiac output.
The factors affecting cardiac output are complex and are interdependent.

of contraction. This property is known as the Frank–Starling phenomenon. It occurs because stretching of the myofibrils results in more efficient creation of cross-bridges between the contractile proteins. Thus, an increase in the distension of the ventricle will result in an increase in the force of contraction sufficient to pump the extra volume. An increase in preload will result in a concomitant increase in cardiac output.

An ability to increase preload is required for animals to be able to maintain a suitable cardiac output in the face of the demands of exercise, systemic vasoconstriction (increased afterload) or cardiac disease. A fixed, low preload restricts cardiac output. This occurs in a number of situations, for example in animals with hypovolaemic or septic shock, or in animals with pericardial effusions which have resulted in cardiac tamponade. Preload may also be too high in certain situations. For example, if there is marked volume overload of the ventricle or poor myocardial contractility which results in a high end-diastolic filling pressure, this will lead to blood 'damming back' into the atria and veins, i.e. congestive heart failure. Diuretics are used to reduce preload and remove the fluid build-up which results from congestive failure (section 6.9.1). Over-diuresis can reduce preload sufficiently that cardiac output is limited and may worsen some of the clinical features of heart failure. Factors which affect preload are summarised in Table 1.1.

Afterload

Afterload is the force against which the ventricles must act in order to eject blood. This is largely dependent on aortic blood pressure, which in turn depends on vascular resistance; however, it also contains a component of myocardial stiffness. Increasing afterload increases myocardial oxygen consumption and may decrease stroke volume. Homeostatic mechanisms usually prevent a fall in blood pressure, which might result from reductions in afterload, by causing vasoconstriction and therefore restoring blood pressure. However, reductions in afterload may also result in an increase in stroke volume and this will maintain blood pressure, within limits. In animals with AV valve regurgitation, there is a reduction in afterload because blood can leak back into the low pressure atria. Thus the total stroke volume will increase, but the forward stroke volume will not change (or may even fall in severe cases). Vasodilators reduce afterload and result in an improved forward stroke volume. Factors which affect afterload are summarised in Table 1.1.

Contractility

The strength of the force of myocardial contraction is dependent on direct autonomic control affecting preload and afterload but also on the contractility of the myocardium. Contractility is a measure of the intrinsic ability of the myocardium to contract to produce a peak tension from a given resting fibre length. This property is independent of loading conditions. It should not be confused with the force of contraction, which is directly affected by preload and afterload. The degree of contractility is also known as the inotropic state. A positive inotropic response is an increase in contractility. Myocardial contractility can be increased directly by sympathetic stimulation, to some extent by a decrease in parasympathetic tone and indirectly by an increase in heart rate.

Table 1.1 Factors affecting preload, afterload, contractility and heart rate

Factors affecting preload
Blood volume
Heart rate
Body position
Phase of respiration (affects intrathoracic pressure)
Respiratory disease (affects intrathoracic pressure)
Muscular pumping of venous blood
Locomotion (affects intrathoracic pressure and venous return)
Atrial contraction
Valvular regurgitation

Factors affecting afterload
Heart rate
Vascular tone (and therefore blood pressure)
Aortic stiffness
Myocardial tension (affected by hypoxia, volume overload)
Metabolic rate
Preload
Valvular regurgitation

Factors affecting contractility
Noradrenaline release from sympathetic nerves (most important)
Increased circulating catecholamines ⎫
Increased heart rate (Bowditch effect) ⎬ increase contractility
Increased afterload (Anrep effect) ⎭
Drugs
Metabolic factors: ⎫
  hypoxia ⎪ increase or
  acidosis ⎬ decrease
  hypercapnia ⎪ contractility
Myocardial disease ⎭

Factors affecting heart rate

Heart disease	Fever
Exercise	Pain
Excitement	Anaemia
Afterload	Systemic disease
Preload	

When contractility is reduced, for example as a result of myocardial disease, stroke volume will fall. This will result in a reflex increase in heart rate and an adjustment in the tone of the peripheral cardiovascular system to ensure that blood pressure is maintained. In the long-term, changes in sodium and water retention will occur, and a high level of catecholamines will be present until an equilibrium is met. To some extent, this will improve contractility via beta receptor mechanisms. Factors which affect contractility are summarised in Table 1.1.

Stroke volume
Stroke volume is the amount of blood ejected by the ventricles per beat. The *ejection fraction* is the proportion of the stroke volume which is ejected (Figure 1.8). Usually this is equal to the *forward stroke volume*, which is the amount ejected into the great arteries. However, when the AV valves leak, some of the

$$\text{Stroke volume} = \text{end-diastolic volume} - \text{end systolic volume}$$

$$\text{Ejection fraction (\%)} = \frac{\text{stroke volume}}{\text{end-diastolic volume}} \times 100$$

$$\text{Regurgitant fraction (\%)} = \frac{\text{total stroke volume} - \text{forward stroke volume}}{\text{total stroke volume}} \times 100$$

Fig. 1.8 Ejection fraction and regurgitant fraction.

blood will flow in a retrograde direction into the atria. The *regurgitant fraction* is the proportion of the end-diastolic volume which flows back into the atria (in the case of AV regurgitation) and makes no contribution to the forward stroke volume. Stroke volume is determined by the volume and pressure of blood filling the ventricles (i.e. preload), the resistance to ejection (i.e. afterload), and myo-cardial cell shortening (i.e. contractility). Long-term changes in stroke volume are mediated by the load imposed on the heart. For example, volume overload as a result of valvular incompetence, or isotonic exercise training, will result in an increase in stroke volume.

Heart rate
Cardiac output is dependent on stroke volume and heart rate. In fact, changes in cardiac output in the horse are usually mediated by changes in heart rate. Pre-load, afterload and contractility alter so that stroke volume can be maintained. The horse has a remarkable capacity to increase cardiac output, by a factor of approximately six-fold from resting values. This is almost entirely due to an increase in heart rate from approximately 24–40 bpm, to a maximal heart rate of the order of 220–240 bpm. Heart rate is controlled by the balance of para-sympathetic and sympathetic innervation. The high vagal tone which is present in normal horses at rest is mediated by the release of the neurotransmitter acetylcholine from parasympathetic synapses. This maintains a slow rate of discharge of the sinoatrial (SA) node and may result in slow or intermittently blocked conduction through the atrioventricular node. It also maintains a rela-tively low inotropic state. The almost instantaneous increase in heart rate to increased demand for cardiac output results from a fall in vagal tone and from the release of noradrenaline from sympathetic fibres, mediated by B1 receptors. The humoral component (adrenaline) takes some minutes to operate, but may have altered in anticipation of an increase in demand for heart rate due to behavioural responses. Catecholamine release also causes an increase in inotropic state. A change in autonomic tone which results in an increase in heart rate is known as a positive chronotropic response. A drug with the same action is known as a positive chronotrope, one with the opposite effect as a negative chronotrope. Factors which affect heart rate are summarised in Table 1.1.

1.4.4 *Control of blood pressure*

Short-term control of blood pressure
The short-term control of blood pressure depends on changes in cardiac output and on vascular resistance and capacitance. Cardiac output is directly affected by

arterial blood pressure, because this is the principal component of afterload. Preload and the force of ventricular contraction are also directly affected by changes in vascular tone, particularly by venous tone. The heart rate is affected by blood pressure via the baroreceptor reflex. In the horse, this is particularly apparent when vagal tone is correlated with aortic pressure. Second degree atrioventricular block often occurs when aortic pressure rises above a level determined by the medulla and the baroreceptors. During the long diastolic interval, the aortic pressure falls, and the cycle is then repeated.

Control of vascular tone
The relative differences in vascular resistance in various tissues dictate the proportion of the cardiac output which perfuses them. This is largely mediated by the tone of the arterioles, which are well supplied by autonomic neurones. Local factors also govern the distribution of the blood flow and, at different times, different organ systems receive more or less blood; however, the brain is always perfused at the expense of other systems. Dramatic changes in muscular and cutaneous blood supply occur during exercise. At this time, blood pressure will fall unless there is an increase in cardiac output. Consequently, despite autonomic control of vascular tone, there is a requirement for a large cardiac reserve in order that demands for an increase in cardiac output can be met. Changes are also mediated by the effects of local vasoactive substances, which act to improve perfusion of hypoxic areas by the systemic circulation. In the lung, however, blood flow to areas of hypoxic tissue is reduced, resulting in a more appropriate distribution of blood in order to maintain gaseous exchange.

In animals with a reduced cardiac output as a result of cardiac disease or hypovolaemia, blood pressure is maintained by an increase in vascular tone. The maintenance of blood pressure under these circumstances requires an increase in systemic vascular resistance (and therefore afterload).

Vascular tone is also important for maintaining preload when there is a demand for an increased cardiac output. Blood pools in the venules and great veins at rest, due to their low muscular tone. At times when blood pressure is in danger of falling, venoconstriction increases venous return and maintains preload. During exercise, skeletal muscular activity increases the return of venous blood from the periphery.

Long-term control of blood pressure
The long-term control of blood pressure is dependent on maintenance of an appropriate blood volume. A complex mechanism involving a number of reflexes and humoral responses centres on adjustments in blood volume mediated by the kidney. For a more detailed description of the mechanisms, readers should refer to specialist texts. In an oversimplified form, the changes which occur when blood volume is decreased can be summarised as follows:

(1) Baroreceptors detect a fall in blood pressure and supply afferent information to the cardiovascular centres.
(2) Volume receptors detect a fall in atrial volume if preload is inadequate.
(3) The juxtaglomerular apparatus detects changes in sodium levels and blood pressure within the kidney.

(4) The thirst centre receives sensory input from osmoreceptors so that water retention can match sodium retention.

(5) Renal blood supply adjusts to a fall in blood pressure by redistribution within the kidney.

(6) Angiotensin levels increase, resulting in an increase in aldosterone secretion by the adrenal cortex and in peripheral vasoconstriction.

(7) Antidiuretic hormone (ADH) levels increase and more water is retained from the collecting ducts by the kidney.

(8) Atrial naturetic peptide (ANP) levels fall in response to changes within the heart, resulting in increased sodium and water retention.

(9) Additional complex changes occur in the kidney, including a change in an unknown factor affecting glomerular filtration.

The overall effect of these mechanisms is to reduce sodium excretion by the kidney. This results in increased retention of water, and maintenance of blood volume. The homeostatic mechanism is well adapted to controlling blood volume. However, inappropriate retention of sodium occurs in congestive heart failure (Chapter 2).

1.4.5 *Myocardial oxygen consumption*

In reviewing the physiological processes involving the cardiovascular system, it is appropriate to consider the oxygen requirements of the heart muscle itself. Oxygen is delivered to the myocardium by coronary blood flow. This flow principally occurs during diastole. Myocardial oxygen requirements are increased by raised heart rate, and high heart rates have the additional effect of decreasing the time available for coronary blood flow. Increased oxygen consumption is also required for conditions in which contractility and afterload are greater than normal. Abnormalities which reduce the capacity of oxygen supply to meet demand lead to an increased wall stiffness, which reduces diastolic filling and increases afterload, and may result in arrhythmias.

1.4.6 *Myocardial wall tension*

Myocardial wall tension is another factor which has an important bearing on cardiac adaptation to physiological and pathological changes in loading conditions. Wall tension is one of the components of afterload, and depends on the distension of the heart by preload. Tension is required to promote contractility via the Frank–Starling mechanism; however, increased tension increases myocardial oxygen consumption.

The long-term response to volume overload is ventricular dilation. Initially, this is a result of changes in the length of sarcomeres. Later the myocytes themselves lengthen and the number of sarcomeres increases. The change in ventricular geometry allows a more efficient contraction and an increased stroke volume can be produced. There is no change in the efficiency of the myocardium until this compensation fails to meet demands and myocardial failure ensues, or if the dilation is sufficient to effect the efficiency of the AV valve apparatus.

A consequence of increased ventricular diameter is increased wall tension.

This relationship is described by the law of Laplace. In a simplified form, this states that wall tension is proportional to the radius of the chamber and the pressure within it, and inversely proportional to the wall thickness. The ventricles therefore respond to increased tension by increasing wall thickness. Pressure overload results in increased wall thickness with no change in the radius of the chamber (concentric hypertrophy) and is rare in the horse. If increased tension is due to volume overload, the ventricle responds (within limits) by increasing in radius without a change in wall thickness. This means that oxygen consumption will not increase unduly and is termed eccentric hypertrophy. The equation summarising the law of Laplace demonstrates this relationship (Figure 1.9). This process of hypertrophy is a normal, healthy response to increased load. In the horse, such loads are normally imposed by exercise training, or by increased preload related to a substantial regurgitant volume. Only at the point of myocardial failure does the wall thickness begin to decrease, resulting in increased tension and oxygen consumption.

$$\text{wall stress } \alpha \frac{\text{internal radius} \times \text{ventricular pressure}}{2 \times \text{wall thickness}}$$

Fig. 1.9 The law of Laplace.
The law of Laplace describes the relationship of the radius of a sphere, the pressure within it, the thickness of the wall and the wall stress.

1.5   The principles of electrophysiology

Normal electrical excitation via the specialised conduction pathway within the heart results in co-ordinated myocardial contraction and relaxation and is essential for efficient cardiac function. Control of the system by internal and higher homeostatic mechanisms results in a normal cardiac rhythm and alters heart rate to maintain an appropriate cardiac output. A knowledge of the anatomy of the normal conduction pathway and the basis of excitation of cells is fundamental to understanding normal and abnormal cardiac function and abnormalities of conduction and rhythm. An appreciation of the differences in the activation process in horses compared with humans and small animals is essential in order that the many misconceptions regarding interpretation of equine ECGs (electrocardiograms) are avoided.

1.5.1   Cellular physiology

The normal activation process within the heart and within each individual myocyte is dependent on specialised cellular physiology. Cardiac tissue has four important characteristics. These properties are present to differing degrees in different cells within the heart.

(1) *Conductivity:* Cardiac cells are joined in a functional syncytium that allows excitation to pass from cell to cell. Specialised cardiac cells have fast or slow

conducting properties which govern the rate of spread of the electrical impulse through them.

(2) *Excitability:* Like nervous tissue, individual cardiac cells exhibit the all-or-none phenomenon, i.e. once a threshold is reached they are completely depolarised by an action potential.

(3) *Automaticity:* Specialised cardiac cells possess automaticity. This means that they will spontaneously depolarise due to the membrane potential gradually becoming less negative until the threshold potential is reached. The rate at which this occurs depends on the type of cardiac tissue and on autonomic nervous control. It is also affected by disease, electrolyte concentrations and by drug therapy.

(4) *Refractoriness:* This property ensures that all cardiac cells have a period after activation during which no level of further stimulus will cause an action potential. It is an important feature of myocardial cells because it prevents tetanic spasm of cardiac muscle. The duration of the refractory period also depends on the type of cardiac tissue, autonomic nervous control, disease states and drug therapy.

These electrophysiological features result from specific properties of the cardiac cell membrane. The membranes contain specialised pumps and channels which selectively concentrate specific ions within the cell and/or remove them from it. The most notable feature is a very high concentration of potassium and low level of sodium within the resting cell. The different concentrations of ions and proteins either side of the membrane result in a potential difference in electrical charge across the cell membrane. The intracellular potential of a resting myocardial cell is −90 mV in comparison with the extracellular fluid. Depolarisation results in a reversal of this potential difference, and is then followed by repolarisation. The process has been divided into five phases, 0–4 (Figure 1.10). During each phase, specific channels and pumps are responsible for movement of different ions, each of which affect the membrane potential. The relative contributions of the different currents which result from this ion movement vary in different tissues within the conduction pathways. This determines the different properties of each specialised cell, and the effects of changes in extracellular ion concentrations, disease and drugs on the cell.

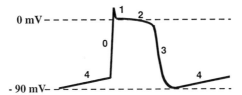

Fig. 1.10 The action potential phases 0–4.
The action potential of myocardial cells has a defined pattern known as phases 0–4. The slope of the phases depends on the exact cell type, autonomic tone, electrolytes, drugs and disease.

1.5.2   The action potential

Depolarisation

Phase 0 represents the depolarisation process, and begins once a cell has reached a certain potential (the threshold potential), spontaneously in the case of pacemaker cells, or as a result of normal depolarisation of adjacent cells in the case of conduction pathway and myocardial cells. In fast-conducting cells such as the Purkinje network and the myocardium, a rapid influx of sodium is responsible for this change in potential. In the slower conducting pacemaker tissues of the SA and AV nodes, the resting potential of the cell membrane is less negative than non-pacemaker cells (around −60 mV). This results in a decreased rate of phase 0 depolarisation and relatively slow conduction. In pacemaker cells, during phase 0 the contribution of the fast inward current carried by sodium is small, and the relatively slow depolarisation process is largely due to movement of calcium ions. Consequently, these tissues are relatively sensitive to changes in calcium concentration and drugs which affect calcium channels.

The plateau phase

The depolarisation phase is followed by a relatively small but sharp drop in potential (*phase 1*) and a plateau phase (*phase 2*), during which a complex interaction of ion movements involving sodium, potassium, calcium, magnesium and chloride, associated with different channels and pumps, results in some decrease of the intracellular potential towards zero.

Repolarisation

After the plateau phase, repolarisation takes place. Sodium is pumped out of the cell in exchange for potassium, resulting in a return of the membrane potential to the resting level (*phase 3*). Repolarisation must occur before another impulse can be transmitted, or before the myocardial cells can contract again. This gives cardiac tissue the property of refractoriness. Abnormalities of the rate of repolarisation (and therefore the degree of refractoriness) have a very important role in the generation of some arrhythmias (section 7.4).

Pacemaker activity

An important property of certain specialised conducting cells and to a lesser extent all conducting tissues within the heart is that they are capable of spontaneous depolarisation and repolarisation independent of external neural stimulation. This property is known as automaticity. The cells with the fastest rate of automaticity are known as pacemaker cells. There is a hierarchy of cells with different rates of automaticity. Under normal circumstances, the SA node has the highest rate and it therefore acts as the pacemaker.

Automaticity depends on *phase 4* of the cardiac action potential. The rate of change in potential is dependent on a time-related change in membrane potassium permeability and is influenced by autonomic tone, electrolytes, drugs and disease. The steeper the slope, the faster the rate of automaticity. Phase 4 is steepest in SA nodal cells but, if these cells fail to depolarise, other tissues which have automaticity will spontaneously depolarise to initiate an impulse. The AV node and junctional tissue also have automaticity and will become the dominant pacemaker if the SA node fails to depolarise. In some disease states, Purkinje tissue may also act as a pacemaker and abnormal automaticity may also occur in other cells.

1.5.3 The conduction process

The conduction network in horses is broadly similar to that found in other species, but there are important differences. The conduction process follows a predictable pathway in the normal heart, passing along specialised conduction fibres, leading to a co-ordinated contraction of atrial and then ventricular muscle (Figure 1.11). The contractile cells of the heart are found in two syncytia, the atria and the ventricles. These syncytia are normally electrically separated except at the atrioventricular (AV) node.

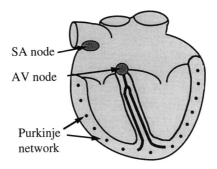

SA node

AV node

Purkinje network

Ventricular activation in horses

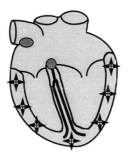
widespread Purkinje network results in depolarisation from multiple points within the myocardium, with small activation fronts speading in all directions (c.f. small animals)

Fig. 1.11 The conduction system and ventricular activation.

The *SA node* governs the rate of the normal heart. The normal rhythm is therefore called sinus rhythm. The SA node is a crescent-shaped structure located at the site where the cranial vena cava enters the right atrium. The impulse is formed in the SA node and spreads across the atria to the AV node. Conduction occurs along specialised fibres; however, the impulse also leads to contraction of atrial muscle. The right and then the left atrium are depolarised. The electrical activity associated with depolarisation of this muscle mass results in a sufficiently large electrical field for it to be detected at the body surface as a P wave.

The *AV node* is found at the junction of the atria and the ventricles, in the interventricular septum (IVS). When the impulse reaches the atrioventricular junction it finds a barrier to further spread. The specialised cells of the AV node conduct the impulse slowly because of their high resting potential, slow phase 0 depolarisation and poor electrical coupling. When the AV node is depolarised, because only a small number of cells are affected, no deflection is seen on the surface ECG. The delay in conduction is represented on the surface ECG by the interval between the P wave and the onset of the QRS complex. The AV node has a slower natural rate of automaticity than the SA node; however, if the SA node fails to initiate an impulse, it can take over as the pacemaker at a slower rate. In the horse, conduction through the AV node is profoundly affected by vagal tone. It is often sufficiently slowed or reduced in amplitude to result in a marked reduction in the normal rate of conduction, or complete abolition of further spread of the impulse (see section 7.7.2).

Once the impulse has passed through the AV node, conduction spreads via specialised fast-conducting fibres within the *bundle of His*, the main *bundle branches* (left and right), and the *Purkinje network*. The Purkinje network ramifies throughout the myocardium. In the horse and other ungulates it is particularly widespread in comparison with humans and small animals. Depolarisation of the Purkinje fibres activates adjacent myocardial cells. Depolarisation of the ventricles is completed rapidly and results in a co-ordinated contraction. Depolarisation of the bundle of His and the Purkinje network is not detected on the body surface ECG. Intracardiac electrodes are required to detect the relatively small change in potential associated with depolarisation of the small number of cells. However, depolarisation of the myocardium results in substantial electrical forces, the net result of which produces the QRS deflection on the surface ECG. The Purkinje tissue has a slower natural rate of automaticity than the SA node or the AV node. If, however, they fail to initiate an impulse, the Purkinje tissues can take over as the pacemaker at a slower rate.

Each cell within the heart repolarises after depolarisation. The sum of the repolarisation processes within the heart can be detected at the body surface in the same way as the electromotive forces of depolarisation. Ventricular repolarisation is seen as the T wave. The change in electrical field caused by atrial repolarisation may or may not be seen. It is termed the atrial T wave, or Ta wave.

1.5.4 *The cardiac electrical field*

When a cardiac cell is depolarising or repolarising, different currents flow across the cell membrane at various points and a potential difference will occur between one part of the cell and another (Figure 1.12). This results in a 'battery' effect with the cell acting as a dipole. During flow of current along the cell surface, an external electrical field is set up around the dipole. However, when the cell is depolarised or repolarised and therefore at a resting potential, the membrane potential is not rapidly changing. Consequently, there is no difference in the membrane potential at different points along the cell surface and therefore no electrical field, despite the potential difference between the inside and outside of the cell.

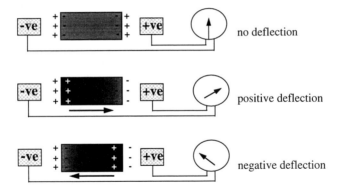

Fig. 1.12 The electrical potential difference across a myocyte.
A myocardial cell can be likened to a battery. When the cell is resting or depolarised there is no net movement of ions and no potential difference is recorded between one end of the cell and the other, but during depolarisation or repolarisation a current is recorded.

The surface ECG

The changes in the electrical field around the heart can be detected by a galvanometer (electrocardiograph) attached to the body surface. The electrocardiograph is simply a voltmeter which records the potential difference between two electrodes. The link between a positive and negative electrode is called a bipolar lead. An electrocardiograph records the potential difference between electrodes placed at various points on the body surface. It does not record the depolarisation of each individual cell, but detects the sum of all the electrical fields which are present at any one time. When an electrocardiogram (ECG) is recorded, it is assumed that the heart can be represented by a single dipole, with the electrical activity producing a simple field around it. This is a major oversimplification, but does not invalidate the use of the technique. The points at which the ECG electrodes are placed are chosen to represent the electrical changes which are occurring in the heart, but a number of factors affect the potential difference between different areas of the body. The position of the heart within the body, the pattern of the spread of activation within the heart, the shape of the thorax, the conductivity of tissues between the heart and the electrodes, and the exact location of the body surface electrodes, all affect the body surface ECG.

Detection of the conduction process

The first electrocardiographers recognised the electrical activity of the heart at the body surface and gave the description P, QRS and T waves to the deflections on their voltmeters (Figure 4.3). These waves and complexes represent the depolarisation and repolarisation of the atria and the ventricles. Identification of these waves allows the clinician to determine that these processes have occurred. The timing of the waves and their duration provides further information about the conduction process.

If conduction follows the normal pathway, the P, QRS and T waves will be recognised and have a normal relationship. If it follows a different pathway, the shape of the complexes, their timing, and the duration of the intervals between them, may change. The rate at which the QRS complexes occur indicates the heart rate. The regularity of the waves and complexes indicates the cardiac rhythm.

The concept of cardiac vector

The ECG voltmeter will have a positive deflection if the net direction of overall activity (vector) is towards the positive electrode of a bipolar lead, and a negative potential if it is away from the positive electrode. The voltage recorded will be largest when the vector is directly towards the positive electrode. If the direction of the maximum potential difference is at an angle to the lead axis, the deflection will be smaller (Figure 1.13). If the electrodes are positioned perpendicular to the vector of electromotive force, no potential difference will be detected. The sum of the electromotive forces changes in magnitude and direction from instant to instant during the course of the depolarisation and repolarisation processes. This is called the instantaneous vector. As the instantaneous vector is difficult to measure, the average direction and magnitude are more commonly recorded. The amplitude of the deflection indicates the magnitude of the vector and is also dependent on the mass of myocardial tissue which is depolarised. Multiple vectors from different groups of cells may cancel each other out when their electrical fields are summated before reaching the body surface.

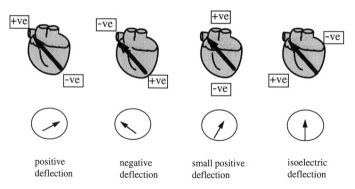

| positive deflection | negative deflection | small positive deflection | isoelectric deflection |

Fig. 1.13 The principle of vectors.
If current is flowing towards the positive electrode a positive deflection will be seen on the voltmeter (ECG). If the vector is directed away from the positive electrode a negative deflection is recorded. If the same voltage current flows along an axis which is oblique to the positive electrode but towards it, a smaller positive deflection is detected. If the vector of depolarisation is perpendicular to the axis of the electrodes there will be no net depolarisation.

1.5.5 ECG lead systems

The process of recording an ECG is discussed in detail in Chapter 4. Over the years a number of lead systems have been developed to record the cardiac electrical field. The aim of these systems is to record each of the waveforms and complexes clearly so that the conduction process can be evaluated. They may also provide information about the direction and magnitude of the cardiac vector. Einthoven's triangle is a system of limb leads which records electrical activity which reaches the body surface in the horizontal (frontal) plane. The heart is assumed to be located approximately in the centre of an equilateral triangle formed by the two forelimbs and the left hind limb. This is the system which is commonly used in small animals and humans. In humans, additional chest leads are useful for detecting areas of abnormal conduction caused by infarcts, a common problem in this species. Chest leads are also useful in some situations in small animals, particularly in animals with congenital heart disease resulting in marked ventricular hypertrophy.

The Einthoven limb lead system can be used in horses and provides useful information about cardiac rhythm and conduction. However, other systems have also been designed to accommodate the fact that in horses the heart is not a point source situated at the centre of a homogeneously conducting triangle formed by the limbs. These systems try to assess the cardiac vector in three dimensions by measuring the electrical field in three orthogonal planes at similar distances from the heart.

1.5.6   The ventricular depolarisation process

The ventricular depolarisation process has been shown to be different in horses (designated along with other ungulates as category B mammals) compared with humans and small animals (category A mammals).

In category A mammals, the Purkinje network carries the impulse to the sub-endocardial myocardium and depolarisation then spreads out from the ends of the fibres, through the myocardium to the sub-epicardial layers, in a series of wavefronts. The initial overall direction of the wavefront is mainly from the left to the right side of the interventricular septum initially, followed by a wavefront which is substantially directed towards the left ventricular apex, and finally towards the cardiac base (Figure 1.14). Because the LV is normally the most substantial muscle mass, the sum of the electromotive force is primarily directed towards the left apex, resulting in a large R wave in lead II of Einthoven's triangle (the lead axis which is approximately parallel to the direction of the wavefront). The main cardiac vector is altered when there is considerable change in the relative proportions of the left and right ventricles. The average of the cardiac vector in the frontal plane is known as the mean electrical axis (MEA).

In category A mammals, increased LV muscle mass can cause a prolonged QRS duration because the wavefront takes longer to spread throughout the enlarged myocardium. In addition, the amplitude of the R wave in lead II is often increased in individuals with hypertrophy of the LV, as a result of the increased muscle mass. RV hypertrophy increases the contribution of the RV to the mean vector and may result in a right axis deviation. These changes are relatively specific for enlargement of the left or right ventricles but are comparatively insensitive. Even in category A mammals, radiography and echocardiography are usually more sensitive techniques for detecting hypertrophy, particularly LV hypertrophy.

In the horse the Purkinje fibres extend throughout the myocardium and ventricular activation takes place from multiple sites. The apical section of the IVS is the first part of the myocardium to be depolarised. This depolarisation often spreads from the left to the right side of the septum, but can be in either direction. Vectors of local electrical activity may even point in both directions, resulting in a cancellation of electromotive forces reaching the body surface and therefore without any deflection on the ECG. The bulk of the ventricular myocardium

Wavefronts spread through the ventricular myocardium
generating a mean vector directed towards the apex

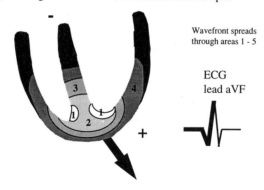

Wavefront spreads
through areas 1 - 5

ECG
lead aVF

Wavefronts only formed in the basal septum and a small
portion of left ventricular myocardium, generating a
mean vector directed towards the base

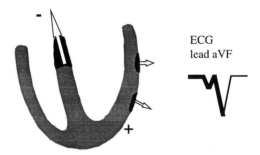

ECG
lead aVF

Fig. 1.14 The ventricular activation process.
The depolarisation of the ventricles is different in category A mammals (man and small
animals) compared with ungulates (including horses) (upper and lower diagrams,
respectively). In horses, the majority of the myocardium is depolarised simultaneously from
multiple points and the voltages from the resulting mini-wavefronts cancel each other out
when measured from the body surface. The surface ECG therefore provides very limited
information about the size of the ventricular myocardium in this species.

depolarises shortly afterwards; however, no large wavefronts are formed
because of the multiple sites from which activation occurs. Because the surface
ECG represents the sum of the electromotive forces within the heart, the overall
effect of the depolarisation of this tissue on the ECG is minimal. Most of the
electrical activity seen at the body surface occurs as a result of the depolarisation
of the basal part of the IVS and a small portion of the LV free-wall. The wavefront spreads towards the heart base so the vector is directed dorsally and
cranially with respect to the body surface (Figure 1.14).

The range of MEA measured in normal horses is extremely wide and MEA is
therefore of very limited clinical value in horses. In addition, the time taken for
the ventricles to depolarise does not depend on the spread of a wavefront
across them so QRS duration is not necessarily related to ventricular size. Thus,
for all practical purposes, ECGs provide little or no information about heart size

in horses, although they do give useful information about heart rate and rhythm.

1.6 The effects of exercise on the cardiovascular system

In an athletic animal such as the horse, it is important to understand the effects of exercise on the cardiovascular system. In human and small animal cardiology, the principal concerns are survival and quality of life in animals with moderate or severe cardiac disease. However, in the horse, clinical cardiology is principally concerned with the effects of relatively minor cardiac disease on athletic performance. Therefore, the adaptations of the equine athlete to exercise training must always be considered when evaluating the cardiovascular system.

Exercise results in profound short-term changes in cardiac output, and to pulmonary and systemic peripheral vessels, and it may also lead to significant long-term changes. Not all of these changes are well understood and this discussion is only brief. Readers are referred to the listed texts for more complete discussion of exercise physiology.

1.6.1 The short-term effects of exercise

The short-term effects of exercise usually begin before the horse has even begun to trot. Excitement plays an important part in preparing the body to cope with the demands of exercise. The sympathetic nervous system will be activated and parasympathetic discharge reduced or abolished, resulting in a tachycardia and vasodilation of the blood vessels supplying skeletal muscle. Blood is diverted from other organs, such as the gut, by local vasoconstriction. Myocardial contractility may increase. Venoconstriction results in an increased venous return, and splenic contraction increases the packed cell volume and oxygen carrying capacity of blood.

During exercise, venous return is also aided by the pumping effect of skeletal muscle on the blood within the venous system, and the changes in intrathoracic pressure associated with respiration. Intrathoracic pressure and venous return are also affected by the alternate compression and decompression of the thoracic cavity by the bulk of abdominal contents moving backwards and forwards during locomotion. Cardiac output is therefore increased due to increased heart rate, preload and contractility and reduced afterload. Of these, increased heart rate is the most significantly altered from the resting value in the horse.

Marked changes in the peripheral cardiovascular system also occur during exercise to allow perfusion of active skeletal muscle and to aid thermoregulation. Although stroke volume increases little during exercise, changes in loading conditions and contractility are required in order to maintain stroke volume in the face of a much increased heart rate and vasodilation in skeletal muscle.

The horse has a tremendous capacity to increase cardiac output, which can rise to six times the resting value. This is more than many other species, including man. The huge cardiac reserve is reflected by the low resting heart rates in horses compared with animals of similar body size, such as cattle, which usually have a resting heart rate of approximately 50–100% higher than that found in horses. Many of the unusual features of the rhythm of the equine heart are related to the high vagal tone which maintains low resting cardiac output in this species.

1.6.2   The long-term effects of exercise

The long-term effects of exercise have not been as well studied as the short-term changes, but a number of adaptations have been observed. Prolonged exercise training leads to eccentric hypertrophy of the LV (and presumably the RV), resulting in an increased stroke volume. The maximum heart rate appears to be similar in trained and untrained animals; however, trained horses appear to be able to maintain stroke volume at high heart rates better than untrained animals, resulting in an increased performance capacity. The distribution of blood flow to skeletal muscles during exercise is assisted by an increase in the ramifications of blood vessels to fibre groups. This results in an increase in the maximal aerobic oxygen capacity of exercise-trained animals. Adaptation due to selective breeding has lead to a difference in the packed cell volume and oxygen carrying capacity of the 'hot blooded' breeds. Fit animals also appear to be able to move faster at the same maximal oxygen capacity. Athletic ability may also be related to the ability to tolerate increased levels of by-products such as lactic acid, which build up in the muscles during exercise, and affect anaerobic exercise capacity.

Chapter 2

Cardiovascular Pathology and Pathophysiology

In order to recognise the clinical signs of abnormal cardiac function and to apply effective treatment strategies, it is essential to understand the changes that take place in heart disease. In its broadest sense, pathology can be approached from the standpoint of pathophysiology, clinical pathology, gross pathology and histopathology.

2.1 Heart disease in horses compared with other species

A wide variety of clinical signs can result from cardiac disease in horses. The exact nature of clinical signs depends on the effects of homeostatic mechanisms and the extent of changes in the distribution of blood supply to tissues. The clinical signs which can be attributed to heart disease must also be distinguished from similar signs which can result from diseases of other body systems.

The term 'heart failure' refers to a situation in which the heart fails to circulate sufficient blood to meet the metabolic requirements of the body for nutrients. In some animals, clinical signs of heart failure are only seen at times of high metabolic demand such as exercise. In other animals, delivery of blood fails to meet even basal requirements and marked disability or death ensues. The clinical signs associated with heart disease in man have been graded on a scale of 1–4 by the New York Heart Association (NYHA). This scale has also been applied to small animals and it is a useful concept in horses.

Class 1   Clinical signs associated with known cardiac disease are not observed or are limited to exercise intolerance during strenuous athletic activity.
Class 2   Clinical signs including tiring and tachypnoea become evident with ordinary levels of exercise.
Class 3   The animal is comfortable at rest, but cannot tolerate any exercise.
Class 4   Clinical signs are severe even at rest.

Horses are usually presented for relatively minor clinical signs in comparison with many small animals. It is relatively uncommon for horses to be presented with overt cardiac failure; the majority of equine cardiac patients fall into classes 1 and 2 of the NYHA scale. There are two principal diagnostic problems for the equine clinician.

One is judging whether heart disease is responsible for signs of exercise intolerance, or if the problem results from abnormalities in other body systems.

The second is whether currently asymptomatic disease may deteriorate and become a problem in the future. The approach to equine cardiology is therefore very different from that in small animal and human cardiology, where the greatest problem is improving the quality of life for patients in class 3 and providing life-saving therapy for patients in class 4 heart failure.

2.2 The pathophysiology of heart failure

Despite the fact that NYHA class 3 and 4 heart disease is relatively uncommon in horses compared with other species, it is helpful to understand the changes which lead to signs of heart failure.

Heart failure may be acute or chronic, compensated or decompensated. The majority of animals with heart failure are in a compensated state in which there is a stable balance between abnormalities and the homeostatic responses to these changes. Treatment of animals with heart disease is aimed at reversing the aetiological factors if possible, in order to return the heart to normality. However, because heart valves cannot be replaced in horses, a complete cure is only possible with some arrhythmias. Treatment of animals with compensated heart disease is therefore based on alleviating clinical signs without reducing cardiac reserve. Treatment of animals with decompensated heart failure is aimed at returning the animal to a compensated state, if the long-term prognosis is sufficiently good for treatment to be worthwhile.

Heart failure has been classified in many different ways, potentially leading to some confusion. Many classifications overlap; animals seldom fall only into one specific category. All of the descriptions are over-simplifications of the pathophysiological processes which occur. However, they are useful concepts because they make one think about the physiological changes which are causing clinical signs.

2.2.1 Congestive heart failure

The processes involved in the development of congestive heart failure (CHF) are complex and as yet are not fully understood. More detailed discussions of the processes involved are contained in some of the recommended reading. In summary, they involve peripheral vascular changes which take place in order to maintain delivery of blood to vital organs, sodium and water retention to increase blood volume, increased heart rate and ventricular hypertrophy (Table 2.1). The homeostatic mechanisms which control cardiac output and peripheral vascular tone, and therefore blood pressure, were described in detail in Chapter 1.

Peripheral vascular changes
The changes which occur in heart failure are similar to those that are responsible for maintaining blood pressure. When cardiac output is reduced, peripheral arteriolar and venous constriction maintains blood pressure until output can be increased by other homeostatic mechanisms. In addition to autonomic changes, accumulation of local vasoactive compounds affects blood flow to some areas. If

Table 2.1 Mechanisms in congestive heart failure

Physiological responses
1. Peripheral vasoconstriction to redistribute blood and maintain blood pressure
2. Increase in preload and heart rate to maintain or increase cardiac output
3. Ventricular hypertrophy to increase stroke volume without increase in preload

Mechanisms of sodium and water retention leading to expansion of blood volume
Detector mechanisms
Baroreceptors
Volume receptors
Juxtaglomerular apparatus
Thirst centre
Renal blood supply

Effector mechanisms
Angiotensin
ADH
ANP
Aldosterone
Autonomic stimulation:
    neural (acute phase, effects reduced in chronic situation)
    humoral
Changes in renal blood flow and distribution
An unknown 'filtration factor'
Change in behaviour (e.g. reduced exercise/activity)

cardiac output is critically low, the periphery will be poorly perfused and cool extremities may be clinically detectable.

Sodium and water retention to increase blood volume
One of the principal responses to a fall in blood pressure is a complex interaction of numerous homeostatic mechanisms which increase sodium and water retention (see section 1.4.4). This results in an increase in blood volume and maintenance of preload. Changes in each of these mechanisms are exaggerated during the development of congestive heart failure (CHF).

CHF develops when volume retention becomes excessive and preload is inappropriately high. This occurs because the homeostatic mechanisms can increase blood volume to such a degree that the heart can no longer pump the required stroke volume, resulting in increased filling pressure. In addition, in severe disease, increased myocardial oxygen consumption makes the ventricles relatively stiff, further increasing filling pressure. The result is that blood dams back in the veins, capillary pressure rises and consequently fluid leaks out into the extracellular space. Oedema formation is one of the principal factors contributing to clinical signs of CHF.

Increased heart rate
One of the principal mechanisms of maintaining blood pressure in the face of decreased forward stroke volume is increased heart rate, mediated by increased sympathetic discharge and decreased parasympathetic tone. This may occur, for example when preload is reduced by haemorrhage. However, a raised heart rate reduces the duration of diastole and therefore limits the time for ventricular filling

and for coronary artery flow and is very energy consuming. In the long-term the tachycardia itself can result in myocardial failure and CHF. In compensated CHF, homeostatic mechanisms compensate so that stroke volume is raised, distribution is efficient and heart rate may return to normal. An increased resting heart rate, in the absence of causes other than cardiac disease, is a strong indicator of the presence of significant heart disease.

Ventricular hypertrophy

Cardiac hypertrophy occurs in response to either pressure or volume overload. Both of these processes increase myocardial wall tension in line with the law of Laplace (see section 1.4.6). Hypertrophy occurs in order to reduce tension.

Concentric hypertrophy is the response to pressure overload. The increase in wall thickness reduces wall tension; the stroke volume of the ventricle remains unchanged or falls. In horses, left ventricular (LV) pressure overload is very rare.

Eccentric hypertrophy is commonly found in horses, both as a normal physiological response to exercise training and as a result of the volume overload in animals with valvular regurgitation. In eccentric hypertrophy, dilation of the chamber results in a proportional increase in stroke volume for the same reduction in myocyte length during contraction. However, the geometrical change which results in increased efficiency also causes an increase in wall tension which must be offset by a concomitant increase in wall thickness. The increased stroke volume gives greater cardiac reserve in athletically trained animals. In volume overload, eccentric hypertrophy occurs in order that a normal cardiac output can be produced at a resting heart rate, without severe changes in peripheral blood supply, although it brings with it the problem of increased myocardial oxygen consumption. Eccentric hypertrophy is therefore one of the first changes which can be measured in horses with heart failure.

2.2.2   Left-sided congestive heart failure

The term left-sided CHF refers to excessive LV filling pressure and consequent increased pressure in the left atrium (LA) and in the pulmonary veins. Acute left-sided CHF results in an increase in the pressure within the pulmonary capillaries and leakage of fluid into the interstitial space. This is called pulmonary oedema. It may result in the appearance of frothy white or blood-tinged fluid at the nostrils. Animals with pulmonary oedema are usually severely exercise intolerant, hyperpnoeic and tachypnoeic.

2.2.3   Right-sided congestive heart failure

The term right-sided CHF refers to increased right ventricular filling pressure and consequent increased pressure in the right atrium (RA) and in the systemic veins. This may result in the formation of ascitic fluid, pleural fluid, and peripheral oedema. In the horse, subcutaneous oedema in dependant areas such as the ventral abdomen, sheath and distal limbs is the predominant sign. This must be distinguished from other causes of oedema formation (Chapter 3, Table 3.3) . In the horse, left-sided CHF usually progresses rapidly to right-sided CHF, because of complex changes in pulmonary vasculature. In many horses, right-sided CHF is the first sign of left-sided heart disease which is noticed by owners. This is in marked contrast to some other species such as dogs in which disease affecting the left side of the heart rarely results in right-sided CHF.

2.2.4 Biventricular failure

The terms right- and left-sided cardiac failure are not strictly accurate, because failure of one side inevitably involves some changes in the function of the other. The term biventricular failure implies that clinical signs of both right- and left-sided CHF are seen.

2.2.5 Oedema formation

CHF may result in clinical signs as a result of a failure to maintain cardiac output, or because of the development of congestive signs. Oedema formation results in a dilutional hypoproteinaemia in the interstitium, reducing the oncotic pressure. After some time, an equilibrium develops and oedema formation becomes self-limiting. However, the position of the equilibrium may be changed if excessive water retention results in a fall in the oncotic pressure of the blood. Other factors may also affect the development of oedema. The left atrium (LA) plays an important role in limiting the effects of mitral regurgitation (MR) which can lead to CHF. With severe MR, end-diastolic pressure rises in the LV resulting in an increase in LA pressure. This in turn increases pressure in the pulmonary veins, resulting in pulmonary oedema. However, the thin-walled atrium can expand to dampen the effects of the increased pressure from the pulmonary circulation. This takes some time (days), but will decrease the tendency for pulmonary oedema formation as a result of MR. For this reason, signs of pulmonary oedema are often most severe when MR develops acutely, for example as a result of ruptured chordae tendineae.

2.2.6 Low output failure

In the majority of animals with heart failure, a stable equilibrium is reached in which homeostatic mechanisms result in compensation and the maintenance of an adequate cardiac output. However, eventually the compensatory mechanisms may not be sufficient to maintain the required cardiac output and signs of cardiac insufficiency such as weakness and weight loss develop. This is known as low output or decompensated failure. This may also occur when cardiac disease develops rapidly, resulting in acute clinical signs.

2.2.7 High output failure

In some situations, cardiac failure will be caused or exacerbated by other systemic changes. For example, the effects of anaemia and pregnancy may precipitate signs of CHF because they result in an increased demand for cardiac output. These are known as high output states. Animals with these conditions may be presented with CHF (high output failure) if they are combined with underlying heart disease. Once the high output requirement is abolished, the signs of CHF may resolve without any change in the underlying cardiac condition.

2.2.8 Myocardial failure

The term myocardial failure implies that there is a reduction in contractility of the myocytes. However, this should not be confused with CHF. Myocardial disease, in which there is a primary problem with contractility, is relatively uncommon. In many cases, CHF is attributable to regurgitant valvular disease and myocardial function is normal. In only a few cases of chronic valvular disease associated with volume overload and tachycardia is contractility reduced.

With the exception of monensin toxicity (see section 6.7.2), there are few reports concerning mechanisms of myocardial failure in the horse. It must be assumed that myocardial failure involves the same cellular processes in horses as in other species, even if the aetiological agent is different. Numerous cellular mechanisms have been implicated. These include abnormal energy metabolism, defective calcium release and resorption by the sarcoplasmic reticulum, abnormal cross-bridge formation and release by contractile proteins, slippage between sarcomeres, down-regulation of beta receptors and exhaustion of synaptic noradrenaline. At the ventricular level, changes such as tachycardia, arrhythmias, hypoxia, fibrosis, and myocyte loss may affect systolic and diastolic function. These changes may be due to primary cardiac disease, or occur secondary to systemic disease or electrolyte disturbances.

2.2.9 Systolic failure

The term systolic failure refers to a limitation to forward stroke volume. Valvular or myocardial disease may result in systolic failure. In the horse, AV valve regurgitation is the most common cause.

2.2.10 Diastolic failure

The term diastolic failure refers to heart failure caused by abnormal ventricular filling. In other species, this may result from stenotic AV valves; however, this abnormality is exceptionally rare in horses. Diastolic failure may also result from pericardial effusion leading to tamponade, constrictive pericarditis and myocardial diseases which prevent normal relaxation. These conditions prevent an increase in right ventricular filling at times of increased demand and therefore limit cardiac output. This may cause exercise intolerance and even collapse. It will also result in increased end-diastolic ventricular pressure which, because the right ventricle has a lower filling pressure than the left, may cause systemic venous congestion and signs of right-sided CHF. Fortunately, these conditions are uncommon in horses.

Diastolic function can also be reduced by diseases which primarily affect the left side of the heart, because increased wall thickness, ventricular dilation, or increased myocardial oxygen consumption can make the ventricles stiff. This may lead to a higher end-diastolic pressure. Arrhythmias can also affect ventricular filling. This is particularly true in the case of atrial fibrillation when the 'pump-priming' action of atrial contraction is absent. Signs are most apparent at high heart rates, when there is less time for ventricular filling.

The causes of diastolic and systolic failure are listed in Table 2.2.

Table 2.2 Causes of systolic and diastolic failure

Systolic heart failure
Mitral valve regurgitation
Severe aortic valve regurgitation
Severe tricuspid valve regurgitation
Myocardial disease
Arrhythmias (supraventricular tachycardias, ventricular tachycardias)
Exacerbated by volume overload, increased myocardial oxygen consumption, high
    demand e.g. exercise, anaemia, pregnancy, fever

Diastolic heart failure
Myocardial disease, especially fibrosis
Pericardial effusion with tamponade
Constrictive pericarditis
Tachycardia > ~ 140 bpm
(Exacerbated by atrial fibrillation and systolic failure)

2.2.11 Forward failure

The term forward failure is used to imply that the clinical signs principally result from a reduced cardiac output, rather than from congestion. This can result from primary cardiac disease, but also from hypovolaemia. Animals with forward failure are weak and exercise intolerant.

2.2.12 Backward failure

Backward failure refers to signs of congestive heart failure. Like the term forward heart failure it is an oversimplification and is not commonly used.

2.2.13 Volume overload

Volume overload is a term which is frequently used in the context of valvular heart disease. In fact, volume overload can occur in other situations, but valvular incompetence is by far the most common cause in horses.

Increased chamber volume results from compensatory mechanisms which increase blood volume so that blood pressure can be maintained (see above), and as a direct consequence of regurgitation. Eccentric hypertrophy results in the ability to pump a greater stroke volume (within limits). In addition, the regurgitant fraction must be accommodated in the receiving chamber (e.g. the LA in the case of MR, the LV in the case of aortic incompetence). The degree of volume overload is a helpful indicator of the severity of valvular regurgitation (see sections 4.2.6 and 6.2.6). Volume overload is also seen in severe myocardial disease.

2.2.14 Pressure overload

Pressure overload is common in humans, as a result of acquired disease such as rheumatic valvular disease and systemic hypertension. In small animals it usually results from congenital heart disease. In horses, pressure overload is very rare. Pressure overload of the right ventricle has been reported in severe pulmonary disease as a result of pulmonary hypertension (cor pulmonale), but is not well recognised as a disease entity in its own right. The most common cause of pulmonary hypertension in horses is left-sided CHF, and this rapidly leads to signs of right-sided CHF.

2.2.15 Decompensated heart failure

The term decompensated heart failure refers to a situation in which homeostatic mechanisms can no longer support an adequate cardiac output and the circulation fails to deliver adequate oxygen to tissues. In a few situations this can be reversed, but usually it leads to an inexorable decline and death.

2.2.16 The pathophysiology of reduced exercise tolerance

In horses, the most significant consideration in heart disease is the effect on exercise tolerance. Unless there is a sudden change in cardiac output, or decompensation of an equilibrium, exercise intolerance is usually the primary presenting sign in horses with heart disease. In addition, once exercise capacity is reduced, long-term changes occur which further reduce the athletic performance of the animal.

Exercise intolerance results from a reduction in the cardiac reserve which is present in normal animals to allow them to cope with increased demand. The reduction in reserve is largely a result of homeostatic mechanisms which maintain blood pressure in the face of cardiac disease. The very nature of these compensatory homeostatic mechanisms results in vital organs being saved from reduced perfusion at the expense of less essential organs such as skeletal muscle, which are relatively underperfused. There may be a reduced preload reserve because the venous tone is increased. This means that there is less scope for increasing cardiac output via the Frank–Starling mechanism and that exercise capacity will be limited. Animals with LV volume overload may develop abnormally high pulmonary artery pressure during exercise, which may reduce the efficiency of gaseous exchange and even cause exercise-induced pulmonary haemorrhage. Alternatively, if cardiac output falls, gaseous exchange cannot take place efficiently, resulting in high blood carbon dioxide levels and low arterial oxygen. In addition to cardiac changes, there are changes in the systemic circulation in animals with significant heart disease. The blood supply to skeletal muscle is reduced at rest and the arterioles may be stiff, preventing the usual increase in blood supply to exercising muscle. In the long-term, the capillary supply to skeletal muscle becomes less extensive. These mechanisms result in decreased muscle efficiency.

2.3   Clinical pathology

A variety of clinical pathological tests are helpful in examination of horses with suspected or proven cardiac disease. In many animals, these tests are helpful because they can reveal abnormalities in other body systems. These abnormalities may indirectly affect cardiac function, or may cause clinical signs which are confused with cardiac disease. Clinical pathological tests which are of particular relevance to heart disease are discussed below. However, for further detail, readers should refer to clinical pathology texts.

2.3.1   Haematology

The main purpose of haematological investigation in horses in the context of suspected or confirmed heart disease is to identify the presence of anaemia and to evaluate the changes in the white cell population which accompany many bacterial and viral infections.

   If an infectious condition such as endocarditis or bacterial pericarditis is suspected, haematological examination may help to confirm the fact that an inflammatory process is present. Bacterial infections often result in an increase in the number of neutrophils (neutrophilia) and identification of immature neutrophils (band cells). Viral infections often result in an increase in the numbers of lymphocytes relative to the neutrophil count. Viral infections are of greatest significance in athletes with reduced athletic performance, either because of the effect of the virus on the respiratory system, or less frequently, due to myocarditis.

   Anaemia can be identified from analysis of the blood haemoglobin and the red cell population. Anaemia may exacerbate existing heart disease by increasing the demand for cardiac output. In severe cases it may result in the auscultation of a cardiac murmur even in the absence of valvular disease (a haemic murmur) because of the reduced blood viscosity and increased cardiac output.

2.3.2   Plasma fibrinogen

Plasma fibrinogen is an acute-phase protein which is raised in animals with inflammatory foci. The exact values depend on the assay used and should be referred to each individual laboratory's normal range. As a general rule, infectious conditions result in particularly high fibrinogen levels. Measurement of plasma fibrinogen is worthwhile in many cases, particularly when endocarditis is suspected. This condition is usually accompanied by a markedly elevated plasma fibrinogen, often in excess of 8 g/l. Fibrinogen assays are a useful screening process which can alert the clinician to the possible presence of an infected focus. This is important because successful treatment of endocarditis requires aggressive use of antibiotics early in the course of the disease. However, it should be remembered that plasma fibrinogen may also be raised in other inflammatory diseases which may complicate heart disease. For example, some horses with pulmonary oedema develop a secondary pneumonia which will result in a raised fibrinogen. Serial fibrinogen assays are helpful for monitoring the progress of inflammatory disease in response to treatment.

2.3.3   Blood culture

Multiple blood culture samples should be taken from an aseptically prepared site in cases in which endocarditis is suspected. Ideally the samples are taken during the rising phase of a fever spike. Often this is not practicable; an alternative is to take daily samples for three days. A large volume of culture medium should be used. Both aerobic and anaerobic cultures should be submitted. Unfortunately, cultures are often negative; however, this does not rule out a diagnosis of endocarditis, or affect the prognosis. Successful culture means that appropriate antibiotics can be selected (see section 6.6.2).

2.3.4   Plasma proteins

Measurement of plasma protein levels is advisable in cases with dependent oedema which cannot be definitively attributed to cardiac disease. This will help to rule out hypoalbumenaemia as a cause of oedema formation. Albumen levels may be slightly low in horses with CHF. Globulin levels may be raised in an animals with an active inflammatory focus.

2.3.5   Viral serology and isolation

Virus isolation and paired serum antibody titres may be helpful to identify the presence of a viral infection and its aetiological agent. Unfortunately, the cardiac manifestations of viral myocarditis are only likely to be apparent some time after the active viral infection when these tests may no longer be helpful.

2.3.6   Electrolytes

Measurement of plasma electrolytes is helpful in cases where arrhythmias are detected. Although abnormalities are seldom detected, they may be very important if present, and usually can be treated simply. Single measurements of plasma electrolyte levels may not be as helpful as multiple samples, or fractional excretion tests which assess the way in which the body is balancing electrolytes. Fractional excretion can be estimated from the following formula:

$$\text{FEE} = \frac{\text{serum creatinine} \times \text{urine electrolyte}}{\text{urine creatinine} \times \text{serum electrolyte}} \times 100$$

where FEE is the fractional excretion of the electrolyte. The normal range should be obtained from the testing laboratory

2.3.7   Cardiac muscle isoenzymes

The value of cardiac muscle isoenzymes in horses is contentious at present. There is little documented evidence which validates their use in horses; however, many anecdotal reports recommend their measurement as an aid to the diagnosis of myocardial disease. The principle of isoenzyme measurements in horses is extrapolated from their use in detecting myocardial injury in humans. Myocardial injury in humans is usually ischaemic in origin and results in much more extensive myocardial cell death than ever occurs in horses, except in a few uncommon conditions such as monensin toxicity. One of the reasons for the popularity of isoenzyme measurment in horses is that there is often no other form of evidence available to confirm or refute a diagnosis of myocarditis. However, there is no evidence that isoenzymes are likely to be of value except where acute myocardial injury has occurred, or in on-going disease. The clinical signs of myocardial damage may only be evident some time after the initial cellular damage occurred, when isoenzyme levels have returned to normal. The extent of myocardial cell death due to myocarditis is seldom likely to be sufficient to result in high levels of cardiac isoenzymes.

Two isoenzymes have principally been used to evaluate myocardial damage in horses. Lactate dehydrogenase (LDH) has five isoenzymes, of which isoenzyme 1 and 2 have been reported by different authorities to originate from myocardial tissue. Creatinine kinase (CK) has two isoenzymes, the MM and MB fractions. It has been suggested that high levels of the MB fraction result from myocardial damage. However, there is a lack of specificity and sensitivity in these assays. Firstly, there is evidence that these isoenzymes can be produced from non-myocardial tissue, therefore raised values are non-specific for myocardial damage. For example, in human athletes the CK MB fraction has been derived from skeletal muscle after hard exercise. Secondly, many animals in which myocarditis is diagnosed from clinical, echocardiographic or electrocardiographic evidence have normal isoenzyme levels, therefore the tests are relatively insensitive. In addition, because the levels seldom rise markedly, cardiac disease is often diagnosed when the isoenzyme level is only marginally outside a 'normal' range, making false positive diagnoses more likely.

With further research, it is possible that these assays will be clinically useful. This would be very helpful, in order that myocarditis could be detected by a routine screening test. However, there is insufficient evidence at present to ensure that the results are reliable and, although there may be individual cases in which elevated cardiac isoenzymes are helpful in pointing towards a diagnosis of myocardial disease, in the author's opinion they should be interpreted with caution.

2.4 Pathology

Pathological examination of the heart should be performed as part of a complete post-mortem (PM) examination. The changes seen at PM in horses with heart disease are usually relatively minor in comparison with other species and are frequently missed unless the examiner has a detailed appreciation of the normal and abnormal features of valves and myocardium. Care should also be taken in interpreting the significance of abnormalities detected at PM. For example, mild degenerative valvular changes are unlikely to be responsible for the sudden death of an animal, even if this is the only abnormality detected at PM.

2.4.1 Gross post-mortem examination of the heart

A complete examination of the body is essential in all cases; however, specific attention must be paid to dissection of the heart when cardiac disease is suspected. A systematic method of inspecting the heart at post-mortem is essential in order that minor changes are not overlooked. In addition, it is very easy to damage structures during dissection so that it is unclear if the lesion is real or iatrogenic. The following protocol is relatively simple to follow.

(1) Note the presence of any pleural or pericardial fluid before the heart is removed from the thoracic cavity.

(2) Inspect the condition of the pericardium.

(3) Examine the epicardial surface of the heart.

(4) Trim fat away from the heart.

(5) Carefully divide the pulmonary artery and the aorta, noting the condition of the ligamentum arteriosum.

(6) Free the pulmonary artery from the atria and cut down its length. Inspect the pulmonary valve. A little gentle washing may be needed at this point to see the valve clearly.

(7) Divide the pulmonary valve by cutting between the leaflets and continue the incision along the junction of the right ventricular free-wall and the inter-ventricular septum, until the incision extends to the base of the tricuspid valve annulus. Inspect the condition of the myocardium, the moderator bands and the tricuspid valve. If a ventricular septal defect is present it may be hidden under the septal leaflet of the tricuspid valve.

(8) Make an incision from the caudal vena cava along the base of the right atrium, and from the cranial vena cava to join this. Extend the incision into the right atrial appendage. Inspect the endocardium of the right atrium for jet lesions.

(9) Cut down the length of the aorta and inspect the aortic valve. Take culture samples at this point if aortic valve endocarditis is suspected. Gentle washing may again be needed at this point to see the valve clearly.

(10) Open the left atrium by cutting between the pulmonary veins and extend the incision into the left atrial appendage. Inspect the endocardial surface for jet lesions and note the position of any lesions relative to the mitral valve leaflets. Jet lesions are rough patches of fibrin deposit on the endocardial surface, but can look like fleshy projections if they are more severe and longstanding (Figure 2.1). Gently wash the mitral valve and note any flailing of leaflets as water fills the ventricle. This can also be done by filling the ventricle via the aortic valve.

(11) Cut down the length of the coronary arteries from the sinus of Valsalva.

(12) Divide the aortic valve between the right and left coronary cusps and cut to the level of the left coronary groove. Divide the myocardium carefully with a scalpel to penetrate into the ventricle without damaging any structures. Extend the incision between the papillary muscles to the base of the mitral valve annulus. Minor moderator bands may need to be cut. Inspect the condition of the myocardium and endocardium. Inspect the aortic valve and the mitral valve. Pay particular note to the origins and insertions of the chordae tendineae. A ruptured chorda tendinea may curl up onto the leaflet or papillary muscle (Figure 2.2). If a ventricular septal defect is present it will usually be just below the right coronary cusp of the aortic valve, right at the top of the septum.

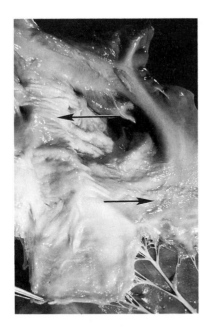

Fig. 2.1 Jet lesions.
Jet lesions on the endocardial surface of the left atrium due to severe mitral regurgitation. The arrows indicate thickened areas of endocardium with a roughened surface.

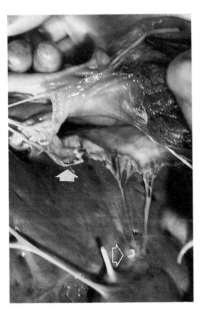

Fig. 2.2 A ruptured chorda tendinea.
The open arrow indicates the tag of chorda left on the papillary muscle. The solid arrow indicates the fibrosed area of the free surface of the mitral valve (right commissural cusp).

(13) Once the chordae have been inspected, divide the caudal mitral leaflet between the chordae from the right and left papillary muscles, leaving the chordae intact. This allows the mitral annulus to be laid out for close inspection of the valve.

2.4.2 Histological examination

Histological inspection of cardiac tissue should be performed by an experienced histopathologist. However, as histology of the equine heart is so seldom requested, interpretation of the findings is often based on general principles and experience in other species. Details of histological changes in valvular and myocardial disease are poorly documented.

If histology it to be performed, sections of atrial and ventricular myocardium, including the endocardium and epicardium, a section at the base of the mitral valve, a section including the region of the AV node and bundle of His, and any areas of obvious gross abnormality, should be taken. These should be placed into 10% formalin solution, but the pathologist should be consulted if any special stains are required because these sometimes require the use of other preservatives.

2.4.3 Valvular changes

The aetiology and pathophysiology of valvular disease in the horse is very poorly understood. Myxomatous change is seen in degenerative valvular disease. It is a relatively common finding, but is not usually as extensive as in the dog. Inflammatory change, with a lymphocytic and or neutrophilic infiltrate has been reported. This suggests that a form of valvulitis may be responsible for the development of valvular incompetence in some cases. Confirmation of this disease process requires further research.

If vegetative endocarditis is present, the endothelium will be broken, with extensive areas of fibrin and thrombus. Inflammatory cells, and in some cases bacteria, may also be seen. Usually endocarditis is obvious on gross examination of the valve. (See section 6.6.6.)

2.4.4 Myocardial changes

Myocardial changes have been reported in a number of diseases, but these reports are very seldom based on large numbers of cases. Consequently, interpretation of minor abnormalities must be tentative, and an expert opinion should be sought. Small white areas of scarring are often seen around the apex of the heart and, unless extensive, may be insignificant.

Chapter 3

Clinical Examination

A thorough and methodical method of history taking and clinical examination is the basis for assessment of horses with suspected cardiac disease. Once these tasks have been performed it becomes possible to select appropriate further diagnostic tests. In equine cardiology, it is particularly important to put the findings in the context of the athletic requirements for the individual animal.

3.1   Background details

The history and background details of the patient are particularly important considerations in the horse because, while the spectrum of disease does not differ widely between different types of animal, the use and consequently the expected exercise tolerance of individual horses differs enormously. As a result, not only the likely diagnosis, but the treatment, prognosis and advice offered may differ depending on individual circumstances.

Important factors to consider are the age, sex, breed and use of the horse. In addition, in some instances the prospective use of the animal, the stage of the athletic season, the ability of the rider and the temperament of the individual horse may need to be taken into account.

3.1.1   Age

Severe congenital heart disease is most often encountered in the neonate. However, many defects go unnoticed until later in life, frequently becoming apparent only when the animal is first put into work, or at a routine examination. Other conditions may complicate the clinical picture in animals with cardiac disease and may be more common in animals of different age. For example, foals are more likely to suffer diseases such as septicaemia and pneumonia than adults. These conditions may cause tachypnoea and tachycardia which can be mistaken for a sign of cardiac disease. In addition, clinical signs may sometimes be incorrectly attributed to heart disease in animals with incidental cardiac murmurs. Valvular heart disease is generally more common in older animals. This is particularly true of aortic valve disease leading to aortic regurgitation. The age of the animal may also affect its use and future use, which may in turn affect the relative significance of cardiac disease. This is usually the most significant consideration.

3.1.2 Sex

In the USA, a higher incidence of cardiac disease has been reported in male Standardbreds than in females. It is unclear whether this relationship is attributable to any difference in athletic requirements in horses of different sex. In other breeds, there is little documented evidence that any cardiac disease processes are more common in either sex. Rupture of the aortic root is reported primarily in aged stallions (see section 6.10.1). However, the influence of the sex of an animal on its use as an athlete or as a breeding animal is a much more significant consideration.

3.1.3 Breed

Some breed predispositions have been reported. Complex congenital heart disease has been noted to have a higher incidence in the Arabian than in other breeds. In the USA, Standardbreds have been reported to have a higher incidence of congenital heart disease, acquired valvular disease and arrhythmias than Thoroughbreds. In the UK, atrial fibrillation has been found to be relatively common in heavy-hunter type animals. This arrhythmia is seldom recorded in ponies. To some extent these findings are biased by the particular populations in the hospitals from which the studies were reported. In the horse, breed is a much less significant factor in the relative prevalence of cardiac disease than in small animals. The influence of breed on a horse's use as an athlete or as a breeding animal is a much more significant factor.

3.1.4 The use of the animal

The prevalence of cardiac disease differs little in animals used for different purposes. However, functional heart murmurs, and arrhythmias which are associated with high vagal tone such as second degree atrioventricular block (2° AVB), are more often noticed in racehorses. Some conditions which might go unnoticed in a pleasure horse may become clinically apparent in a performance animal. For example, racehorses cannot perform normally with atrial fibrillation, but animals which are not required to perform rigorous exercise may have the condition without obvious clinical signs before it is discovered as an incidental finding.

The significance of cardiac disease may vary enormously depending on the use of the animal. A condition which renders an animal unsuitable for racing may not prevent it from performing normally as a hunter or, if it progresses further, from use as a hack. Rigid rules of thumb are inappropriate and the clinician should consider every case individually, in the light of the demands of the rider. Even the rider's ability and experience and the animal's temperament may need to be considered.

3.1.5 The prospective use of the animal

Inevitably, the clinician will be asked to give an opinion on the likely effect of cardiac disease on the animal's suitability for work in the future. This is a particularly difficult problem at a pre-purchase examination (see section 8.1.3). It is seldom possible to give an accurate assessment of the likely future course of events; however, prognostication is aided by serial assessments and the use of diagnostic aids such as echocardiography.

It may also be important to consider the potential effect of a problem, such as a cardiac murmur, on the resale value of a horse, or on any difficulties which might be encountered in insuring it. It is likely that exclusion clauses will be placed on the insurance of such animals and this should be pointed out to owners and prospective owners.

3.1.6   The stage of the athletic season

The training programme of an animal may have an important bearing on advice and treatment. For example, an animal with atrial premature complexes may be treated with steroids or given a prolonged period of rest. If the problem occurs towards the end of the season, it may be preferable to adopt a conservative approach because there is insufficient time for treatment to be effective and for training to resume. In other instances, there will be pressure to get an animal back in training in preparation for a specific event, and steroid treatment may have to be considered (see section 7.8.3).

3.2   History

A thorough history is very useful both in establishing a diagnosis and in assessing the significance of heart disease. A number of historical details should be established, and these are summarised in Table 3.1.

3.2.1   Management

It is helpful to find out the duration of ownership, or the time during which the horse has been in the present training establishment. If an animal has only recently been acquired, important details about the animal's previous history may not be known and only a limited amount of performance record data may be available.

The previous, current and prospective use of the animal are very important factors to establish. This may affect whether mild disease has been clinically evident, and the significance of the condition for future use.

3.2.2   Previous evidence of cardiac disease

It is important to ask whether any evidence of cardiac disease was noted at previous clinical examinations. This may be known to the veterinarian if he or she has regular contact with the animal. It is important not only to ask whether any abnormalities have been detected, but also whether normal auscultatory findings were reported.

3.2.3   General medical history

A variety of previous problems may provide evidence of other conditions which

Table 3.1 Check list for clinical findings in horses with cardiac disease

Backgrounds details
Age, sex, breed, use
Insurance, prospective use, prospective sale

History
Management, e.g. bedding – straw/shavings/paper
Feeding, e.g. dry or soaked hay, concentrates, supplements
General health considerations e.g. vaccination, worming
Previous/current medical problems:
   viral infection in individual or in-contact animals
   cough
   URT noise
   epistaxis
   tachypnoea/dyspnoea
   myopathy
   weight loss
   appetite and water intake
Performance history
Main presenting signs
Duration of presenting signs
Treatment if any
Date of last auscultation

Clinical examination
Environment
Body condition, demeanour
Check approximate age
Mucous membranes: CRT, colour
Arterial pulse: rate, rhythm, quality, consistency
Head and neck: nasal discharge, lymph nodes, larynx, scars from previous surgery
Jugular vein: patency, distension, pulsation
Ventral abdomen, sheath, distal limbs: oedematous filling
Respiratory pattern and rate
Respiratory sounds (including re-breathing bag)
Cardiac area: palpation, auscultation, percussion

may complicate, or which may have been mistaken for signs of cardiac disease. Therefore, a general medical history should always be recorded. In addition, specific signs of potential cardiac disease which may be recognised by the owner should be known. These include exercise intolerance or prolonged recovery after exercise (see below), peripheral oedema formation, and even a pounding heart or irregular heart rhythm noted by the rider.

Respiratory signs are a particularly important subject for detailed questioning. It should be established whether a cough has been present at any stage. Although coughing is a relatively uncommon sign of cardiac disease, it can be seen in animals with pulmonary oedema, and may also have been caused by respiratory infections which can be associated with subsequent myocardial disease. For this reason, it should be established whether a viral illness has affected that individual or other horses in close proximity. Other infectious conditions such as bacterial pneumonias may also affect the animal and be mistaken for signs of cardiac disease. Allergic small airway disease is still an under-recognised cause of signs varying from coughing to poor athletic performance, and owners should be closely questioned about air hygiene. Dyspnoea and tachypnoea may be seen in animals with left-sided congestive heart failure (CHF) and pulmonary oedema, but can also result from respiratory disease. Epistaxis has been reported in a number of animals with cardiac disease. It is most commonly associated with arrhythmias such as atrial fibrillation and atrial premature complexes in athletic animals. However, exercise-induced pulmonary haemorrhage usually occurs without underlying heart disease.

Musculo-skeletal problems are a very significant cause of poor athletic performance, and should not be forgotten even in a horse which is suspected to have a cardiac disease. Mild bilateral lamenesses are most commonly overlooked. Myopathies associated with exercise are a potential cause of poor athletic performance (see section 8.2.1). Aorto–iliac thrombosis is an uncommon cardio-vascular cause of ischaemic myopathy (see section 6.10.5).

Other problems such as colic, diarrhoea and any recent weight loss should also be noted. Occasionally these may result from cardiac disease. Diarrhoea and weight loss are often seen in animals with CHF. Weight loss is a common feature of endocarditis and may be the primary presenting complaint. Questioning about vaccination status and worming history may be important in some instances, for example where viral illness is suspected or when anaemia results in a haemic murmur.

3.2.4 Performance history

One of the best indicators of the significance of heart disease is its effect on athletic performance. If a horse has had a problem, for example a relatively quiet murmur of mitral regurgitation, for a long period of time, but has a good performance record, it is quite likely that the significance of the condition is minor. However, if athletic performance has been disappointing, then it is more likely that the valvular regurgitation is significant and that this is responsible. Nevertheless, even when mitral regurgitation is present, other causes of poor performance should also be considered (see section 8.2.4). It is therefore important to find out whether the horse has ever performed well, or whether the performance level has dropped off in the recent past. For example, it may be possible to infer that the onset of a problem such as atrial fibrillation was likely to be at the time of the deterioration in performance. This may be helpful in advising about the chances of successful treatment (see section 7.8.5). There are occasions on which successful sale of an animal may depend on a satisfactory working record after the point at which the problem was detected. However, the value of a performance history depends on the horse performing at a level which is similar to that which it is intended to do in the near future. For example, it may be difficult to establish the duration of atrial fibrillation in an animal which has been rested for a prolonged period.

3.3 The clinical examination

The clinical examination described below places particular emphasis on the cardiovascular system. A check list for significant findings in horses with suspected cardiac disease is included in Table 3.1. However, a complete general clinical examination is also required. The examination depends on careful observation and a knowledge of the wide variation of normality which may be encountered. The findings should be accurately recorded so that they can be used for future reference. A wide range of clinical signs may be seen in animals with cardiac disease. These range from no signs, to poor athletic performance, to signs of CHF (Table 3.2).

Table 3.2 Clinical signs of cardiac disease

Mild disease	no clinical signs
	reduced exercise tolerance
Moderate disease	tachycardia
	tachypnoea
	dyspnoea following exercise
	abnormal arterial pulse
	jugular distension
	oedema over ventral abdomen
	oedema in distal limbs
	pathological arrhythmias
Severe disease	cool extremities
	weight loss
	reduced capillary refill time
	cough (left-sided failure)
	dyspnoea at rest
	collapse

3.3.1 The patient's environment

It is important to take note of the stable conditions. Other diseases, such as chronic obstructive pulmonary disease, which may be relevant to the case, may be influenced by these conditions.

3.3.2 Patient attitude and condition

Animals with marked CHF and particularly those with endocarditis frequently appear depressed and may lose weight. Excited animals are usually tachycardic.

3.3.3 Mucous membranes

Abnormal mucous membrane colour is a non-specific and insensitive indicator of cardiac dysfunction. However, some horses in low-output heart failure will have pallor or peripheral cyanosis and animals with right to left shunts such as tetralogy of Fallot may have central cyanosis. Evidence of anaemia may be accompanied by a physiological ('haemic') murmur and a high cardiac output. Injected mucous membranes are found in some animals with endocarditis or severe systemic disease.

Capillary refill time (CRT) is also an insensitive indicator of peripheral perfusion and can even appear to be normal in a recently dead animal! However, CRT should be assessed in all cases. It may be increased in high-output conditions such as febrile illnesses, or decreased with low-output failure, hypotension or shock. It can be a valuable indicator for monitoring the effects of drug treatment.

3.3.4 Arterial pulse

The pulse should be palpated to assess rate, rhythm and quality. Pulses can usually be easily palpated from the facial artery, but pulsation of the transverse facial, median or digital arteries, or arteries in the skin, can also be detected. However, the facial artery is the most relaible because it is less frequently affected by other local factors.

The pulse quality reflects the difference between the systolic and diastolic pressures rather than the absolute or mean arterial pressure. The facial pulse profile usually has a double peak which can be easily detected at resting heart rates. It may be markedly biphasic at normal heart rates in resting animals. Weak pulses can be misleading because the absolute strength of the pulse is quite variable. Pulse quality is stronger in an excited animal. It is well worthwhile palpating arterial pulse quality in as many normal horses as possible, in order to become familiar with the range of normality. One situation in which assessment of the pulse quality is particularly useful is in aortic regurgitation, when it may become strong but short lasting ('water-hammer pulse') if the condition is advanced (see section 6.5.2). 'Pulsus alternans' may occur in animals with myocardial depression. In this situation there is an alternatively strong and weak pulse, despite a regular sinus rhythm. Pulse deficits may occur when there is a premature beat, or a very short R–R interval in an animal with atrial fibrillation. Because the ventricles contract prematurely, they have not have time to fill normally, so the stroke volume is small. In addition, end-diastolic aortic pressure is still relatively high, so the difference between systolic and diastolic pressure is small.

3.3.5 General inspection of the head and neck

A thorough examination of this region is important before moving on to the thorax. If a nasal discharge is present, it is important to note whether it is unilateral or bilateral, mucoid, mucopurulent or sanguinous, foul smelling or odourless. The owners should be questioned about its duration. Palpation of lymph nodes may reveal important information. The larynx should be palpated for evidence of muscle atrophy, and examined for scars indicative of previous surgery.

3.3.6 The jugular vein

The jugular vein acts as a manometer of central venous pressure and can provide very useful information. Patency of flow should be assessed on both sides. The jugular filling time can be measured from the time taken for the vein to fill to the level of the jaw when occluded, and it can be delayed in some animals with heart failure. However, it is a very crude guide to cardiac output and can be very variable in normal animals.

Some 'pulsation' of the vein is observed at the thoracic inlet in the normal horse, because it is so close to the right atrium. The normal variation in pressure in the jugular veins is described as a series of 'waves' and 'descents' (Figure 3.1), which are related to the changes during the cardiac cycle (see section 1.4.1). The *a* wave marks right atrial contraction. This is followed by the *x* descent, when the atria relax. The *c* wave occurs at the time of ventricular systole, and is relatively small. It may be difficult to distinguish it from pulsation of the adjacent carotid artery, which occurs simultaneously. This is followed by the *x'* descent, when the ventricles pull the atrioventricular (AV) valves towards the apex, resulting in a fall in pressure within the atria. Because the *c* wave is often small, the *x* and *x'* descents are sometimes regarded as one phase. The next positive wave is termed the *v* wave. This is due to the increase in right atrial pressure caused by filling during the latter half of ventricular systole. This is followed by the *y* descent, which occurs when the AV valves open and the stored blood rapidly fills the ventricles in early diastole. The waves and descents are more easily seen in most horses than in other species because they have relatively superficial veins, a thin hair coat and a slow resting heart rate.

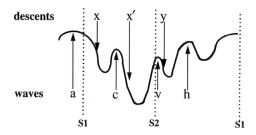

Fig. 3.1 Jugular pressure contour.
Changes in jugular filling reflect changes in central venous pressure and can be useful indicators of normal and abnormal cardiac function.
Key: **a** wave is due to right atrial (RA) contraction; **c** wave is due to closure of the tricuspid valve (TV) at the onset of systole; **v** wave is caused by a rise in RA pressure during systole due to continued venous return while the TV is closed; **h** wave is caused by a rise in RA pressure during diastasis due to continued venous return; *x* descent is due to RA relaxation; *x'* trough is caused by the ventricle pulling the AV valve ring towards the apex resulting in reduced pressure in the RA; *y* descent is due to the drop in RA pressure when the TV opens in early diastole.

Observation and palpation of the vein may help to identify the atrial contraction wave. Its presence or absence provides valuable information about conduction of the electrical impulse through the heart. It is often particularly prominent in the horse because the ventricles have usually almost completely filled before atrial contraction, and the ventricular pressure at this point is relatively high. Right atrial contraction therefore contributes relatively little to ventricular filling at low heart rates and the pressure wave is transferred to the jugular veins. Identification of the *a* wave therefore indicates that atrial contraction has taken place. It will be absent in horses with atrial fibrillation, and present in the absence of the *v* wave and *x* and *y* descents in 2°AVB (see section 7.7.2).

Some confusion exists over the term 'jugular pulse'. Pulsation may occur in three situations:

- Tricuspid regurgitation, with a raised venous pressure.
- Atrioventricular dissociation.
- Right-sided CHF.

Only the first two of these result in a true jugular pulse. In tricuspid regurgitation, the contraction of the ventricles forces blood up the jugular vein in a retrograde fashion through the incompetent valve. The *a* wave and the *v* wave may merge to produce one large pressure wave. The *x* descent is lost and a prominent *y* descent is seen. Just one large rise and fall in jugular filling is therefore seen. This is almost invariably accompanied by a raised central venous pressure. In AV dissociation, pulse waves will be seen in the jugular vein when the atria contract against a closed tricuspid valve, during ventricular systole. They fail to generate sufficient pressure to open the AV valves and the contents of the atria are forced in a retrograde fashion. These are called 'cannon' or 'giant *a*' waves.

Right-sided CHF may result in distension of the jugular vein due to an increased right ventricular end-diastolic pressure and subsequently an increased central venous pressure. In this situation the vein is continuously distended rather than distended by a pulsation. However, pulsations may be superimposed owing to incompetence of the tricuspid valves which often accompanies the volume overload of the right side of the heart, or because the pulsation of the carotid artery is transmitted through the filled vein. The latter is not a true jugular pulse.

To check whether a jugular pulse is present, the vein should be occluded and blood milked from the point of occlusion towards the thoracic inlet. If a true jugular pulse is present, the vein will fill from the thoracic inlet.

The observation of a distended jugular vein is a very important finding. However, the position of the head will alter the degree of distension. The jugular vein will fill in a normal animal when it lowers its head because the vein is then ventral to the right atrium. One or both jugular veins may also be distended when venous return is impaired by a thoracic mass, or even when there is a large pleural effusion.

3.3.7 *Dependent oedema*

Signs of dependent oedema may be associated with CHF or a number of other conditions. Oedema is most often found in the distal limbs and ventral abdomen (Figure 3.2). In males, the prepuce may fill with fluid. The finding of dependent oedema due to cardiac disease is a poor prognostic indicator, so it is important to rule out other potential causes. Differential diagnoses in this situation are summarised in Table 3.3. Mild degrees of filling of the distal limbs and sheath are common in normal horses which are inactive, and can also be affected by diet.

3.3.8 *Palpation and percussion*

In addition to palpation of arterial and jugular pulses, the cardiac impulse should also be palpated over the area of its maximal intensity (the apex beat area). This

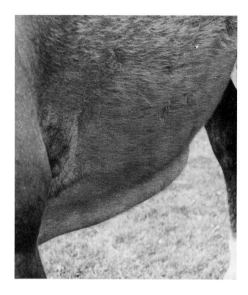

Fig. 3.2 Ventral oedema.
A plaque of oedema is visible on the ventral aspect of the abdomen and thorax. A number of differential diagnoses should be considered (Table 3.3).

Table 3.3 Causes of dependent oedema

Congestive heart failure (right-sided or biventricular)
Mitral regurgitation (commonly)
Aortic regurgitation (less commonly)
Tricuspid regurgitation (uncommonly)
Myocardial disease (rare)
Pericardial effusion (rare)
Constrictive pericarditis (rare)

Hypoproteinaemia
Protein-losing enteropathy (may be neoplastic, parasitic, bacterial or inflammatory
  in origin)
Liver failure
Protein-losing nephropathy

Vasculitis
Purpura haemorrhagica
Equine infectious arteritis
Equine infectious anaemia
Drug hypersensitivities

Local obstruction to venous and lymphatic return
Tumour
Abscess
Trauma
Cellulitis
Late pregnancy

is the point at which the ventricle contacts the chest wall, rather than the true cardiac apex. The apex beat results from twisting of the ventricle at the onset of systole and helps to identify the timing of systole and diastole. It can also be a useful guide to the position of the heart in the thorax, and is of value in identifying the position of the valve areas. Gross cardiomegaly may be detected when the apex beat is displaced caudally. The cardiac apex may also be abnormally positioned when the heart is displaced by a mass in the chest. The force of the cardiac impulse should be noted; however, this alters markedly depending on the cardiac output and the thickness of the chest wall. The impulse will therefore be relatively weak in fat, thick-chested animals and strong in an excited Thoroughbred. The apical impulse will also be reduced in animals with myocardial failure or a pericardial effusion.

3.4   Auscultation

Auscultation provides invaluable information about the events of the cardiac cycle and blood flow. A methodical approach allows the maximum amount of information to be derived from auscultation. The novice clinician should take every opportunity to auscultate normal animals, so that the wide range of normal sounds is appreciated.

3.4.1   The generation of the heart sounds

Four transient heart sounds, associated with vibrations occurring during the normal cardiac cycle, are heard in the horse. Two, three or four of these sounds may be heard in a normal animal. The two sounds which mark the beginning and end of systole, and which are heard in all normal animals, are the first and second heart sounds. In many animals, the third heart sound will be heard shortly after the second. In most, the fourth heart sound will be heard immediately before the first heart sound. The heart sounds are described as transient sounds, in order to distinguish them from murmurs. Murmurs can be defined as protracted noises heard during a normally silent period of the cardiac cycle. Because the transient sounds are related to the electrical and mechanical events of the cardiac cycle, it is useful to identify them. They provide information on the timing of the cycle and the presence or absence of some of these events. Usually the mechanical events on the left and right sides of the heart occur almost simultaneously. Often the interval is so short that it could only be detected using phonocardiography, however, there are circumstances under which the interval is long enough for it to be detected on auscultation. If the interval between the events on the left and right sides is sufficient (> 30 msec), the sound can be 'split' into two elements.

The intensity of the transient sounds varies in different animals. They are best heard in fit thin horses and in foals, but may be very quiet in fat, barrel-chested ponies. They are louder in an excited animal, or during tachycardia. Sounds may be muffled by fluid in the thoracic or pericardial cavities. Solid tissue such as tumours, abscesses or consolidated lung, which displace the heart or are present between the heart and the chest wall, may result in the sounds being reduced or increased in intensity, depending on the position of the heart valves in relation to the body surface.

3.4.2 The first heart sound

The first heart sound (S1) is a relatively low frequency sound usually described as a 'lub'. It marks the beginning of mechanical systole and therefore starts some time shortly after the beginning of the QRS complex of the ECG. The sound is caused by a number of mechanical events including opening of the semi-lunar valves, motion of the ventricular walls and acceleration of blood into the great arteries. In some cases, closure of the atrioventricular valves also contributes to the sound, but in normal animals, at normal heart rates, the AV valves have already closed at the time of the onset of the pressure rise within the ventricles at the beginning of systole.

The first heart sound is loudest over the apex beat area on the left side of the chest and in the corresponding area on the right. It may be accentuated in cases when the ventricles begin to contract while the AV valves are open. This may occur with premature beats, atrial fibrillation or AV dissociation. The intensity of S1 may be reduced when there is poor myocardial contractility, or poor transmission of sound.

A split S1 is an unusual finding, and may or may not be associated with any pathological condition. It is important that the fourth heart sound (S4, or atrial contraction sound) is not mistaken for a split S1, because identification of S4 is an important part of the assessment of the cardiac rhythm as it identifies atrial contraction (see below). The finding of a split S1 is not usually significant, except when it is mistaken for S4 in an animal with atrial fibrillation and an incorrect diagnosis is made. The characteristic irregularly irregular rhythm would be another important clinical finding in this situation. Where doubt exists it is a wise precaution to record an ECG.

3.4.3 The second heart sound

The second heart sound (S2) is a relatively high frequency sound, usually described as a 'dup' or 'dub'. S2 is shorter in duration than S1. It marks the end of systole and usually occurs shortly after the T wave of the ECG (the T wave is labile and therefore does not have a fixed relationship with mechanical events). The sound is principally caused by deceleration of blood in the great arteries just after the closure of the semi-lunar valves, at the incisura.

The intensity of S2 is reduced when the stroke volume is reduced, either as a result of a premature supraventricular or ventricular contraction or due to myocardial disease. This is because the deceleration of blood at the end of systole is reduced.

In the normal horse, S2 is frequently split. This can be best appreciated if the stethoscope is placed cranially over the heart base, corresponding to the pulmonary valve area. The aortic component of S2 (A2) precedes the pulmonary component (P2) in most horses, although P2 can precede A2 in normal animals. Respiration increases the degree of splitting because the pulmonary valve closes later during inspiration due to increased right ventricular stroke volume and increased ejection time. Pulmonary valve closure may be delayed in animals with a significant left to right shunt such as a large ventricular septal defect for the same reason. Pulmonary hypertension may result in an increase in the intensity of P2, making S2 sound louder than normal.

3.4.4   The third heart sound

The third heart sound (S3) is a transient sound which is heard in some horses. It is low in frequency, with a short, thudding quality. It is best heard over the apex beat area just ventral to the point where S1 is loudest. It is most often heard in fit athletic animals and is a less common finding in older horses and ponies. S3 is also loud in animals with significant left ventricular (LV) volume overload as a result of moderate to severe mitral regurgitation. The reason that the sound is loud in these animals is that it is created by the rapid deceleration of blood in the LV at the end of passive early diastolic filling. When the volume of blood filling the ventricles in early diastole is large, the deceleration of blood as the ventricles reach their elastic limit is marked. Supportive evidence for the source of the sound can be produced by recording a simultaneous phonocardiogram and M-mode echocardiogram. S3 occurs at the end of early diastolic filling, when the early diastolic dip of the septum seen on echocardiography indicates rebound of the ventricular walls.

The third heart sound varies in intensity at different heart rates. It may summate with the fourth heart sound at high heart rates to produce a gallop sound.

3.4.5   The fourth heart sound or atrial sound

The fourth heart sound (S4) is a transient sound which is heard immediately prior to S1. The sound is associated with the movement of blood cause by atrial contraction. Because of its timing, the sound has been called the atrial sound, atrial contraction sound, or 'A' sound. In the author's view, this is a less confusing terminology than S4, because at normal heart rates it is perceived as the first of the transient sounds in a group of four. The author uses the term A sound rather than atrial contraction sound because the sound may not be caused entirely by contraction of the atria. Phonocardiographic studies show the sound to have two components, S4 and S4'. The first of these is associated with the acceleration of blood at atrial contraction, the second with closure of the AV valves after the contraction is over. The second of the sounds is the louder, but the PR interval needs to be greater than 0.30 seconds for it to be heard. It is most clearly heard during a period of 2°AVB.

The A sound is best heard just dorsal to the apical beat areas. Sometimes it is more easily heard on the right side of the chest. It is best heard at slow heart rates and may be difficult to distinguish from S1. In some horses the interval between the A sound and S1 may be occupied by a presystolic murmur, but it can be difficult to distinguish a presystolic murmur and a loud A sound in some cases. This may be because they are both caused by the sound of AV valvular leakage which occurs just as the valve leaflets close. The jet of blood associated with this is easily detected on pulsed wave Doppler examination and is most apparent in animals with loud A sounds and presystolic murmurs. No pathological abnormality seems to be associated with a loud *A* sound or a presystolic murmur.

3.4.6 *Heart rate and rhythm*

It is essential that a suitable period of time is spent in assessing cardiac rhythm by auscultation because some significant arrhythmias are intermittent. It is also important to measure the heart rate when the horse has settled. Many horses will have a raised heart rate for some minutes and some may never have a true resting heart rate in the presence of the clinician. The horse's attitude should be taken into account because accurate measurement of heart rate is extremely useful. A tachycardia is one of the important signs of significant cardiac disease, although it is not seen in all cases. A true resting heart rate above 45 bpm should be regarded as abnormal and a cause should be identified, all be it that excitement is the most likely factor.

3.5 Cardiac murmurs

There are two important steps in the evaluation of a cardiac murmur. The first is to identify the source of the murmur, the second is to judge its significance. The significance of the murmur cannot be established with any accuracy without a specific diagnosis. It is therefore very important to identify clearly and classify the murmur or murmurs heard and, if necessary, then to consider the use of diagnostic aids. The situation in the horse is complicated by the common finding of murmurs associated with normal blood flow.

Murmurs are generated when there is turbulent blood flow which causes vibration of cardiovascular structures. Turbulence is generated in fluids under a number of circumstances. Low fluid viscosity, large diameter vessels, and high velocity flow are factors which increase the likelihood of turbulent flow. Turbulence in blood flow is common in the horse because of the large stroke volume and large ventricles, atria and great vessels. These factors mean that high velocity blood flow occurs in the aortic and pulmonary artery roots in early–mid systole. Murmurs are frequently associated with this flow and are therefore called 'flow' murmurs. Because early–mid systolic flow murmurs are associated with ejection into the great arteries, they are also called 'ejection-type' murmurs. The term 'functional' is also used for murmurs associated with normal blood flow. In addition, a murmur can result from low blood viscosity, for example due to anaemia. This is termed a haemic murmur. Physiological situations which are associated with a relatively high cardiac output may also result in a high blood flow velocity. This is the case in anaemia, septicaemia, and peripheral arteriovenous fistulae. These murmurs can be called physiological.

Abnormal communications within or around the heart often lead to high velocity flow and turbulence. The most common example is when murmurs result from blood leaking back through valves. If a small hole or leak between leaflets is present, a pressure gradient across the valve will result in a jet flowing through the communication, similar to a fountain. The intensity of the murmur generated by the turbulence will also be affected by the volume and velocity of the jet, so a number of factors may potentially affect murmur intensity. Valvular regurgitation is usually due to a valvular abnormality, but some leakage may occur in the normal heart at the moment when the valves close. Usually any turbulence associated with this is inaudible. Abnormal communications are also formed by structural defects in the myocardium, such as a ventricular septal defect, or by shunting vessels such as a patent ductus arteriosus.

In humans and small animals, murmurs are often associated with flow through abnormally narrow (stenotic) valves. This narrowing results in an increase in the velocity of blood flow through the valve and generation of turbulence. This situation is rare in the horse.

Auscultation of murmurs is easiest when the heart sounds are well conducted to the body surface. A small amount of turbulence occurring in the heart and great vessels may not produce sufficient vibration for them to be heard using a stethoscope. Intracardiac phonocardiography demonstrates that most horses have murmurs generated in the great arteries, but that they are insufficiently loud to reach the body surface.

3.5.1 Classification of cardiac murmurs

Murmurs are classified in order to aid their identification and as a useful reference for subsequent examinations. Functional murmurs and murmurs associated with various pathological conditions have certain characteristics. Classification of murmurs helps to identify functional from pathological murmurs and to distinguish between the different types of pathological murmur. The classification is according to the timing and duration of the murmur, its quality (pitch, change in intensity), intensity (loudness), point of maximum intensity and radiation.

Timing and duration
Murmurs should be identified as being systolic or diastolic (or rarely, continuous). The duration of systole and diastole can then be subdivided into the following categories:

(1) Early, mid or late (proto, meso or telo) systolic or diastolic.
(2) Pansystolic (from the beginning of S1 to the end of S2).
(3) Holosystolic (from the end of S1 to the beginning of S2).
(4) Holodiastolic (from the end of S2 to the beginning of S1).
(5) Presystolic (between the A sound and S1).

Diagrammatic representation of these murmurs helps to clarify their timing and acts as a useful reference for subsequent examinations (Figures 3.3–3.10).

Character
The term 'character' or 'quality' of a murmur refers to its change in intensity, pitch and other subjective qualities. The changes in intensity of a murmur depend on the change in velocity of flow and, therefore, on the pressure gradient which is generating flow. The change in intensity is best illustrated by phoncardiography; however, it can also be appreciated on auscultation. Murmurs associated with AV valve regurgitation usually have a fairly constant intensity throughout systole because the pressure gradient between the ventricles and atria remains

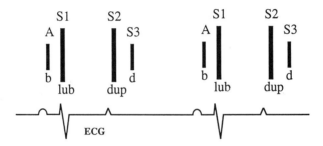

Fig. 3.3 Normal heart sounds.
Key: **A**, atrial contraction sound (**S4**); **S1**, first heart sound; **S2**, second heart sound; **S3**, third heart sound; solid lines represent the transient sounds and the shaded areas represent the timing and shape of a murmur as it would be seen on a phonocardiogram.

high throughout systole, and are termed plateau-type or band-shaped murmurs. The murmur associated with aortic valve incompetence gradually declines during diastole because the pressure gradient between the aorta and the LV falls away due to run-off into the systemic circulation and ventricle. These are termed decrescendo murmurs. In the great arteries, the velocity of blood flow rises and falls rapidly, and is greatest in early–mid systole. Consequently, murmurs associated with normal flow in these vessels increase and then decrease in intensity, are loudest in early–mid systole and are termed crescendo–decrescendo murmurs (although the crescendo period is short and can be difficult to identify clearly on auscultation). The murmur associated with a patent ductus arteriosus (PDA) is described as a waxing and waning murmur because of the changes in intensity caused by variation in the pressure gradient across the shunt.

Descriptive terms such as harsh, soft or musical can be used to describe a murmur. Additional characteristics such as variability in the intensity of a murmur at different heart rates may also be noted. The majority of murmurs are noises, i.e. they are a mixture of different frequencies of sound. A musical murmur is not a vague descriptive term, but a specific description of a murmur in which a specific frequency or frequencies of sound are detected. Musical murmurs are usually caused by resonating structures such as valve leaflets which vibrate and produce a a pure note of sound.

It is also possible to classify a murmur according to its variablity during the course of auscultation. Some murmurs vary in intensity or quality on a beat to beat basis, others may vary depending on the heart rate.

Intensity
The intensity of a murmur is graded on a scale of 1–6 (or 1–5). Each grade should be given in relation to the range used (e.g. grade 3/6). The grades are:

Grade 1: A quiet murmur that can be heard only after careful auscultation over a localised area.

Grade 2: A quiet murmur that is heard immediately once the stethoscope is placed over its localised PMI.

Grade 3: A moderately loud murmur.

Grade 4: A loud murmur heard over a widespread area, with no thrill palpable.

Grade 5:   A loud murmur with an associated precordial thrill.
Grade 6:   A murmur sufficiently loud that it can be heard with the stethoscope raised just off the chest surface.

In general terms, loud murmurs are more likely to be significant than quiet murmurs. However, some murmurs are not associated with a large volume of abnormal flow but are very loud. This most often occurs when a structure is made to vibrate rapidly in the jet of abnormal blood flow. Often these murmurs are musical. Theoretically, a large abnormal communication may carry a substantial amount of low velocity blood flow generating a murmur which may be of low intensity, or even absent. However, this is rare and clinical signs are usually very severe before this stage is reached in the horse.

Point of maximal intensity and radiation

Confusion has arisen over the position of the point of maximal intensity (PMI) of sounds associated with the different valve areas. The point at which sounds are loudest does not correspond accurately with the anatomical position of the valves because sounds have to be transmitted to the body surface to be heard. Systolic sounds associated with the AV valves are best heard towards the apex beat area because they are transmitted by the stiff ventricular wall to the point at which it touches the chest wall. However, external anatomical landmarks are a rough guide to the location of underlying cardiac structures. The mitral valve area is located in the fourth or fifth intercostal space on the left side of the chest just dorsal to the level of the olecranon. The aortic valve area is located in the fourth intercostal space on the left side of the chest just below the point of the shoulder. To hear sounds in this area, the stethoscope must be pushed forward under the triceps muscle. The pulmonary valve area is located in the second or third intercostal space on the left side of the chest just ventral to the aortic valve area. The tricuspid valve area is located in the third or fourth intercostal space on the right side of the chest approximately midway between the level of the olecranon and the shoulder. Sounds associated with the tricuspid valve may also be heard on the left side of the chest in the second intercostal space at a similar level in some animals. These areas reflect the cranio–caudal orientation of the LV and the right–left orientation of the right ventricle (see section 1.2.1).

Although external landmarks are a general guide to the position of valves, there is a slightly variable relationship between these landmarks and the position of the heart. In addition it is not always easy to identify the exact intercostal space on each occasion. For this reason, it is helpful to identify the location of the valves by identifying the characteristic sounds heard in each area. The mitral valve area is defined as the area where S1 is loudest, on the left side of the chest. The heart base is the area where S2 is most easily heard, although S1 may still be relatively loud in this area. The same principles apply on the right side of the chest. The tricuspid valve area is usually well cranial to the caudal aspect of the triceps muscle, if the horse is standing level. The stethoscope should be advanced well into the axilla, with the right leg ideally positioned in advance of the left.

The radiation of murmurs can be a helpful guide to their origin and is a rough guide to the severity of the condition. Functional murmurs are usually localised to a limited area. Murmurs associated with pathological processes can be localised or widespread. In general terms, the more widespread they are, the more significant the degree of valvular incompetence. The radiation of a murmur often reflects the direction of the jet. The holodiastolic murmur of aortic regurgitation usually radiates ventrally on the left side of the chest, but may also radiate to the right side in some animals if the jet projects towards the interventricular septum. Murmurs of mitral regurgitation may radiate dorsally and caudally if the jet runs up the caudal aspect of the left atrium, dorsally and cranial if they are running up the cranial wall. In the latter case the PMI may appear to be towards the base of the heart because the jet is causing vibrations along the atrial wall where it borders the aorta.

In some cases, a fine vibration of the chest wall will be apparent on palpation. This is known as a precordial thrill. A thrill is associated with a high velocity jet, and is most commonly found in animals with a ruptured chorda tendinea of the mitral valve, when the jet may strike the left side of the left atrial wall (see section 6.4.1 and 6.4.2) with aortic regurgitation, and in animals with a ventricular septal defect (Chapter 5). A precordial thrill is indicative of significant disturbed flow.

Using the classification described above, it is possible to categorise each murmur so that its probable origin can be decided. There are a limited number of conditions which commonly affect the equine heart, so a few, typical murmurs will usually be found (Figures 3.3–3.11). The identification of murmurs is summarised in Table 3.4.

3.5.2 Functional cardiac murmurs

Early–mid systolic ejection-type murmurs

Early–mid systolic ejection-type murmurs are heard in up to 60% of normal horses. They occur in all breeds and types, but are often louder in athletic horses and foals. There is no evidence that they are associated with any abnormality. They are caused by high velocity blood flow during the ventricular ejection phase. They are classically described as crescendo–decrescendo, however, the crescendo element may be lost in S1. In some animals the murmurs sound like a rather long and fuzzy S1. The most important features in detecting these murmurs are that:

(1) They finish before S2, so a silent period can be heard between the end of the murmur and the beginning of S2 (Figure 3.4).
(2) They are usually medium- or high-pitched in character.
(3) They are loudest over the heart base.
(4) They are localised in radiation.
(5) They may be variable in intensity at different heart rates, different R-R intervals and on different occasions.

These murmurs are most often heard on the left side of the chest, but may also be heard on the right side.

Table 3.4 Classification of functional and pathological murmurs

Timing	Duration	Character	Intensity	PMI	Radiation	Diagnosis
Systolic						
	early–mid	crescendo-decrescendo	1–3/6	basal areas	localised	functional murmur
	pansystolic	plateau	gd 2–6	L apical area	dorsal and cranial/caudal	mitral regurgitation
	pansystolic	plateau	gd 2–6	tricuspid area	dorsal and cranial/caudal	tricuspid regurgitation
	pansystolic	plateau	gd 3–6	usually right sternal border	to left +/–left basal	ventricular septal defect
	holosystolic	plateau	gd 2–6	L apical area	dorsal and cranial/caudal	mitral regurgitation
	holosystolic	plateau	gd 2–6	tricuspid area	dorsal and cranial/caudal	tricuspid regurgitation
	late systolic	crescendo	gd 2–5	L apical area	dorsal and cranial/caudal	mitral regurgitation (? prolapse)
	late systolic	crescendo	gd 2–5	tricuspid area	dorsal and cranial/caudal	tricuspid regurgitation (? prolapse)
Diastolic						
	early	short 'whoop'	gd 1–3	basal or AV areas	localised	functional murmur
	presystolic	grating	gd 1–3	AV region	localised	functional murmur
	holodiastolic	decrescendo	gd 1–6	left basal area	ventral +/– right	aortic regurgitation

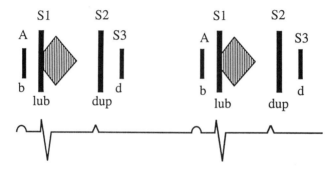

Fig. 3.4 Early–mid systolic ejection-type murmur.

Early diastolic murmurs

A distinctive functional murmur can be heard in early diastole in some horses. This is most often found in fit young animals and has been described as a 'two-year-old squeak'. The murmur is squeaky is quality, but can be found in any age of horse. The exact cause of the murmur is unclear. It may be related to rapid early diastolic flow, to a small leak at the aortic valve as the valve closes, or to another unknown cause. The murmur is high-pitched, with a distinctive 'whoop' sound. It may be more obvious at slightly increased heart rates, and for this reason may be detected after light exercise in some animals when it was absent at rest. The important features which identify it and distinguish it from pathological diastolic murmurs are that it is very short in duration, occurring between S2 and S3 (Figure 3.5). It may be heard on the left or right side of the chest, or both. There is no evidence that it is associated with any valvular or myocardial abnormality.

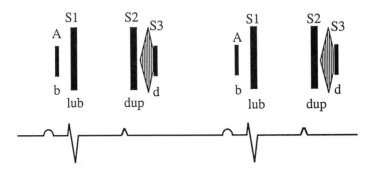

Fig. 3.5 Early diastolic murmur.

Presystolic murmurs

The phase of presystole occurs between atrial systole and ventricular systole. Because this period is relatively short, the murmur may be difficult to distinguish from the A sound and S1 (Figure 3.6). The murmurs are short and grating in quality, and may be heard on either side of the chest. The cause of presystolic murmurs is unclear. Evidence from Doppler echocardiography suggests that they may be due to leakage of blood into the atria at the time of AV valve closure. The amount of blood leaking at this time is of no physiological significance, so they are not considered to be a cause for concern.

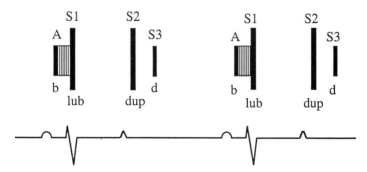

Fig. 3.6 Presystolic murmur.

3.5.3 *Cardiac murmurs associated with pathological conditions*

Holosystolic and pansystolic plateau-type murmurs

Holosystolic and pansystolic plateau-type murmurs are associated with blood flow between two chambers when there is a fairly constant pressure gradient throughout systole. This occurs with AV valve regurgitation and ventricular septal defects (VSDs). In both of these situation, blood flows from a high-pressure chamber to a low-pressure chamber and produces a murmur of relatively constant intensity ('plateau' or 'band' type). A holosystolic murmur is one which lasts from the end of S1 to the beginning of S2 (Figure 3.7). A pansystolic murmur is one which lasts from the beginning S1 to the end of S2, and therefore obscures these heart sounds (Figure 3.8). The difference between them is academic in terms of the diagnosis. Pansystolic murmurs are often louder and more significant.

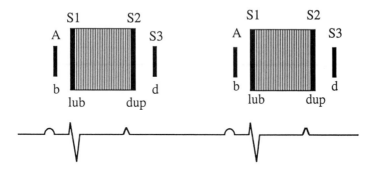

Fig. 3.7 Holosystolic plateau-type murmur.

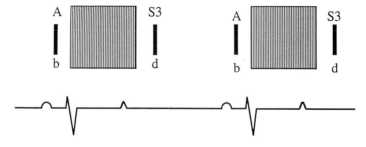

Fig. 3.8 Pansystolic plateau-type murmur.

Late systolic crescendo-type murmurs

Late systolic crescendo-type murmurs are associated with AV valve regurgitation when the valve does not become incompetent until well after the beginning of systole. They may be associated with valve prolapse. They often have a musical element (Figure 3.9).

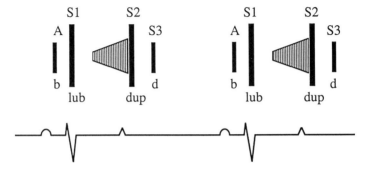

Fig. 3.9 Late systolic crescendo murmur.

Holodiastolic murmurs

Holodiastolic murmurs last from the end of S2 to the beginning of S1 (Figure 3.10). They are associated with incompetence of the semi-lunar valves. Because the pressure gradient between the great arteries and the ventricles gradually falls during diastole, the murmurs fade in intensity and are decrescendo. Blood flow through an incompetent pulmonary valve seldom generates sufficient vibrations for a murmur to be heard at the body surface so, when a holodiastolic murmur is heard, it is almost certainly caused by aortic valve insufficiency. The PMI is over the left base, and the murmur usually radiates ventrally. It may be heard on the right side of the chest also. The character of the murmur can be quite variable. It may be low or high in pitch, and frequently has a musical element. It often has a cooing, rasping, blowing or buzzing nature. The murmur may have a distant

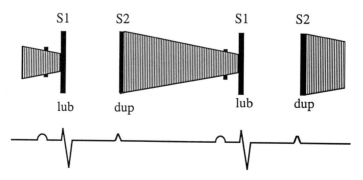

Fig. 3.10 Holodiastolic decrescendo murmur.

quality. In some cases there will be an increase in intensity at the time of atrial contraction, associated with the jet of blood striking the anterior septal leaflet of the mitral valve (see section 6.5.3).

Continuous machinery murmurs

Continuous machinery murmurs are associated with blood flow through a ductus arteriosus. Usually this flow has ceased within a few days of birth; if it is patent after this period it is known as a PDA (see section 5.10). The murmur waxes and wanes in intensity during systole and diastole and is continuous because of the persistence of a variable pressure gradient between the aorta and the pulmonary artery throughout the whole of the cardiac cycle (Figure 3.11). The PMI of the murmur is over the left heart base, but the murmur can be almost as loud over at the right heart base. If a ductus arteriosus remains patent, it may lead to CHF. As pulmonary hypertension develops, the diastolic element of the murmur is lost because the diastolic pressures in the aorta and the pulmonary artery begin to equilibrate. The murmur is quite common in neonates, but PDAs are very rare in animals over a few days of age.

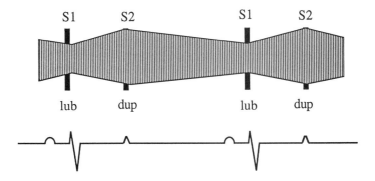

Fig. 3.11 Continuous machinery murmur.

Murmurs in horses with colic

Murmurs typical of MR and functional murmurs may also be detected in horses during episodes of colic. The reason for this is not clear; however, it seems likely that it is related to altered fluid balance rather than to myocardial depression or primary valvular disease. In some cases, the murmur may have been present but undetected for some time. It is wise to re-examine animals in which murmurs are detected in these circumstances, after other clinical problems have been resolved, before any judgement is made as to their significance.

3.5.4 Other abnormal heart sounds

Systolic clicks

Systolic clicks are short, sharp sounds heard in mid-systole. They are uncommon. Clicks are usually of unknown significance, although they are seldom associated with significant disease. There are a variety of causes including minor abnormalities of the chordae tendineae and AV valve prolapse. If a systolic click is heard, an echocardiographic examination may be helpful, in order to rule out significant cardiac disease.

Pericardial friction rubs

Pericardial disease is uncommon in the horse and there are few specific clinical findings which indicate its presence. However, a pericardial friction rub is a specific indication of the presence of pericardial disease, although not indicative of its severity. The sound is fairly distinctive and has been likened to the creaking of a door or the branch of a tree. It may be a single sound but it is usually biphasic or sometimes triphasic, occurring in systole and diastole. Subjectively, it sounds extracardiac, but it is in time with the cardiac cycle. It is caused by rubbing of the visceral pericardial surface with the epicardium. If a pericardial rub is heard, echocardiography is indicated as the most specific method of diagnosis of pericardial disease.

Gallop sounds

Gallop sounds are a combination of the third and fourth heart sounds, resulting in a three component sound to the cardiac cycle similar to the sound of the footfall of a galloping horse. While these sounds are abnormal in humans and small animals, in which they usually indicate the presence of significant myocardial disease, they are normal at higher heart rates in the horse.

3.6   The practice of auscultation

It is important that auscultation is performed in a methodical manner and that sufficient time is allowed for rhythm and rate to be assessed, and for the heart sounds to be heard over the entire cardiac silhouette, on both sides of the chest, at a true resting heart rate.

The stethoscope should first be placed over the apex beat. The beginning of systole can be recognised by movement of the stethoscope by the apical impulse. In the apex beat area, S1 will be clearly heard. S3 is best heard just ventral to this area. It may be helpful to establish the rhythm and rate of the heart initially, and then identify the beginning of systole and diastole. Then it is helpful to inch the stethoscope cranially and dorsally until it is over the cardiac base, where S2 will be heard best. As the stethoscope is moved, it may help first to concentrate on the heart sounds, then on systolic murmurs and then on diastolic murmurs. It is sometimes useful to 'listen-in' to different frequencies so that one can concentrate on low-pitched sounds and then on high-pitched sounds. The bell of the stethoscope transmits low-pitched sounds best and should be used in addition to the diaphragm. Once the cardiac area has been completely covered on the left side of the chest, the same process can be completed on the right. It is common for inexperienced clinicians to fail to advance the stethoscope far enough into the axilla and consequently they may miss important sounds. It may be helpful to make the horse stand with the leg advanced on the side of auscultation, if it is well tolerated.

After careful auscultation, it is helpful to make a note of the findings in the form of diagrams, as shown for the different murmur classifications, annotated onto an anatomical drawing of the cardiac area (Figure 3.12). This can be combined with case details and history into a clinical record sheet (Figure 3.13).

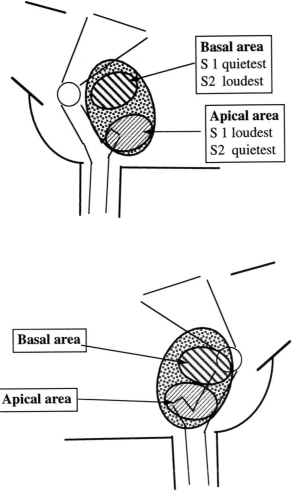

Fig. 3.12 Auscultation areas.
Auscultation areas over the left hemi-thorax (upper diagram) and right hemi-thorax (lower diagram), from which the point of maximal intensity can be localised.

3.7 Examination of the respiratory system

Auscultation of the lung fields is an important part of the clinical examination of the horse with suspected cardiac disease. It is important to identify changes which may be a result of cardiac disease, particularly the presence of pulmonary oedema due to left-sided heart failure. More commonly, pulmonary disease will be a complicating factor in an animal with cardiac disease. Alternatively, the signs of respiratory disease may be mistaken for those of heart disease.

Equine Cardiology Record Sheet

Date
Owner's name   Tel. No.
Horse's name
Age   Sex
Breed   Use
WT   Colour
Demeanour   Condition
M. memb   Pulse
Nasal discharge   Rate
Jugulars   A
Peripheral oedema   S1
Rhythm   S2
ECG   S3

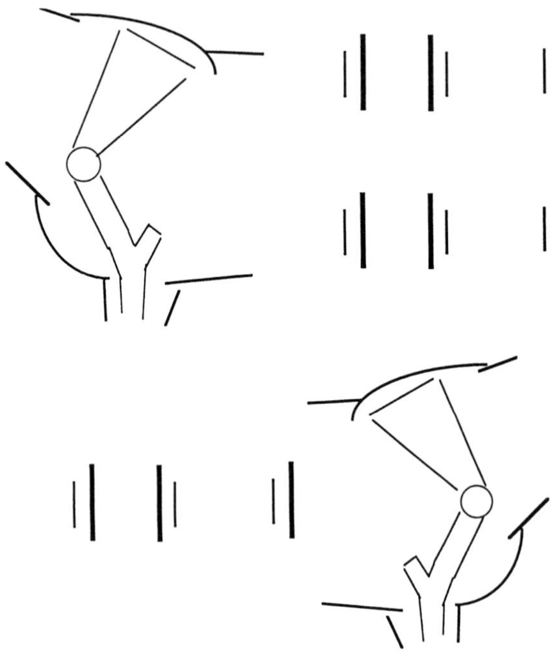

Fig. 3.13 A case record sheet.
This case sheet is used by the author to record case details including the characteristics of murmurs.

In addition to auscultation, examination of the lower respiratory tract (LRT) should also include percussion to establish the extent of the lung fields and the presence or absence of pleural fluid or air. The upper respiratory tract (URT) should also be examined. A nasal discharge may indicate URT disease such as sinusitis, URT infection, pharyngeal dysfunction with associated dysphagia, or LRT conditions such as viral or bacterial infection or chronic obstructive pulmonary disease. Laryngeal dysfunction due to recurrent laryngeal neuropathy is a very important cause of poor athletic performance and palpation of the larynx should form part of a routine clinical examination. Endoscopy is extremely useful for evaluation of both the upper and lower respiratory tract and clinicians who expect to see animals with suspected cardiac disease need to become familiar with the technique.

3.7.1 Auscultation of lung fields

Auscultation of respiratory sounds requires quiet surroundings because abnormal sounds may be very subtle. Sounds may be harsh and dry, or suggestive of fluid movement within airways. Frequently, the most obvious abnormal sound is that of air flowing over a pool of fluid in the trachea at the thoracic inlet; it is important to include this area in auscultation.

An invaluable aid to auscultation is the use of a re-breathing bag. This simple technique results in much deeper respiratory movements than normal and accentuates sounds. A large plastic bag is placed over the nose and twisted so that there is a tight air seal. The bag should be held so that it does not occlude the nares during inspiration. The horse will start to breathe more deeply because of the build-up of carbon dioxide in the exhaled air which it re-breathes. The technique is tolerated remarkably well. Coughing and large quantities of muco-pus are produced on occasion, which illustrates to owners the effects of the lung disease.

3.8 The effects of exercise

Cardiac disease is of most importance in the context of its effects on exercise tolerance. It is therefore logical to assume that examination of the animal during exercise is of value in assessing the significance of cardiac disease. Unfortunately, examination of animals during and even after exercise is complicated by a number of factors. Only a limited range of tests can be performed during exercise. There is also a tremendous difference in the fitness levels of different animals, and it is often unwise to assume that cardiac disease is responsible for apparent exercise intolerance. Nevertheless, so long as the limitations are considered, examination of the horse during and after exercise is of considerable value in selected cases. In addition, in the UK, examination of horses after exercise forms part of the pre-purchase examination and may correctly or incorrectly lead to the suspicion of cardiac disease.

Very few veterinarians in practice will have the opportunity to subject animals to controlled exercise programmes such as those which are possible using a high-speed treadmill. In the field, facilities for evaluating horses at exercise may limit the value of any tests. There is little purpose in examining a racehorse which has poor racing performance in a small muddy field. The principal purpose of examinations at exercise is to evaluate any abnormal cardiac rhythm rather than to assess the exercise tolerance of the animal.

3.8.1 Arrhythmias

The most common situation in which exercise is of use in clinical evaluations is to see whether arrhythmias detected at rest persist at higher heart rates and whether exercise induces arrhythmias. Vagally mediated arrhythmias such as 2°AVB and sinus block are usually abolished by reducing parasympathetic tone and increasing sympathetic tone. This is easily detected on auscultation after trotting the horse in hand. However, some arrhythmias, which were infrequent or absent at rest, may become more frequent, paroxysmal or sustained during exercise. It is important that these are detected and characterised because they are often associated with poor athletic performance. Occasionally arrhythmias which may be associated with pathological conditions, such as ventricular premature beats, are no longer apparent at higher heart rates. While this makes them less likely to be a significant problem, it is important that they are recognised. Thus, the abolition of an arrhythmia by increasing heart rate is not in itself a diagnosis of a vagally mediated arrhythmia, all arrhythmias should also be recognised by their other characteristics and if necessary by electrocardiography.

Recording exercising ECGs is particularly useful if an arrhythmia is present only during exercise, or if the effects of high intensity exercise on its frequency need to be assessed (see sections 4.1.6, 7.8.3, 7.8.6 and 7.8.8). Portable ECGs, rushed to the side of an animal after exercise, may also give valuable information, but are less satisfactory than radiotelemetric recordings during exercise.

3.8.2 Murmurs

It is a commonly held belief that murmurs which are inapparent after exercise are insignificant. In the author's view, this rule of thumb, while not wholly without foundation, is dangerous. Functional murmurs associated with ejection of blood through the semi-lunar valves are often variable in intensity at different heart rates. They are dependant on stroke volume and afterload, consequently they may vary if there is a change in heart rate. Sometimes these murmurs increase in intensity after excitement or exercise and may even become apparent in animals which are excited or exercised although they were absent at rest. Often auscultation after exercise is hampered by extraneous noise and respiratory sounds. Under these circumstances it is possible to miss murmurs which may be of significance to the future performance of the horse. For example, a quiet holosystolic plateau-type murmur associated with mitral insufficiency may be difficult to hear at higher heart rates. While a quiet murmur of this type may not always be significant at the time of examination, it is important that it is detected and not attributed to normal flow.

High-pitched early diastolic murmurs are particularly likely to be increased in intensity at heart rates in the range of 36–60 bpm. Sometimes murmurs will be less apparent after exercise, but it is not clear whether this is due to more difficult auscultatory conditions, particularly respiratory noise and wind blowing on the stethoscope if the examination is performed outside. Decreased murmur intensity may also be related to other changes such as increased blood viscosity due to splenic contraction.

It is important that all the characteristics of a murmur are considered in evaluating its origin and significance. If murmurs are characterised according to the guidelines described above (see section 3.5.1) it should be possible to identify the source of most cardiac murmurs, to make a specific diagnosis, and then to make a reasoned judgement of the significance of the condition.

3.8.3 Heart rate

The heart rate during exercise and recovery is relevant to the significance of a cardiac condition; however, it also depends on numerous variables such as the fitness of the horse, the state of the ground and presence of other abnormalities. Prolonged recovery following exercise may result from significant pulmonary or cardiac disease. As a rough guide, the heart rate should return to within 15% of the normal level within 15 minutes of the end of light exercise and within 30–45 minutes for more rigorous exercise. Horses with pulmonary disease may remain tachypnoeic for a prolonged period during which the heart rate has fallen at a normal rate.

Within the limits of the numerous factors which affect heart rate, a rough guide to the rate which would be expected after prolonged exercise at different gaits in a fit horse is of some value. Approximate values are:

	beats per minute
Trot	80
Canter	110
Fast canter	140
Gallop	180
Maximal heart rate	240

In some instances it may be helpful to establish what level of exercise can be achieved before reaching maximal heart rates. This may indicate the amount of work which the horse could reasonably be expected to perform.

3.8.4 Standardised exercise tests

Standardised treadmill exercise tests which allow graded exercise have been developed as a method of investigating exercise physiology and causes of poor athletic performance in racehorses. The level of fitness is often more predictable and uniform in these animals than in pleasure horses. The heart rate (and often ECG) can be monitored during the exercise while the speed and incline of the treadmill are altered in a series of steps. Signs of decreased exercise tolerance which may be shown on these tests are a high maximal heart rate, a short time taken to reach maximal heart rate, a low maximal oxygen uptake and a prolonged recovery time with slow return of heart rate to normal. However, some of these findings can result from musculo-skeletal problems, upper airway obstruction or lung disease; they are not specific for cardiac dysfunction. Therefore, although standardised exercise tests can be helpful in establishing that a problem is present, they are less useful for identifying the specific cause of poor performance.

Chapter 4

Diagnostic Aids in Equine Cardiology

The most important part of investigation of the cardiovascular system in all species is clinical examination and in particular auscultation. Following this, further diagnostic aids are used to provide additional information about disease processes and their effects. An increasing number of diagnostic aids are available. Thanks to the advent of new technologies it is now possible to obtain objective data about cardiac function which help to identify abnormalities and aid judgement of their severity. The use of these techniques is at the centre of continuing research into cardiovascular physiology and disease and is a rapidly developing field. However, in this chapter the emphasis is on the use of these techniques as practical aids to diagnosis and prognostication in clinical cases.

4.1 Electrocardiography

4.1.1 Principles

The principles of electrocardiography were described in detail in section 1.5. Physiological principles should be understood because they affect the way in which electrocardiography is used and its interpretation. Misconceptions about the value of the technique in horses are commonplace and erroneous extrapolations are often made from small animal and human electrocardiography.

4.1.2 Equipment

Equipment suitable for recording ECGs in horses is readily available and relatively cheap. Because the principal purpose of recording ECGs is to evaluate the cardiac rhythm rather than examine complex size and conformation in different leads, a single-channel machine is ideal. These are now small and light enough to be held in one hand. They are usually battery powered so they can be used in the horse's stable, or even used where the animal is exercised. The only advantage to using a multi-channel machine is that movement artefacts, which may be evident on two leads only, might be misinterpreted as an abnormal complex when only one channel is recorded. Multi-channel recordings can also be useful in the rare situation when a clear P wave is not seen using the bipolar leads commonly used in the horse (see below), in which case a different lead system may show the waveform more clearly. However, in the vast majority of cases, a single-lead recording is all that is required.

A large number of single-channel machines are available. Unfortunately the clips supplied by the manufacturer are often inadequate and it is worth purchasing silver-nickel crocodile clips, filing down the teeth and bending the jaws so that they are atruamatic but still remain firmly attached to the horse. Spare leads can be taped together so that they do not tangle. Careful storage of the recording is advisable because it will spoil if it is allowed to get wet or is exposed to direct sunlight. Envelopes provide a cheap and convenient filing method.

4.1.3 Recording an ECG

Recording an ECG in a horse is simple. All that is required is a clear trace in which the P waves and QRS complexes are easily seen. Limb leads, particularly lead two, are often adequate. However, horses have a strong panniculus reflex when clips are attached to their upper limbs and movement will result in artefacts on the recording. A much simpler method is to record from the trunk of the body. Because the mean vector of ventricular depolarisation recorded on the body surface ECG is directed mainly cranially and dorsally, the largest signals are recorded with a bipolar lead placed in a ventro-dorsal or cranio-caudal plane. The two lead systems which are commonly used are a base-apex lead and a Y lead.

A *base-apex lead* has the positive electrode positioned over the apex beat area of the heart (i.e. on the chest wall just behind the left olecranon) and the negative electrode over the cardiac base. The left or right jugular furrow, or the loose area of skin just cranial to the scapula, are suitable as the position for the basal electrode.

A *Y lead* has the negative electrode attached over the manubrium at the thoracic inlet and the positive electrode over the xiphoid.

In both these systems the QRS complex is largely negative because the cardiac vector is directed cranially and dorsally, away from the positive electrode. If the electrodes are attached the wrong way round the QRS complex will be largely positive, which does not prevent assessment of cardiac rhythm but can be confusing.

On most machines, in order to obtain a bipolar lead it is convenient to use the leads marked 'right arm' (usually coloured red in the UK) and 'left arm' (usually coloured yellow in the UK). If the lead selection dial is turned to record lead one the right arm lead will be negative and the left arm lead positive. A neutral electrode is required if a mains-powered machine is used (use the electrode labelled 'right foot', which is usually black). The thoracic inlet is a convenient site for a base-apex neutral lead, the neck for a Y lead.

When a trace is recorded, a paper speed of 25 mm/sec is usually appropriate, although a faster speed is required if a tachycardia is present. The amplitude of deflection should be marked on the trace at the beginning of the recording. The standard deflection used is 10 mm/mV; however, the amplitude of the QRS complex may be too large to fit on the paper, particularly with a base-apex recording, and 5 mm/mV may be preferable. With most machines, the thickness of the baseline is determined by the stylus heat. This can be turned up or down as appropriate. Paper is marked in either blue or black. Black traces duplicate better if they are to be photocopied or sent by facsimile. Electrode gel provides the best electrical contact; however, spirit can also be used.

The lead systems which are used in the horse are shown in Figure 4.1 and Table 4.1. The limb leads and chest leads are shown only because they are sometimes required by overseas veterinarians at pre-purchase examinations; however, in the view of the author, they very seldom aid diagnosis. If a rechargeable machine is used, it is worth remembering that it should be recharged after use and not left switched on.

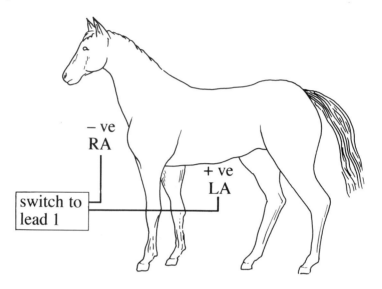

Fig. 4.1   Recording a base-apex or Y lead ECG.

4.1.4   Interpretation of an ECG

Evaluation of an ECG ('reading' an ECG) should be carried out in a thorough methodical manner. It is helpful if a consistent system is adopted so that errors are not made. A check list for assessing ECGs is shown in Table 4.2. The identification of specific arrhythmias is described in detail in Chapter 7. A typical normal ECG is shown in Figure 4.2. Identification of the waveforms and interval measurements are shown in Figure 4.3 and Table 4.3.

Heart rate

Heart rate is easily calculated by counting the number of complexes in a known period, for example counting the number within a 12 second interval and multiplying by 5. Alternatively, the rate per minute can be calculated by dividing 60 by the R–R duration in seconds. ECG paper is divided into small boxes (of 1 mm) and large boxes (of 5 mm). At a paper speed of 25 mm/sec, each small box represents an interval of 0.04 seconds, and each large box therefore represents 0.2 seconds. If accurate measurements of durations are required then a faster paper speed (50 mm/sec) aids measurement. Often the paper is marked with

Table 4.1 The lead systems which can be used for recording an ECG

Base-apex lead	Right arm electrode (red in UK, white in US) cranial to the right (or left) scapula
	Left arm electrode (yellow in UK, black in US) over the apex beat on the left side (level with the olecranon)
	Record 'lead I'
Y lead	RA electrode over manubrium
	LA electrode over xiphoid
	Record 'lead I'
Limb leads and augmented leads	
Lead I	Potential difference (PD) between left fore leg (+ve) and right fore leg (–ve)
Lead II	PD between left hind leg (+ve) and right fore leg (–ve)
Lead III	PD between left hind leg (+ve) and left fore leg (–ve)
aVR	PD between right fore leg (+ve) and the left fore and left hind legs (–ve)
aVL	PD between left fore leg (+ve) and the right fore and left hind legs (–ve)
aVF	PD between left hind leg (+ve) and the right and left fore legs (–ve)
Chest leads	
CV6LL	PD between the left sixth ics, level of the olecranon (–ve) and the central terminal
CV6LU	PD between the left sixth ics, level of the shoulder (–ve) and the central terminal
CV6RL	PD between the right sixth ics, level of the olecranon (–ve) and the central terminal
CV6RU	PD between the right sixth ics, level of the shoulder (–ve) and the central terminal
V3	Approximately = CV6LL
V10	PD between the point of the withers in the mid-line (–ve) and the central terminal, also called a Z lead

Table 4.2 Interpretation of an ECG

1. Assess the *quality* of ECG. Check the calibration of the amplitude of deflection, the paper speed and whether the filter was on or off. Look for artefacts.
2. Calculate the *heart rate*. Establish whether it is fast, slow or normal, and whether it is variable.
3. Assess the *overall rhythm*. Establish whether changes in rhythm are intermittent or persistent and whether they are induced or terminated by excitement or any procedures such as a vagal manoeuvre (e.g. ocular pressure or carotid sinus massage).
4. Assess each *wave/complex* in turn. Measure the duration and amplitude of the P wave and QRS complex and the duration of the intervals. Establish whether all the complexes are similar or not.
5. Examine the *relationship between the complexes*. Check whether each P wave is followed by a QRS complex, and whether there is a P wave before each QRS complex.
6. Define the *heart rhythm* and a *plan* for further diagnostic investigations and treatment if necessary.

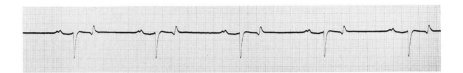

Fig. 4.2 A typical normal ECG recorded with a base-apex lead.

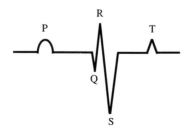

Fig. 4.3 Identification of the waveforms of the ECG.

Table 4.3 Measurements of the normal complex and interval duration

	Guideline normal values for ECG wave and complex durations and intervals (Y lead)	
	Duration (sec)	No. small boxes (25 mm/sec)
P wave	< or = 0.16	4.0
PR interval	< or = 0.5	12.5
QRS complex	< or = 0.14	3.5
QT interval	< or = 0.6	15.0

lines above the divisions on the trace which represent one second intervals when a paper speed of 25 mm/sec is used. Some ECG machines will mark one second intervals on the paper.

Mean electrical axis

Calculation of the mean electrical axis from the limb leads is of little clinical value in horses because the vector in the frontal plane is extremely variable and because the use of Einthoven's triangle is less appropriate in horses than in small animals (see section 1.5.5). From a practical standpoint, the amplitude of the complex is not a useful guide to heart size. However, the amplitude may be reduced if there is a pleural or pericardial effusion, and increased during exercise, or if the animal is excited, or if a complex has a ventricular origin.

Waveforms

It is important to be able to recognise normal complexes. P waves are small deflections of a few millivolts which are usually positive in a base-apex or Y lead recording. They are often notched and may have a positive and a negative component (biphasic). The QRS complex is usually a larger deflection (up to 3–4 mV in a base-apex lead). The first negative deflection is the Q wave, the first positive deflection is the R wave, and the second negative deflection is the S wave. The T wave follows and is very labile in size and orientation (see below).

Interval duration

The ECG should be examined to determine the duration of the intervals between complexes. The principal purpose of this process is to determine heart rate, although interval duration is also dependent on the conduction process and may be affected by autonomic tone, electrolyte levels and drugs. Unfortunately, the effects of electrolyte disturbances on wave morphology and interval duration are less predictable in the horse compared with small animals, therefore evaluation of the ECG is not a particularly useful method of assessing abnormalities in electrolyte levels.

Artefacts

It is important to be able to recognise artefacts so that they are not interpreted as abnormalities and, ideally, to be able to eliminate them. The most common artefacts are due to movement, either of the horse or of the leads or clips. Any such movement should be kept to a minimum. It is helpful to hold the leads close to the clips so that they do not swing. Movement artefact is particularly difficult to avoid when recording an ECG in an exercising animal. These artefacts are seen as sharp deflections which are haphazard but may occasionally resemble a QRS complex. Muscle tremor may produce a fine motion of the baseline of lower amplitude. Large undulations in the baseline may be caused by exaggerated respiratory motion. This may be less marked on a Y lead than a base-apex lead.

Interference from electrical mains hum is a common cause of artefact, especially with mains-powered ECG machines. This is apparent as regular waves at a frequency of 50 Hz. Mains interference can be reduced by ensuring that all the leads have good electrical coupling with the horse. A neutral electrode should be used. Standing the horse on a rubber insulating mat will help. Turning off other electrical appliances in the room, including fluorescent lights, also reduces the interference. The ECG machine and the mains supply should be properly earthed. Battery-powered machines pick up more interference when they are running low on power. If electrical artefact is still present, switch the ECG filter on. This is specifically designed to cut out high-frequency noise such as AC interference.

T-wave morphology

T-wave morphology is extremely variable and is particularly dependent on heart rate. Even beat to beat changes in the R–R interval often affect the size and polarity of the T wave. T-wave changes may also be seen in animals with cardiac disease, electrolyte disturbances and systemic disease. However, the changes are extremely variable and non-specific and they are therefore of little use in making a specific diagnosis. Some veterinarians have attached a lot of significance to T-wave changes. It has been suggested that these abnormalities are suggestive of myocarditis or heart strain, and that they are related to poor athletic performance. The pathophysiological basis of the condition described by the term heart strain is unclear, indeed it is difficult to establish what is meant by this term. T-wave changes may occur in myocarditis; however, since the T-wave changes are not specific and it is difficult to define a normal T-wave, in the author's opinion they are not helpful in the diagnosis of myocarditis. Recently, it has been shown that T-wave changes are a common finding in horses in training which have a normal performance record, although they are less commonly found in animals which are being rested.

4.1.5   Heart score

The measurement of heart score was popularised in Australia by Steel and co-workers in the 1960s and is still widely used in the southern hemisphere. It is measured by calculating the mean duration of the QRS complex in the three-limb leads. Steel found the measurement to correlate closely with athletic performance and heart weight. However, later studies have failed to find a strong correlation between these factors. The method has little basis in electrophysiology because the majority of the myocardium is electrically silent at the body surface (see section 1.5.6). In addition, precise measurement of the duration of the QRS complex is difficult because the ST segment is slurred in many normal animals. There are a number of reasons why the measurement may be increased in athletic animals. However, in the author's view, measurement of heart score is a misleading technique in individual horses and has no clinical value.

4.1.6   ECGs recorded during exercise

Many horses have arrhythmias at rest which result from the high vagal tone which is found in this species. These arrhythmias are usually abolished by the fall in vagal tone and increase in sympathetic tone which accompanies excitement or exercise. Auscultation is usually sufficient to detect resolution of the arrhythmia. Only a slight increase in heart rate is usually required, so the rhythm can also be recorded by performing a standard ECG examination once the animal comes to rest.

It is more difficult to detect arrhythmias which occur during high heart rates at peak exercise, or which may occur at exercise more or less frequently than at rest. This is particularly important in the case of atrial premature complexes (APCs), ventricular premature complexes (VPCs), and paroxysmal atrial fibrillation. To evaluate these arrhythmias, which are often associated with poor athletic performance, it is very helpful to record an ECG while the animal is actually exercising. To do this the horse can be run on a treadmill and attached to the ECG machine by wires ('hard-wired'). Alternatively, radiotelemetry can be used with the horse exercised in its usual environment, or on a treadmill. With radiotelemetry, there is less chance of wires pulling on the electrodes and causing interference. For outdoor use, a battery-powered machine is useful. The range of the transmitter and receiving unit ideally should be at least 100 m.

The main problem with ECGs recorded at exercise is poor electrical contact which results in artefacts and makes interpretation of the ECG trace difficult. This is best avoided by placing the electrodes in small perforated chamois leather pouches sewn on to a girth strap. The leather pouches are soaked in water or saline and the strap is pulled very tight. The best contact is found when the animal starts to sweat. Alternatively, the electrodes can be attached to a shaved area of skin with adhesive. Electrodes are usually placed either side of the chest. Trial and error may be required in order to find the electrode positions which produce the largest QRS complex but least artefact due to movement and poor electrical contact in different individuals.

Radiotelemetry is also useful for monitoring animals with arrhythmias while they are being treated with anti-dysrhythmic drugs, or for the monitoring of any acute-care patient. It is particularly useful for monitoring animals during treatment for atrial fibrillation (AF). If these animals are suddenly excited or are moved for an ECG to be recorded, and are already hypotensive, they have been known to collapse. In addition, because an ECG can be recorded continuously, significant changes in the cardiac rhythm such as the development of an atrial tachycardia can be seen and appropriate action taken before clinical signs deteriorate.

4.1.7 *Heart rate monitors*

Heart rate monitors can be useful in some situations, such as measuring heart rate at different levels of exercise. The main factor in determining heart rate at any level of exercise is fitness. However, animals with heart disease may have an inappropriately high heart rate. Because the degree of fitness is so variable in different animals, no precise rate should be expected. However, in animals with heart disease, knowing what level of exercise can be performed before maximal heart rates (usually around 220–240 bpm) are reached, can be helpful. For example, in a horse with AF which fails to respond to treatment, or an animal with valvular disease, the level of exercise which is required to raise the heart rate to an arbitrary level such as 180 bpm, may be a good guide to the amount of work which the animal can safely be expected to perform. Radiotelemetry will also provide this information.

4.1.8 24-hour ECG monitoring

One of the principal problems with standard ECG recording is that the cardiac rhythm is only recorded for a very short period of time. Consequently, a significant arrhythmia may not be detected during the examination, particularly if it is intermittent. In addition, when the animal is truly at rest, a different rhythm may be observed than when the clinician is present.

A 'Holter' monitor can be used to record the ECG signal on magnetic tape over a 24-hour period. The electrodes are attached with adhesive and can be bandaged in place or held by a tight girth. Some horses will require a roller to stop them rolling and displacing the electrodes. The tape is then played through a computer which is programmed to detect specific arrhythmias. Although the recording monitors themselves are relatively cheap, the computer system is very expensive and the tapes are usually sent to a human hospital for analysis. The computer must be programmed to search for parameters suitable for equine rather than human arrhythmias.

There are a number of situations in which a 24-hour ECG recording is helpful. In animals which collapse intermittently, arrhythmias are often suspected. Since animals seldom collapse when the clinician is present, and an arrhythmia may not be present at the time of the clinical examination, a 24-hour ECG may be of benefit. However, even then it may only be helpful if the animal actually collapses during the period of the recording (see section 8.3.2). 24-hour ECGs are perhaps more useful in detecting paroxysmal bouts of arrhythmias such as atrial or ventricular tachycardia. Atrial premature beats may be found in animals with poor athletic performance related to myocarditis. Animals which have repeated bouts of AF, which either resolve spontaneously (paroxysmal AF) or have been successfully treated, may have APCs during the remission of AF. In this instance, the chances of recurrence of AF are increased and the animal should be rested (see section 7.8.5).

When atrial or ventricular premature beats are detected during a routine ECG, it may be difficult to decide how significant they are. They may be only very occasional, in which case they are unlikely to be significant. However, there is the possibility that they are occurring with increased frequency at times other than the period of examination and may be of clinical significance. Vagally mediated arrhythmias and bradycardia are much more frequently detected during a 24-hour recording than during a standard examination. Although it may be difficult to interpret the findings, these recordings give clinicians valuable information which would not otherwise be available.

4.2 Echocardiography

In human and small animal medicine, radiography and electrocardiography provide useful information about cardiac chamber size. In the adult horse, these techniques are of little value for this purpose. Echocardiography is a non-invasive diagnostic technique which allows images of cardiac structure to obtained, the size of cardiac chambers and vessels to determined, and quantitative and qualitative information about cardiac function to be derived. Previously, this information required invasive techniques or post-mortem examination. It is no exaggeration to say that echocardiography has revolutionised equine cardiology. It has allowed clinicians not only to identify cardiac lesions, but to make objective assessments of the effects of these lesions. It has improved our understanding of normal cardiac function and cardiac disease in the horse and has allowed non-invasive assessment of the effects of drugs and exercise training on the heart.

Echocardiography is a technique that is now within the financial reach of some practices and is likely to become more widely available in the future as prices fall further. Practitioners who do not have access to equipment suitable for equine echocardiography should understand the uses of the technique so that they can decide which cases would benefit from referral to a specialist centre. Anyone with an interest in cardiology should be encouraged to see real-time echocardiography because it provides a clearer understanding of cardiac anatomy and function in normal and diseased animals than is possible from clinical examination and reading of literature alone.

4.2.1 The principles of echocardiography

2DE and M-mode echocardiography

A understanding of ultrasound physics and the control settings of ultrasound machines is required if good quality images are to be obtained. Ultrasound is high-frequency sound which is produced when a piezoelectric crystal, mounted in a transducer, is stimulated by an electrical current. The sound waves are too high in frequency to be audible. They are thought to be harmless to tissue at the intensities used in diagnostic imaging. The passage of sound waves depends on the acoustic impedance of body tissues. Sound is reflected by interfaces between materials of different acoustic impedance.

The majority of the ultrasound waves pass through structures on to other structures lying further from the surface, but reflected sound returns to strike the crystal, deforming it and producing electric signals which correspond to the degree of deformation. This electrical information is transformed by electronics in the ultrasound machine so that it can be displayed on a cathode-ray tube as pulses of light. Because the speed of sound within the body is relatively constant, the depth of the tissue interface can be known and reflected echoes are displayed on the screen on a depth scale.

In echocardiography, sound is directed into the body and is reflected by interfaces between tissues of different acoustic impedance such as myocardium, valves and blood. Blood reflects little sound so it appears relatively black (hypoechoic, or anechoic) compared with the myocardium which reflects more of the ultrasound and therefore appears relatively white (hyperechoic or echogenic). The endocardium and valves are the most echogenic structures. Ultrasound does not pass through air or bone. Because the heart is surrounded by lung over the majority of its surface and is contained within the bony cage of the thoracic cavity, the ultrasound beam must be aimed through gaps (which are known as acoustic windows), in order to produce images of the heart.

Frequencies of 2–10 MHz are used in diagnostic ultrasound. The lower end of this range is used in transducers designed for equine echocardiography because low frequency sound penetrates a greater depth of tissue. A trade-off in the use of low frequency transducers is that there is a loss of image detail because the increased wavelength results in reduced resolution.

M-mode echocardiography and two-dimensional echocardiography (2DE) are the two techniques which are usually used to produce images of the heart in real-time. In M-mode echocardiography (motion mode, or time-motion mode), the crystal is stationary and the beam produced is a pencil-beam of sound. The signal is produced almost continuously. Echoes are displayed on the screen on the Y axis, with time displayed on the X axis (Figure 4.4). This produces an almost continuous image of the position of the cardiac structures which are in the line of the beam.

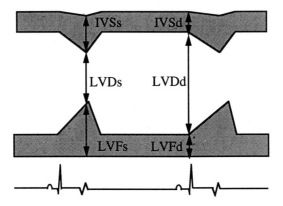

Fig. 4.4   A diagram of an M-mode echocardiogram (right parasternal short-axis, chordal level) showing measurement of left ventricular dimensions.

Echocardiography has become more popular since the advent of 2DE, which produces an image of cardiac structure. 2DE images are also referred to as B-mode images (brightness mode). Originally, static B-mode images were produced, but improvements in technology allowed the image to be rapidly updated resulting in a real-time image. 2DE images are more easily understood than M-mode traces because of the greater spatial detail. A comparison has been made between the two techniques and different ways of illuminating a room. M-mode is the equivalent of looking round a dark room with a narrow-beam torch. 2DE is the equivalent of using a floodlight.

A 2DE image can be produced in one of three ways. The first and simplest is to have multiple crystals mounted in line to produce a 'curtain' of sound. This method is known as linear array and is used in many rectal probes in current use in veterinary medicine. The problem with the use of this technology for echo-cardiography is that it is difficult to aim the curtain of sound through the acoustic windows, so some of the heart is likely to be obscured from view and only a limited number of views can be obtained. This prevents a complete echo-cardiographic investigation, although it may allow detection of gross abnormalities such as a pericardial effusion, very poor myocardial contractility, or large vegetations on the heart valves.

To be able to examine the heart in a large number of image planes, a point source is required with a sector or 'fan' of sound produced by sweeping the sound in an arc. Transducers which produce this arc of sound are called sector scanners. The sector can be produced by rotating or oscillating the crystal mechanically; this type of transducer is called a mechanical sector scanner. Alternatively the sector can be produced by using an array of crystals which are electronically stimulated in sequence to produce a fan-shaped beam. These are known as phased-array transducers. Because the beam has to be swept through an arc, a finite time is taken to produce each sector image. The arc is then repeated and the image is updated. The quality of the image therefore depends on how many lines of data are displayed per arc and how often the image is updated. The rate at which the image is updated is known as the frame rate.

One of the main problems in equine echocardiography is the great depth which is required for the whole heart to be displayed on the screen. Because the transducer has to wait longer for the sound to be reflected back from tissue interfaces at greater depth, the whole arc takes much longer to produce than those with less depth, and the frame rate is relatively low. Fortunately, the significance of this is offset to some extent by the slow resting heart rate in the horse, which means that the number of frames per cardiac cycle is much the same in equine echocardiography as it is in human echocardiography.

Doppler echocardiography

The principles of Doppler echocardiography (DE) are somewhat more complex than those of ultrasound imaging. DE has been used in equine medicine since the late 1980s and has proved particularly valuable in evaluation of congenital heart disease and acquired valvular heart disease. It is used to provide information about blood flow, following evaluation of the structure and the size of the heart using 2DE and M-mode studies. DE is also very useful in a research setting for assessment of cardiac function. A thorough DE examination requires rigorous technique and is extremely time-consuming. Equipment for DE is still relatively costly and the technique is likely to remain limited to referral centres for the foreseeable future. Recently, colour-coded DE has become available to a few institutions. This technique reduces the time required for Doppler examinations and makes them easier to perform, but has the same physical limitations.

The Doppler principle is evident to anyone standing by a railway line or a busy road as traffic moves past: the pitch of the sound of an engine drops as the vehicles pass. This is because sound waves are compressed as a source of sound moves towards an observer and are therefore higher in frequency than those emitted when the source is travelling away from the observer (Figure 4.5). The principle also applies to sound which is reflected off a moving target. The change in frequency of the sound is proportional to the velocity of the target in relation to the source of the sound.

DE involves the emission of ultrasound waves of known velocity which are reflected from interfaces and return to the transducer, in the same way as for echocardiographic imaging. The equipment detects changes in the frequency of the reflected sound in comparison to the emitted sound. In DE, the most important interfaces which reflect the sound are red blood cells (RBCs). Thus, if the emitted ultrasound is reflected off RBCs moving towards the transducer the reflected sound will be of a higher frequency (and shorter wavelength) than the emitted sound. The change in frequency (frequency shift) is proportional to the

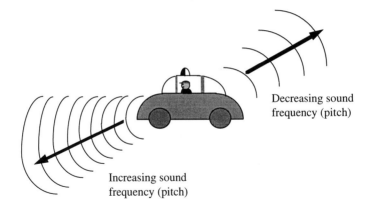

Fig. 4.5 The Doppler effect.
The sound emitted by a car is perceived as higher in pitch if the car is moving towards an observer than if it is moving away. The change in pitch is proportional to the velocity of the car. The same principle applies to sound reflecting from red blood cells back to an ultrasound transducer (see text).

velocity of the cells towards the transducer. A computer inside the Doppler unit calculates the velocity of the moving blood from the Doppler shift equation (Table 4.4). The calculated velocity is displayed on a velocity/time graph with blood flow towards the transducer displayed above a baseline and flow away displayed below it. This form of display is known as spectral Doppler (Figure 4.6). The standard form of DE, in which the transducer emits and receives sound waves simultaneously, is known as continuous-wave (CW) Doppler.

A critical feature of the Doppler shift equation is the effect on the angle of the beam to blood flow (Figure 4.7). If the cells are moving in a direction oblique to the line of the ultrasound beam, the velocity calculated will be an underestimate of their true velocity unless this angle is known and can be included in the calculation. Unfortunately, the exact angle is seldom known. Estimating it and using the angle correction software which is available on many machines usually only adds to the potential inaccuracy of the method. This means that, at all times, every effort should be made to keep the line of the ultrasound beam parallel to blood flow. In practice, angles under 15° either side of parallel are acceptable because the error will be less than 4%.

Initially, DE was performed independently of echocardiographic imaging. Later, it became possible to display Doppler information at the same time as an image, a technique known as duplex imaging. This allows the echocardiographer to guide the position of the Doppler beam within the heart. Another advance was the development of pulsed-wave Doppler (PWD). With standard CW Doppler, the frequency shift in the reflected ultrasound can come from anywhere along the course of the beam. However, it is often helpful to obtain information about blood flow in specific parts of the cardiac chambers and great vessels. PWD sends a pulse of known, short duration, and then records returning echoes for a limited period some time later. By limiting the period during which returned echoes are detected, the distance from the transducer of the targets which return the echoes is known. The 'gated' period can be displayed on the

Table 4.4 Doppler equations (Doppler shift equation, Bernouilli equation, Nyquist principle, calculation of cardiac output)

Doppler shift equation

$$\text{Frequency shift} = \frac{2FV \cos \alpha^0}{C}$$

where
F = emitted frequency
V = velocity of the reflecting target (blood cells)
α^0 = the angle between the ultrasound beam and the direction of blood flow
C = is the velocity of sound in the body (1560 m/sec)

Bernouilli equation (modified)

$$P = 4 \times (V_2^2 - V_1^2)$$

where
P = the pressure gradient across the narrowing (e.g. valve or VSD)
V_1 = the initial velocity
V_2 = the maximum velocity in the narrowing
Usually when Doppler measurements of velocity are made, velocity is high and V_1 is negligible, so P can be approximated to $= 4 \times (V_2^2)$

Nyquist principle
Nyquist limit = PRF/2
i.e. aliasing occurs when Doppler frequency $> \frac{1}{2}$ pulse repetition frequency

Calculation of cardiac output
Stroke volume = velocity time integral × internal area of vessel
(Velocity time integral (VTI) = area within envelope of spectral Doppler trace)
CO = stroke volume × heart rate

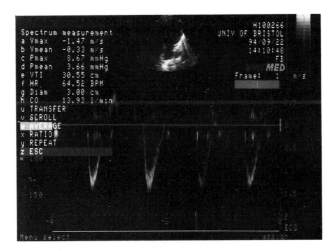

Fig. 4.6 A spectral Doppler display.
A line has been traced around the signal recording blood flow through the aortic valve (the envelope). The display is below the baseline because the blood is flowing away from the transducer. The envelope is clear because the blood flow is laminar, i.e. the cells are all moving at the same speed. Note that the velocity of flow is greatest in the early–mid systole.

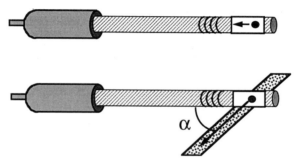

Fig. 4.7 Effect of angle on Doppler measurements.
In order to measure the true velocity of flow the Doppler beam must be parallel to blood flow. If the beam is oblique:

measured velocity = actual velocity × cos α° (see text).

screen as a small box known as the sample volume. This corresponds to the area of the heart from which the Doppler signals are received. The time taken for the PWD sound-wave to reach the near end of the sample volume can be termed T1. The time taken for it to reach the far end of the sample volume can be termed T2. The machine starts to listen to returning echoes after T1 × 2 and stops after T2 × 2 (Figure 4.8). The sample volume can be guided into specific areas of interest such as the atrial side of atrioventricular (AV) valves to detect regurgitant blood flow, or the right ventricular side of a ventricular septal defect (VSD) to detect blood flowing through the defect. Thus DE can be used to detect blood flow, to identify the direction of flow, and to calculate the velocity of flow.

One of the problems with the use of PWD is that the rate at which the pulses of sound are produced is limited by the fact that a new pulse cannot be sent until the preceding one has been received. The number of pulses which can be sent per second is known as the pulse repetition frequency (PRF). The greater the depth

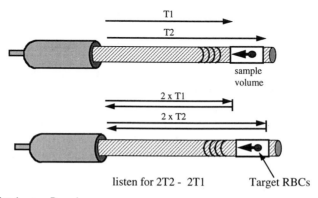

Fig. 4.8 Pulsed-wave Doppler.
Pulsed-wave Doppler echocardiography allows measurement of blood flow in a specific anatomical site. The velocity of sound in soft tissue is known so the distance from the transducer can be calculated. The Doppler beam is 'range gated' by sending a short pulse of known duration and recording recorded signals a set period of time later. The transducer will begin receiving after (T1) × 2 and stop after (T2) × 2.

of the sample volume, the lower the PRF. The PRF becomes a limiting factor when measuring the frequency shift associated with high velocity jets. This is because of a physical factor known as the Nyquist principle. This states that frequency shift (and therefore velocity) can only be measured accurately when the sampling rate is twice or more than twice that of the frequency shift being measured (Table 4.4). When the Nyquist limit is exceeded, the flow of blood will be displayed in the opposite direction to its true direction (aliased) which can be confusing. Aliasing is a particular problem in horses because the depth of many areas of interest means that PRF is relatively low, while the velocity of jets associated with valvular regurgitation or a VSD are usually quite high. For this reason, quantitative data about high-velocity jets is best derived from CW Doppler, which is not affected by aliasing.

When a PWD sample volume is placed in an area of laminar flow, for example the flow which is usually found in the pulmonary artery, a clear line will be displayed on the velocity/time graph indicating that the majority of the blood cells are moving at the same speed. Where this clear line is seen it is described as an 'envelope' (Figure 4.6). A line can be drawn around the envelope, and the area under the line is the velocity/time integral (VTI). The VTI is directly proportional to the stroke volume ejected through the valve and, if the area of the vessel is accurately measured and the VTI is the maximum which can be recorded from the site (i.e. the ultrasound beam is parallel to the line of blood flow), the stroke volume can be calculated. Cardiac output is then simply calculated by multiplying the stroke volume by the heart rate (Table 4.4).

The clarity of the envelope of a PWD signal depends on the range of blood flow velocities within a sample volume. When the sample volume is placed in an area of turbulent flow associated with a regurgitant jet which is causing a cardiac murmur, a range of RBC velocities will be seen because blood is flowing in different directions relative to the transducer. It may even be displayed either side of the baseline.

The principles of physics can be put to good use by clinicians. An example is the use of DE to estimate pressure gradients, a task which previously required invasive catheterisation techniques. Once accurate measurements of the frequency shift associated with a jet of blood flowing between two chambers have been made, it is possible to estimate the pressure gradient between these chambers using a derivative of the Bernouilli equation. A simplified version of this equation is suitable for use in most instances (Table 4.4). An example of the use of this principle is estimation of the pressure gradient between the left ventricle (LV) and right ventricle (RV) in an animal with a VSD. This is estimated from CW Doppler measurement of the velocity of blood shunting through the defect. If the RV pressure is raised then the defect is likely to be of clinical significance and may affect the horse's athletic ability (see section 5.5.5).

Colour-flow Doppler mapping
Colour-flow DE (colour-coded DE) is a form of PWD which is subject to exactly the same physical limitations as standard PWD. The direction of flow in a large number of individual sample volumes is measured and colour-coded. Usually, flow away from the transducer is coded blue, flow towards the transducer is coded red. The colour scale is usually displayed on the side of the screen. The

tone of the colour depends on the velocity of flow and its brightness on the intensity of the signal (i.e. on the number of RBCs reflecting sound). The colour-coded pixels are displayed in a sector superimposed on a 2DE image so that the location of the flow within the heart is known. It is important to restrict the angle of the 2DE image and colour sectors as much as possible because the information requires time to be collected and may produce this result in a very slow frame rate, particularly if the depth display is large. As with PWD, aliasing occurs; with colour-flow Doppler the blood will be encoded with the opposite colour from that expected. Some machines code areas of turbulent or disturbed flow with a 'variance' pattern in green.

4.2.2 Equipment

Many veterinary practices now have ultrasound equipment for pregnancy and tendon scanning. Unfortunately this equipment is seldom suitable for echo-cardiography. As discussed in the previous section, equine echocardiography is best performed with a low-frequency sector scanner. A frequency of 2.0–3.0 MHz is suitable, although a 3.5 or 5.0 MHz transducer may be best for echocardiography of foals because the penetration is adequate and resolution is improved.

A number of other features are important considerations in selection of suitable equipment. These are summarised in Table 4.5. Most practices will be forced to compromise when selecting an ultrasound machine, but a suitable

Table 4.5 Features of an ultrasound machine required for equine echocardiography

Essential
Sector scanner
2DE and M-mode echocardiography
Transducer frequency < 3.0 MHz
Depth display > 24 cm

Highly desirable
Transducer frequency 2.0–2.5 MHz
Long focus transducer
Depth display 30 cm
ECG timing
High quality video recorder
Cine-loop facility
Angle of beam 70–100°
Flexible gain setting
Measuring software
Doppler (steerable CW, stand alone CW, pulsed-wave Doppler, high PRF
    pulsed-wave Doppler)
Foot switch for freeze frame and 2DE/M-mode/Doppler change
Portability
Hard copy facility such as a video printer or a multi-format camera

Often promoted by manufacturers, but seldom helpful
Cardiac software package
ECG triggered freeze frame

frequency and depth display are essential if effective echocardiography is to be performed. Ultrasound machines used for echocardiography should have an M-mode facility which can be selected rapidly rather than via a complex menu. Machines should also be equipped with ECG leads and ECG display. This is particularly valuable for making measurements at specific times of the cardiac cycle and for interpreting spectral Doppler. A foot pedal for freezing frames or for switching from 2DE to M-mode is very helpful.

Ancillary equipment is also important. The most important of these is a good quality video recorder which is required unless a cine-loop facility is available on the ultrasound machine. A video tape recording is the best means of recording hard copy for later analysis or comparison with other studies because the real-time image is much easier to interpret than a still frame. Other forms of hard copy are also available. Equipment for Polaroid photography is relatively cheap but each image is quite expensive. Multi-format cameras provide good quality images but are expensive both in terms of capital and running costs. A video printer is cheaper if more than a few images are to be made and is ideal for most practices.

4.2.3 *Practical use of echocardiography*

Echocardiography is a skill which must be learned and for which there is no substitute other than practice. However, it is important that even the most experienced echocardiographer follows a standardised examination technique so that oversights are avoided. The examination is facilitated by effective restraint of the animal and thorough patient preparation.

Animals must be suitably restrained so that they do not damage expensive equipment, but most horses accept the feel of the transducer after a few seconds. It is important that animals are treated calmly so that they become used to the presence of the echocardiographer and equipment; excitement-induced tachycardia will not help assessment of the examination. In fact, in some horses the heart rate falls during the echocardiographic examination to a value below that recorded during the initial clinical examination. This true resting rate may itself be useful information. Stocks are useful in the majority of cases, although they may not be suitable for some horses. It may be possible to position a fractious animal next to a stable door so that the machine is kept at a safe distance (long transducer leads are a useful feature). Chemical restraint is best avoided if at all possible. Alpha$_2$ agonist sedatives such as detomidine and xylazine result in a marked reduction in systolic function, although diastolic measurements may still be of some clinical value after sedation with low doses if examination is precluded without the use of sedatives. Acepromazine may be the best sedative from the point of view of effect on quantitative echocardiography, but even this should avoided if possible.

Because ultrasound will not pass through air, coupling gel is applied to produce good contact between skin and transducer. In most animals it is easier to obtain a good image if hair is clipped from the axillae. In thin, fine-haired animals such as racehorses in training this is not necessary so long as the coupling gel is worked well into the coat. In other animals, clipping is essential, even if this means that fractious horses have to be sedated some hours before the echocardiographic examination in order to allow the effects of the sedative to wear off. Cleaning of the skin with soapy water and/or spirit prior to the application of coupling gel removes grease and dirt and allows the gel to soak the hair and skin. It is helpful to use low viscosity gel for application to the skin and a thicker gel on the transducer as this stays on the transducer head longer. Only once good acoustic contact between the transducer and body is established can a good quality examination begin. Often a few minutes are required for the gel to soak into the skin before the best image is obtained.

Right parasternal views are most easily obtained using the left hand to hold the transducer, with the examiner facing in the same direction as the horse, so that the transducer can be angled into the axilla. Similarly, left parasternal views are most easily obtained using the right hand. Subdued lighting is required to see the screen clearly.

4.2.4   The echocardiographic examination

M-mode echocardiography can produce an infinite number of one-dimensional 'ice-pick' views of the heart; 2DE can produce an infinite number of image planes. There is therefore a need for standardisation of beam position to aid recognition of landmarks and facilitate communication between workers. In quantitative studies, regardless of the type of measurement, a standardised approach is needed so that accuracy and reproducibility are optimal. This will allow consistency of method both between different horses, in the same horse on different occasions and between different echocardiographers. Meticulous attention is required in order to obtain correctly oriented imaging planes in relation to internal landmarks. In clinical situations, planes of view can be lesion oriented, but if this approach is adopted exclusively, abnormalities may be missed. A standardised examination procedure should therefore be followed routinely.

The orientation of M-mode views is traditionally directed by recognition of the characteristic motion of valves and chamber walls and a knowledge of cardiac anatomy, imaged from a fixed transducer location. However, most machines allow the M-mode cursor to be positioned on a 2DE image in order to facilitate identification of landmarks for M-mode imaging. Measurements can therefore be made directly from the 2DE image, or from guided M-mode traces.

For optimal image quality, it is important that the gain and post-processing controls are suitably altered. The brightness of the echoes displayed on the screen will depend on the power setting (usually near 100%), the difference in the acoustic impedance of the two structures at the interface which is reflecting sound and the gain setting. The intensity of the ultrasound is reduced by tissues so that at greater depths less sound will be reflected from comparable interfaces. The gain setting can be adjusted to allow for reduced strength of signals from deeper structures by amplifying the echoes from structures further from the transducer. Post-processing controls allow the operator to alter the contrast of the image by altering the grey scale. For echocardiography, the settings are usually quite high because identification of the endocardial borders and the valves is more important than fine detail of myocardial texture. This is the opposite of the situation in ultrasonography of most soft tissue structures such as tendons or liver.

Imaging planes and transducer position

In comparison with man and small animals, the positions from which 2DE views of the adult equine heart can be obtained are limited. The principal limitation is that the apex of the heart rests on the sternum and this precludes a true apical view and prevents measurement of the length of the LV. Consequently, the only views of the heart obtainable in the adult are parasternal (sometimes called paracostal), with the long axis of the heart either perpendicular or oblique to the axis of the beam.

Transducer positions required to obtain specific views can be guided by internal cardiac landmarks or the position of the transducer on the chest wall. The transducer needs to be located in the correct position and then angled and rotated to different degrees to obtain the standardised image planes. The transducer location is defined as left or right parasternal, ventral or dorsal and cranial or caudal.

In order to be sure of the position of the ultrasound beam in relation to one's hand, it is helpful to place one's thumb on the guide mark on the transducer so that the plane of the beam runs parallel with the palm of the hand. With most machines, if the guide mark and the thumb are positioned dorsally, dorsal structures are displayed on the right of the screen. This is the conventional method of display.

Standardised imaging planes and transducer location

A number of standardised views for 2DE and M-mode imaging have evolved over the last decade. It is helpful to obtain these views before looking specifically at structures of special interest by angling, rotating or moving the transducer to image lesions. Angled views are usually required for Doppler echocardiography, so that the beam can be positioned as close as possible to parallel with blood flow. This is largely governed by the spectral Doppler signal rather than the exact anatomical position, although the 2DE image is helpful to guide positioning of the cursor and to identify areas when PWD is used to map out jets of regurgitant blood flow. The views described below and the transducer location required to obtain these images are summarised in Table 4.6.

Right long-axis views

Right long-axis view optimised for left ventricle and atrium 'reference view' The right parasternal long-axis view is optimised to image the ventricular inlets when the axial beam (the centre of the sector) transects the basal portion of the interventricular septum (IVS) and the chordae tendineae of the posterior mitral leaflet, with the long axis of the ventricle approximately perpendicular to the axial beam. The structures imaged in this plane are the RV, right atrium (RA), tricuspid valve (TV), IVS, interatrial septum, and the majority of the LV, mitral valve (MV), left atrium (LA) and LV free wall (Figure 4.9). The view is usually best obtained from the 4th intercostal space with the transducer positioned just dorsal to the olecranon, but the exact position should be adjusted to allow for individual

Table 4.6 Transducer positions

Views	Location	Angulation	Rotation	Structures visible	Guidelines
Right long-axis 'reference' optimised for LV and LA	Right parasternal reference	0 dorso–ventral 0 – + caudal	None	RA, TV, IVS, LV LA, MV	Axial beam crosses basal IVS and CT of caudal mitral leaflet. Long axis of LV perpendicular to beam
Right long-axis 'reference' optimised for LVOT and AOV	Dorsal to reference	0 – + dorsal 0 – + caudal	+20 – +30°	RA, TV, RV, IVS, LVOT AoV, Aorta, (LA, PA)	Axial beam transect AOV base Long axis of LV perpendicular to beam
Right long/oblique axis (RV inflow/outflow view)	Dorsal to reference	+ dorsal + – ++ cranial	–30 – +10°	RA, TV, RV, PV, PA AoV, (LA)	Axial beam transects right coronary artery AoV seen in oblique section
Right short-axis papillary level	Ventral to reference	0 – ventral + caudal	–80°	LV, IVS, (RV)	M-mode cursor crosses between papillary muscles, LV lumen as circular as possible Most basal level with no CT seen
Right short-axis chordal level	Reference	0 dorso–ventral + caudal	–80°	LV, IVS, CT, RV	LV lumen as circular as possible M-mode cursor bisects IVS CT seen, MV not seen
Right short-axis aortic level	Dorsal to reference	0 – + dorsal + cranial	–60 – –30°	LV, IVS, CT, RA RV, TV, AoV, LA	Axial beam transects of AoV Mercedes-Benz sign of AoV, AoV circular
Left long-axis optimised for LV and LA (reference view)	Reference	0 dorso–ventral 0 – + caudal	0 – +10°	LV, MV, CT, LA	Axial beam between papillary muscles and mitral valve Long axis of LV perpendicular to beam
Left long-axis optimised for LA	Dorsal to reference	0 dorso–ventral 0 – + caudal	0 – +10°	LV, MV, CT, LA	Axial beam bisects MV annulus Long axis of LV perpendicular to beam
Left short-axis papillary level	Ventral to reference	0 dorso–ventral 0 – + caudal	–100 – –90°	LV, IVS, RV, RVFW	LV lumen as circular as possible Axial beam crosses junction of IVS and LVFW
Left short-axis chordal level	Reference	0 dorso–ventral + caudal	–100 – –90°	LV, IVS, RV, RVFW, CT	LV lumen as circular as possible Axial beam crosses junction of IVS and LVFW, ventral to LVOT

Key: Angulation: 0, none; +, slight; ++, marked. Rotation: +, clockwise; –, anticlockwise. (See also List of Abbreviations, page ix.)

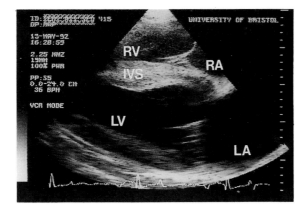

Fig. 4.9 Right parasternal location, long-axis reference view.
It is convention to display dorsally positioned structures on the right side of the screen.
From the right parasternal location, right-sided structures are closest to the transducer and
therefore displayed at the top of the screen.
Key: **RA**, right atrium; **RV**, right ventricle; **IVS**, interventricular septum; **LA**, left atrium; **LV**,
left ventricle.

variation. This view has been described as the 'reference' view and it acts as a
guideline from which other views can be obtained. It helps to gain an initial
impression of the overall motion and size of the chambers. Gross structural
defects and valvular lesions can be seen.

**Right long-axis view optimised for left ventricular outflow and aortic
valve** From the reference location the transducer can be moved slightly dorsally for a view optimised for the aortic valve in long axis. In this view, the axial
beam transects the base of the aortic valve, with the long axis of the LV outflow-
tract perpendicular to the axial beam. The structures imaged in this plane are the
RV, RA, TV, IVS, aortic valve and portions of the LV, MV, ascending aorta and
LA (Figure 4.10). In small horses, or with machines with sufficient depth display,
the pulmonary artery (PA) may be visible in cross-section, dorsal to the LA and
deep to the aorta. This view shows the structure and motion of the aortic valve,
although abnormal motion is more easily seen on M-mode. The size of the RV,
RA and aorta can be assessed. This view is usually the best in which to identify a
VSD, positioned just below the aortic root. The transducer can be tilted slightly
dorsally for Doppler assessment of the tricuspid valve.

Right long/oblique-axis view optimised for pulmonary valve From the
reference location, with the plane of the beam in long axis, the transducer can be
angled cranially for a view which is often described as a right ventricular inflow/
outflow view. A wide range of angulations produce similar views with different
degrees of obliquity. The axial beam transects the right coronary artery, with the
aorta in an oblique section. The structures imaged in this plane are the RA, TV,
RV, PV, PA, aorta, and a portion of the LA (Figure 4.11). This view allows an
overall impression of RV size to be made and the structure of the TV and PV to
be assessed. The size of the PA can be measured.

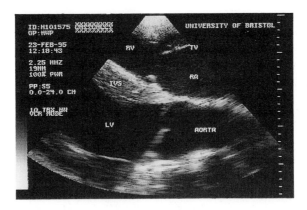

Fig. 4.10   Right parasternal location, long-axis LV outflow view.

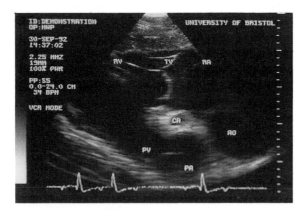

Fig. 4.11   Right parasternal location, oblique-axis RV inflow/outflow view.
Key: **CA**, coronary artery; **PV**, pulmonary valve; **PA**, pulmonary artery; **Ao**, aorta.

Right short-axis views   These 2DE views are principally used to guide the position of the M-mode cursor so that LV dimensions can be measured and the motion of the MV and IVS can be assessed. The transducer is rotated through approximately 90° from the long-axis position to produce short-axis views. The author finds anti-clockwise rotation more comfortable than clockwise rotation, but it results in cranial structures being displayed on the left side of the screen which breaks convention. So long as the same method is always used, the cranial and caudal aspects of the LV should not be confused. The cross-sectional views can be obtained at various levels of the LV.

Right short-axis view, chordal level   Measurements of LV diameter are conventionally made at the chordal level. At this level, the papillary muscles are no longer visible indenting the LV lumen, but chordae tendineae are clearly seen (Figure 4.12). Neither the characteristic 'fish-mouth' appearance of the MV in 2DE or 'M'-shape excursion on M-mode or the LV outflow-tract come into view. The position and angulation of the transducer should be adjusted to try to make

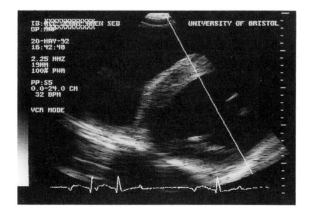

Fig. 4.12 Right parasternal short-axis location, chordal level, with the M-mode cursor positioned across the middle of the ventricle in order to record an M-mode trace for measurement of LV dimensions (Fig. 4.13).

the LV lumen appear as close to circular as possible to ensure that the true short-axis is obtained. The M-mode cursor can then be placed across the maximum diameter of the LV, bisecting the IVS. Consistent positioning of the transducer and M-mode cursor is essential if accurate measurements are to be made. The M-mode trace at this level has a characteristic appearance and is useful for assessing the motion of the IVS (Figure 4.13). M-mode is preferable to 2DE for measurement of LV diameter because it is easier to identify end-systole and end-diastole from the M-mode trace than to freeze the 2DE image at exactly the right time.

Many papers quote values for thickness of the RV free-wall and RV diameter, made from M-mode recordings at this level. However, unless these are grossly abnormal, they are of little value because there are no suitable landmarks for accurate measurements. In addition, the surface of the RV is irregular and trabeculated and the measurements made from M-mode cannot allow for this.

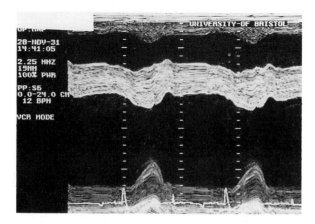

Fig. 4.13 M-mode trace recorded from the right parasternal location, chordal level.

Right short-axis view, mitral valve level At the mitral valve level, a characteristic 'fish-mouth' appearance is seen on 2DE. The 'M' shape excursion of the valve seen on M-mode corresponds with the opening and closing of the mitral valve in early and late diastole. The points of motion of the valve on the M-mode trace have been given letters to identify each phase of the cycle (Figure 4.14). The relative size of the waves of motion and their timing provides information about blood flow. High frequency motion such as that associated with aortic regurgitation is particularly well seen in this view. The presence or absence of characteristic motion is helpful to identify some arrhythmias.

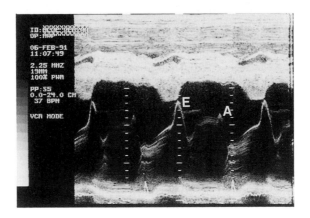

Fig. 4.14 M-mode right parasternal location, mitral level, showing the E wave and A wave of the mitral valve.

Right short-axis view, aortic valve level The aortic valve level is the level at which the aortic valve is seen in circular cross-section, with the valve leaflets creating a 'Mercedes–Benz' sign in diastole (Figure 4.15). An M-mode recording

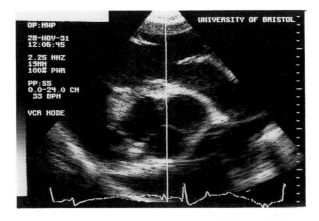

Fig. 4.15 Right parasternal short-axis location, aortic valve level, showing the position of the M-mode cursor for recording aortic valve motion (Fig. 4.16).

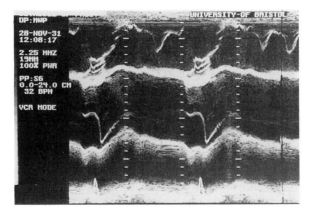

Fig. 4.16 An M-mode trace recorded from the right parasternal location, aortic valve level. The right ventricle and atrium are closer to the transducer at the top of the screen, the aorta runs across the middle of the screen, and the left atrium is seen in the far field. The aortic valve can be seen to open shortly after the R wave of the ECG.

is made by placing the cursor across the middle of the valve (Figure 4.16). M-mode traces may show high frequency motion. Lesions on the valve are often more easily seen on 2DE images in this view than in the long-axis view. In some animals with a VSD, the defect is more easily seen just below this level in short-axis rather than in the long-axis view.

The ratio of the aortic root and left atrial diameter has often been measured from an M-mode trace recorded at this level. However, this is fraught with error because the angle at which the cursor bisects the LA is very variable. In fact, the cursor actually crosses the left atrial appendage, rather than the body of the atrium itself. Left atrial diameter is best measured from the left long-axis parasternal view in 2DE (see below). M-mode aortic root : LA ratios are only of any value if the atrium is very dilated.

Left long-axis views In all but the largest animals or those with very dilated ventricles, with suitable equipment, the whole of the heart can be seen from a right parasternal position. However, examination from the left side allows the heart to be examined in a different plane than from the right side and may provide additional information. For example, rupture of the MV chordae tendineae often involves the right commissural cusp, and this is more easily seen in long axis from the left parasternal view than from the right. Examination of the LA, and measurement of its diameter is also routinely performed from the left parasternal long-axis view. The transducer is placed in a slightly more dorsal position than for the view centred on the LV, with the axial beam transecting the base of the MV (Figure 4.17). The size of the LA is maximised and the right atrium appears as a small round chamber directly deep to the MV annulus precluding measurement of LV diameter. The measurement calipers are positioned at the base of the valve, rather than more dorsally where there is a risk that they will be placed into a pulmonary vein.

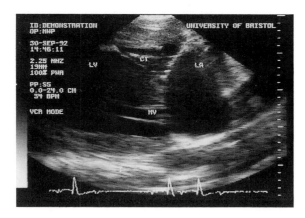

Fig. 4.17 Left parasternal location, long-axis LV/LA view.
Key: **CT**, chordae tendineae.

Left short-axis views Short-axis views can be used to measure the size of the LV; however, this is in a plane which is perpendicular from that measured from the right parasternal location. The M-mode cursor, should be placed through the junction of the LV free-wall and the septum (Figure 4.18). This view can be useful for assessing LV size and the structure and motion of the MV.

In animals with thick chest walls or a dilated heart, or when using equipment with limited depth display, the LV free-wall may be beyond the range of display from a right parasternal view, precluding measurement of LV diameter. Measurement from the left parasternal view offers an alternative. However, it should be remembered that this is not exactly the same measurement as from the right parasternal view, and values are slightly different.

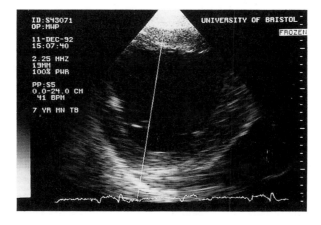

Fig. 4.18 Left parasternal short axis location, chordal level, with cursor in position crossing the junction of the IVS and LV free wall for measurement if LVD cannot be measured from the right parasternal location.

4.2.5 Indications for performing an echocardiogram

Echocardiography can be used to investigate cardiac structure, size and motion; from these an assessment of cardiac function can be made. DE provides further information on blood flow and pressures within the chambers and great vessels.

The decision to perform an echocardiogram is usually made to:

- investigate the source and the significance of a cardiac murmur;
- investigate underlying heart disease and the effects of a cardiac arrhythmia;
- investigate the presence and significance of myocardial disease;
- investigate the presence and significance of pericardial disease;
- evaluate the heart in cases in which cardiac disease is suspected but is not apparent from clinical examination, such as endocarditis in an animal with recurrent pyrexia, or myocardial dysfunction in a case of known exposure to monensin toxicity.

By far the most common of these is investigation of the source and, even more importantly, evaluation of the significance of a cardiac murmur. Although echocardiography, especially DE, is helpful to identify the source of a murmur, in particular whether a murmur is functional or is related to cardiac disease, the main purpose of echocardiography is to assess the effects of the disease. The most significant feature is measurement of volume overload which results from valvular regurgitation. Salient features of the echocardiographic examination are described below. Echocardiographic features of each of the common valvular conditions are described in sections 6.2.6, 6.3.3, 6.5.3 and 6.6.2.

4.2.6 Interpretation of an echocardiogram

Measurement of cardiac dimensions

Echocardiography allows an objective quantitative assessment of the effects of cardiac disease, exercise training, physiological changes and drugs. It is most useful to measure the degree of volume overload associated with valvular heart disease, so that its significance can be assessed and an accurate prognosis for athletic use given. However, the value of quantitative methods depends on rigorous adherence to measurement guidelines, in particular obtaining the appropriate image plane for any one measurement. Measurements which are made without reference to these guidelines are positively unhelpful because they may lead to an incorrect judgement. The usefulness of measurements also depends on a suitable range of measurements from normal animals to compare with those made in the patient. Published normal ranges are now available for adult Thoroughbred horses, but are limited for other breeds. Cardiac dimensions tend to be greater in larger and more athletic breeds. However, as a general rule there is a weak relationship between heart size and body weight within each breed.

The most useful measurements are of LV and LA diameter, although LAD cannot be measured with as much accuracy as LVD. RV and RA size have to be assessed subjectively, with the aorta acting as a useful guide for comparison. Occasionally measurement of PA and aortic diameter can be helpful. Guidelines for measuring cardiac dimensions and a range of values obtained in normal adult Thoroughbred horses are shown in Table 4.7.

Table 4.7   Guidelines for measuring cardiac dimensions and a range of values obtained in normal adult Thoroughbred horses

All measurements made using leading-edge to leading-edge technique (cursor placed at transducer side of the thin hyperechoic endocardial echoes for near and far endocardial surfaces) except PV, AoV and LAD measurements (inner edge of endocardial surface). Five measurements of good quality frames which strictly meet measurement criteria should be measured at resting heart rates in unsedated animals, and the mean value calculated. Evaluation should not be made on measurements alone. If measurements cannot be certain to be accurate they should be interpreted with caution.

Dimension	Image plane	Measurement guidelines	Average (cm)	Max	Min
LVDs	RCSx M-mode (Figs 4.4, 4.12 and 4.13)	Standard R chordal M-mode image with cursor through mid-point of ventricle from nadir of septal motion to LVFW	7.5	9.1	5.8
LVDd	RCSx M-mode	Standard R chordal M-mode image IVS–LVFW at onset of R wave	11.9	13.5	9.7
IVSs	RCSx M-mode	Standard R chordal M-mode image IVS thickness at nadir of septal motion	4.2	5.2	3.2
IVSd	RCSx M-mode	Standard R chordal M-mode image IVS thickness at onset of R wave	2.9	3.7	2.3
LVFWs	RCSx M-mode	Standard R chordal M-mode image Greatest LVFW thickness	3.8	4.6	3.2
LVFWd	RCSx M-mode	Standard R chordal M-mode image LVFW thickness at onset of R wave	2.2	2.6	1.7
LAD	LLx 2DE (Fig. 4.17) RLx 2DE (Fig. 4.10)	Maximal dimension of left atrium dorsal to valve annulus at end-diastole	12.8	14.5	11.3
AoV	RLx 2DE (Fig. 4.10)	Width at sinus of Valsalva, at end-diastole	8.7	9.7	7.8
PV	ROx 2DE (Fig. 4.11)	Width at base of valve at end-diastole	6.1	8.0	5.2
LVDs	LCSx M-mode (Fig. 4.18)	M-mode cursor through junction of IVS and LVFW smallest dimension, minimum ventricular diameter	7.4	9.5	5.7
LVDd	LCSx M-mode	M-mode cursor through junction of IVS and LVFW onset of R wave, maximum ventricular diameter	12.0	14.2	10.5
FS% (R)	R C M-mode	(LVDd–LVDs)/LVDd × 100	36.9	45.0	28.0
FS% (L)	L C M-mode	(LVDd–LVDs)/LVDd × 100	38.0	47.0	27.0

Key: LVDs – Left ventricular diameter at end-systole, LVDd – Left ventricular diameter at end-diastole, IVSs – Interventricular septal thickness at end-diastole, LVFWs – Left ventricular free-wall thickness at end-systole, LVFWd – Left ventricular free-wall thickness at end-diastole, LAD – Left atrial diameter at end-diastole, AoV – Aortic valve diameter, PV – Pulmonary valve diameter, FS% – Fractional shortening, RCSx – Right chordal short-axis, LCSx – Left chordal short-axis, LLx – Left long-axis, RLx – Right long-axis, ROx – Right oblique-axis, 2DE – Two-dimensional image.

Adapted from Long, K.J. (1992) Two-dimensional and M-mode echocardiography. *Equine Vet,* **4:** 303–10, and Patteson, M.W. (1993) *Echocardiographic studies in the horse.* PhD thesis, University of Bristol. Maximum and minimum values are derived from 78 clinically normal Thoroughbred and Thoroughbred-cross horses; values outside this range are not necessarily abnormal but are uncommon.

Fractional shortening

Measurement of cardiac dimensions allows calculation of figures which are a guide to cardiac function. The most commonly used echocardiographic parameter of ventricular performance is fractional shortening (FS%); which is calculated from the formula shown in Figure 4.19. Fractional shortening is used as an estimate of myocardial contractility. However, this is only a guide and is very dependant on the loading factors which affect the contraction of the heart (see section 1.4.3). If the ventricle does not fill normally during diastole the FS% will be reduced. FS% is particularly sensitive to changes in afterload. An increase in systemic blood pressure or an increase in myocardial stiffness will therefore reduce FS%. FS% can also be influenced by the heart rate. Excitement may result in an increased FS% as a result of catecholamine release. Valvular heart disease will affect ventricular function before any change in myocardial contractility occurs. For example, mitral regurgitation will result in a decreased afterload because it acts as a let-off valve during systole. In addition, if the valvular disease is severe enough to have resulted in volume overload, preload may be increased. These factors increase FS% by decreasing systolic dimensions and increasing diastolic dimensions respectively. Once myocardial failure develops, FS% will fall.

$$\text{Fractional shortening (\%)} = \frac{\text{LVDd} - \text{LVDs}}{\text{LVDd}} \times 100$$

LVDd = left ventricular diameter at end-diastole
LVDs = left ventricular diameter at end-systole

Fig. 4.19 Calculating fractional shortening.

Some ultrasound machines have software which can calculate stroke volume and ejection fraction from echocardiographic measurements. Unfortunately, these estimates are only as accurate as the original measurements, and depend on the use of appropriate formulae. They should not be regarded as accurate measurements, but may be a helpful guide in some circumstances.

Evaluation of the cardiac chambers

The overall shape of the ventricles and atria should be examined. The chambers become more globular in animals with marked volume overload. The septum may bow away from the enlarged chamber. The apex of the LV has a more rounded appearance in volume overload, although this can be created artefactually if the beam does not transect the true long axis of the ventricle.

The structure of the cardiac chambers is examined to ensure that no defects are present. By far the most common defect is a VSD. This is most often recognised as a gap between the base of the IVS and the base of the aorta. It is usually seen in the long-axis view but may be more easily seen in the short-axis view or oblique views in some animals. Atrial septal defects (ASDs) are much less commonly recognised. Drop-out of the interatrial septum is a common artefact and must be distinguished from true defects. ASDs may occur at different levels within the septum. If they are real, the edges of the septum either side of the defect usually appear rather echogenic and thickened.

Analysis of myocardial texture is seldom helpful. The echogenicity of the myocardium is very dependant on the gain and post-processing settings of the machine, the angle of the beam, the depth of the tissue and the acoustic impedance of structures between it and the transducer. For example, in the right parasternal reference view, the middle of the IVS may appear more echogenic than other areas because it is perpendicular to the plane of the beam. The papillary muscles normally have a rather heterogeneous appearance and are more echogenic in comparison with the rest of the myocardium. Hypoechoic areas may be seen if there is dissection of blood into the myocardium, for example in the case of a rupture of the aortic root.

Masses within the chambers are unusual. Vegetations on the endocardium as well as valves may be seen in animals with endocarditis. However, unlike some other species, thrombi within the atria are seldom seen in the horse.

Where precise measurement of the size of chambers is not possible, a subjective assessment of their relative size is helpful. The aortic root only changes in size slightly during systole, and acts as a baseline for comparison with other structures. However, the root can be dilated by an aneurysm or the presence of a VSD and may be smaller than usual in low-output cardiac failure. Subjective comparison of RA and RV diameter with the size of the aorta and LV is particularly useful in assessing volume overload of the right side of the heart.

An important consideration in animals with severe left-sided heart disease resulting in pulmonary hypertension is measurement of pulmonary arterial size. Dilation of this vessel can terminate in rupture, resulting in sudden death. Animals with a dilated pulmonary artery are unsafe to ride.

Valvular lesions

The most significant echocardiographic feature of valvular lesions is their effect on cardiac dimensions and performance. However, lesions can be seen and may be significant findings. The most striking are the large vegetations found in most animals with endocarditis (Figure 4.20). The aortic valve is most commonly affected, although the MV is also affected in a significant number of cases.

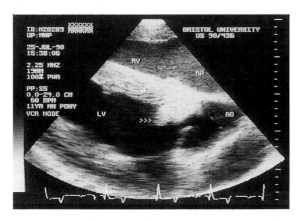

Fig. 4.20 Vegetative endocarditis.
The chevrons point to a large echogenic vegetation on the right coronary cusp of the aortic valve (cf, the shape of the left coronary cusp which is normal).

Vegetative lesions are seldom seen because endocarditis is very uncommon. More often, a slight increase in the thickness and echogenicity of the AV valves is seen, or small nodular thickenings on the aortic valve may be present. The apparent thickness and echogenicity of valves is markedly affected by the settings on the machine, in the same way as was described earlier for changes in myocardial texture.

Valves normally have areas which are more echogenic than others because they are more perpendicular to the line of the beam. For example, the tip of the left coronary cusp of the aortic valve often looks thicker and more echogenic than the rest of the valve. Absence of obvious thickening or nodules on a valve does not eliminate it as a site of disease and regurgitation and the AV valves quite frequently appear normal even when they leak. Nodular thickening of the valve, particularly the aortic valve (Figure 4.21), does not always result in valvular insufficiency.

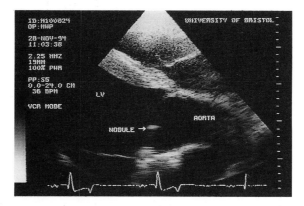

Fig. 4.21 Aortic valve nodule.
A nodule can be seen on the left coronary cusp of the aortic valve in a long-axis view.

Evaluation of the motion of valves and chamber walls

Abnormalities of the valves may be apparent only because of changes in their motion. Prolapse of the valve is defined as billowing of a leaflet into the chamber which it guards. It can be created artefactually if the plane of the beam does not truly bisect the valve; however, it can be real (Figure 4.22). Prolapse of the aortic valve is considered by some cardiologists to be the cause of high-pitched early diastolic murmurs. Prolapse of the MV is associated with late systolic murmurs, and may be the cause of systolic clicks. It may occur in the same individual on one occasion and not on the next. In the author's experience it is seldom associated with severe mitral regurgitation and volume overload, although moderate levels of regurgitation can occur. Prolapse of the TV is quite common and may not be clinically significant if it does not result in volume overload.

Occasionally a portion of a valve can be seen curling back into the preceding chamber. This is known as flail and results from ruptured chordae tendineae to the AV valves and torn semi-lunar valves. Most commonly these are seen on the left side of the heart. Ruptured chordae tendineae most often affect the right commissural cusp of the MV. Flail of this leaflet is best seen from a left para-

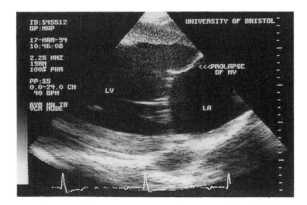

Fig. 4.22 Prolapse of mitral valve.
The mitral valve can be seen to bow into the left atrium (*arrowed*) rather than forming a rounded dome shape with the concave side towards the atrium (cf. Fig. 4.17).

sternal long-axis view, when a portion of valve will be seen curling into the LA against the far wall (Figure 4.23). If the flail is not entirely in the line of the beam only an echogenic dot is seen in the LA during systole. A cine-loop facility or good quality video for slow replay are very helpful in identifying prolapse and flail because they are best appreciated on 2DE.

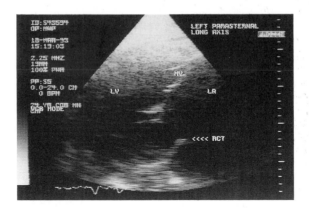

Fig. 4.23 Flail of the right commissural cusp of the mitral valve.
A portion of the mitral valve can be seen to move into the left atrium during systole due to rupture of a supporting chorda tendinea (marked by chevrons).

Flail leaflets frequently vibrate, resulting in very loud and often musical murmurs. This high-frequency vibration is best seen on M-mode echocardiography. Vibration of a valve, IVS or ventricular free-wall may occur when it is struck by a high velocity jet of blood. This is most commonly found in animals with aortic regurgitation (AR), when the regurgitant jet strikes the septal mitral leaflet (Figure 4.24). It may even result in an apparent reduction in the extent to which the MV opens. Vibration of the aortic valve is also seen in many animals with AR (Figure 4.25).

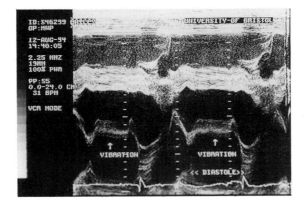

Fig. 4.24 Vibration of the mitral valve.
The septal leaflet of the mitral valve can be seen to vibrate during diastole in many horses with aortic regurgitation.

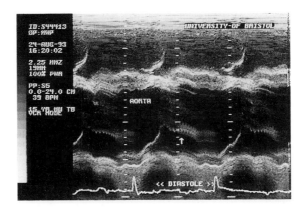

Fig. 4.25 Vibration of the aortic valve.
The aortic valve itself can vibrate (*arrowed*) during diastole in some horses with aortic regurgitation.

Abnormal motion of the valves may be seen with some arrhythmias. For example, the A wave of the MV will be absent in animals with atrial fibrillation. Undulations of the valves and myocardium occur normally in animals with sinus or atrioventricular block. In horses with myocardial failure, abnormal motion of the walls may be seen. The IVS and LV free-wall may fail to contract synchronously, a feature known as dyskinesis. Septal motion is often exaggerated in animals with severe volume overload (Figure 4.26). The IVS may give the impression of bowing towards the RV with severe AR or mitral regurgitation (MR) (Figure 4.27). In RV volume or pressure overload, the IVS will appear flat or may bow into the LV (Figure 4.28). In severe cases, paradoxical septal motion may become apparent, with the IVS moving towards the LV free-wall during diastole and away during systole.

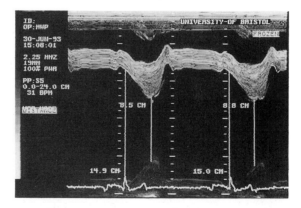

Fig. 4.26 Exaggerated septal motion.
Motion of the IVS is dramatic in many animals with left ventricular volume overload due to valvular disease (as in this Arab-cross pony with severe mitral regurgitation).

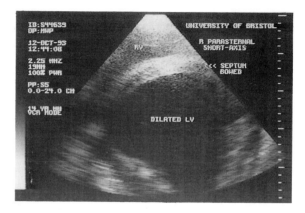

Fig. 4.27 Septal bowing into RV with LV overload.
Bowing of the IVS into the RV can occur in some animals with LV volume overload, depending on the pressures within the RV and LV.

Spontaneous contrast

In many animals, a grey haze will appear in the cardiac chambers when the heart rate is slow. This is known as 'smoke'. It is usually most marked in the RA and RV. It may occur in normal horses and it is particularly obvious in sedated animals, but also occurs in horses with valvular or myocardial disease. However, horses with severe disease will have more marked spontaneous contrast because they have slow intra-cardiac blood flow. There is no clear cut-off between normal and abnormal. Spontaneous contrast is unusual in other species and it is regarded as significant in horses by some veterinarians. However, in the author's opinion, it is a common finding in fit horses and by itself should not be taken to be a sign of abnormality. Its intensity is also very dependent on the settings of the ultrasound machine and monitor and the quality of the image. Larger 'particles' of echogenic material have been reported to be more common in animals which

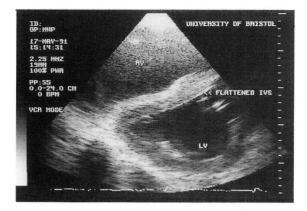

Fig. 4.28 Septal bowing into LV with RV overload.
Bowing of the IVS into the LV can occur in some animals with RV volume overload. This can indicate severe RV disease or can be secondary to primary LV volume overload and failure, (as in this Connemara pony with severe mitral regurgitation and congestive heart failure).

suffer from EIPH than in normal horses. These particles can also be seen in some normal animals, particularly immediately after deep inspiration.

Pericardial disease

The pericardium is a fibrous structure and, although it is very thin, it appears as a bright white line surrounding the heart on echocardiography. Usually it is in contact with air-filled lung, so no structures will be seen beyond this line. Occasionally it acts as a mirror to echoes, with reverberation artefact producing a mirror image of the heart in the lung beyond the pericardium.

A pericardial effusion appears as an anechoic band surrounding the heart, between the moderately echogenic myocardium and the echogenic pericardium (Figure 4.29). A pericardial effusion becomes most significant when it results in a sufficiently high pericardial pressure to restrict venous return, a situation called tamponade (see section 6.8.1). The first echocardiographic sign of tamponade is collapse of the RA. When it is more severe it may cause partial collapse of the RV during diastole. IVS motion may appear abnormal, partly because the heart can swing from side to side within the pericardium. Strands of fibrin may appear as echogenic fronds within the pericardial space in bacterial pericarditis. Very echogenic particles may result from gas bubbles indicating the presence of an anaerobic infection. These findings indicate the need for aggressive treatment even if tamponade has not occurred. Ultrasound may be helpful to guide drainage of the effusion to relieve the tamponade and analyse the fluid.

Constrictive pericarditis is much more difficult to diagnose echocardiographically. The pericardium may appear thickened. If there is sufficient fibrous tissue, restriction of diastolic flow may occur, with flow checked midway through early diastolic filling resulting in a step in the early diastolic motion of the MV on the M-mode trace.

The pleural space

Accumulation of fluid within the pleural space may be seen in animals with right-

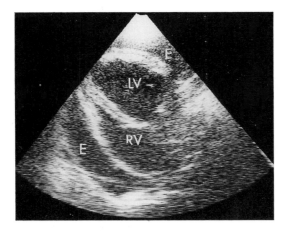

Fig. 4.29 Pericardial effusion.
A pericardial effusion seen from a left parasternal long-axis view. The anechoic space (**E**) between the transducer and the left ventricle (**LV**) on the far side of the right ventricle (**RV**) is due to fluid collecting in the pericardial sac.

sided heart failure, or pleural disease. An anechoic or hypoechoic space can be seen between the pericardium and the chest wall. Further investigation of pleural fluid accumulations is required because it usually indicates severe disease.

A protocol for 2DE and M-mode echocardiography is shown in Table 4.8.

4.2.7 The use of Doppler echocardiography

In a clinical setting, DE is primarily used for confirming a diagnosis of valvular incompetence based on auscultatory findings, for mapping the area of the jet or regurgitant blood in order to estimate the severity of the condition, and for measuring the velocity of blood shunting through a VSD in order to determine the pressure gradient between the ventricles.

In a research setting it is a very useful, non-invasive method of estimating stroke volume and cardiac output. Further information on the use of DE for haemodynamic investigations is found in specialist texts and references given in the list of further reading.

DE allows identification of the timing of blood flow during the cardiac cycle if an ECG is recorded simultaneously. It enables the echocardiographer to determine the direction of blood flow, provided that aliasing does not occur (see section 4.2.1). This is usually sufficient information to confirm the diagnosis. Using pulsed-wave Doppler echocardiography this can be combined with spatial information from the 2DE image so that the location of blood flow within the heart can be documented.

The duration of the jet may not appear to last throughout the period during which regurgitation takes place. This may be because the jet moves out of the line of the ultrasound beam during the cardiac cycle. In addition, the heart swings towards the apex during systole so the position of the sample volume relative to the valve and chamber alters during the cardiac cycle.

Table 4.8 A protocol for 2DE and M-mode echocardiography

Preparation
Consider suitable restraint of the horse and protection of equipment
Clip hair from the axillae except in very fine-haired animals
Clean dirt and grease away with soap/spirit
Apply acoustic gel
Attach the ECG clips
Alter the gain settings and post-processing as appropriate

Examination
Start with *right parasternal long-axis view*
Assess: image quality, must be adequate for thorough examination
           overall size and shape of left ventricle
           overall size and shape of right ventricle
           overall size and shape of right atrium
           relative size of aorta, LV and left atrium
           IVS especially just below the aortic root (site of most VSDs)
           tricuspid valve structure
           mitral valve structure
           aortic valve and aortic root structure
           LV, IVS, mitral valve and aortic valve motion

Rotate transducer to obtain a *right short-axis view*
Assess: aortic valve structure
           IVS structure
           LV and IVS motion

Position the *M-mode* cursor across the middle of the LV (bisecting the chordae) and switch to M-mode
Measure LVD at end-diastole and end-systole
Calculate FS%
Assess: high frequency motion, velocity and pattern of IVS, mitral valve and aortic valve
           motion (can measure systolic time intervals)

Rotate and angle the transducer to image the pulmonary valve (*RV inflow–outflow view*)
Assess: tricuspid valve structure
           tricuspid valve motion
           pulmonary valve structure
           pulmonary valve motion
Measure the size of pulmonary artery using 2DE

Switch to *left parasternal position*, examine in *long-axis*
Assess: overall size and shape of left ventricle
           structure of mitral valve
           motion of LV, IVS, mitral valve and aortic valve
Measure the LA diameter using 2DE (maximise diameter and measure at the base of the annulus)

Rotate transducer to obtain a *short-axis* view
Assess the motion of LV and IVS
Position M-mode cursor across LV
Measure LVD at end-diastole and end-systole
Calculate FS%

Adjust the plane of the beam to identify specific lesions as necessary during the examination

Pulsed-wave Doppler mapping

Mapping of the area of the jet within the receiving chamber is a time consuming and laborious process, which must be thoroughly performed if it is to be of value. DE in the horse is hampered by the limited number of views which can be obtained. Satisfactory 2DE and M-mode views can be obtained from parasternal views because the chambers lie perpendicular to the line of the beam and therefore return strong signals. When using DE to measure blood flow, the line of the beam should be as close to parallel with blood flow as possible, and this is seldom achievable. A second problem is that many jets of regurgitant blood flow, particularly mitral regurgitation, do not flow in predictable patterns and can be difficult to detect. With experience, auscultation is probably just as accurate a method of identifying regurgitant blood flow. Nevertheless, PWD mapping is a useful method of assessing the severity of valvular disease.

For evaluation of MR, a left parasternal long-axis view is obtained, and the transducer is then moved slightly ventral and angled steeply dorsal so that the LA is in the far-field and the MV is as near perpendicular to the valve as possible. An angle of around 45° to the valve is usually achievable. The sample volume is then placed behind the valve and moved along the atrial side of the valve until a regurgitant jet is detected. The area of the origin of the jet is mapped out if possible, and then the sample volume is moved gradually further and further into the atrium. The process should be repeated with the image plane slightly altered, remembering that the jet and the atrium are three-dimensional. Using colour-flow Doppler, the process is far less time-consuming, but multiple image planes should be examined. Jets of MR often run up the walls of the atrium, or sometimes run straight into it. The echocardiographic features of MR are summarised in Table 4.9.

For examination of tricuspid regurgitation (TR), a right parasternal long-axis view optimised for the LV outflow tract is obtained. The transducer is then tilted slightly dorsal and the sample volume is placed on the atrial side on the tricuspid valve. Jets usually run down the atrial wall where it borders the aorta. The echocardiographic features of TR are summarised in Table 4.10.

Mapping of jets of AR is less helpful than for AV valve regurgitation. It is difficult to get a good angle on the valve and the whole of the LV at the same time. A tilted left parasternal long-axis view with the transducer aimed cranially and dorsally is best. The echocardiographic features of AR are summarised in Table 4.11.

One of the problems in interpreting DE is that most valves leak to a degree in normal horses. Jets of regurgitant flow which are detected at or close to the valve in early systole (AV valves) or diastole (semi-lunar valves) can be regarded as normal. There is no clear cut-off point between normality and abnormality, particularly in the case of tricuspid regurgitation. As a general rule, significant jets are much more extensive and are more easily detected. They may be graded from mild to severe on the grounds of the extent of the jet (Figure 4.30). This is an estimate rather than a quantitative method because other factors may influence the size of the jet, including the control settings of the ultrasound machine and the quality of the Doppler unit.

Table 4.9 Summary: Echocardiographic features of mitral regurgitation

Aims of echocardiographic examination
Use 2DE to evaluate valvular structure:
   gain subjective impression of volume overload
   measure left atrial dimension
Use M-mode to measure left ventricular diameter at end-diastole and end-systole
Use pulsed-wave Doppler to detect and map area of jet

Technique
Right parasternal long-axis view for overall assessment of cardiac function
Right parasternal short-axis view for positioning of cursor for measurement of LVD
Right and left parasternal views for assessment of left atrial structure and motion
Left parasternal long-axis view for measurement of left atrial diameter
Tilted left parasternal long-axis view for pulsed-wave Doppler mapping

Common findings
Mild/no gross valvular abnormalities
Degrees of:
   increased LVDd due to volume overload
   increased left atrial dilation due to volume overload
   increased fractional shortening due to regurgitant fraction
   regurgitant flow detected on pulsed-wave Doppler mapping

Other significant findings
Diffuse or localised valvular thickening
Valve prolapse
Flail leaflet
Arrhythmias
Other cardiac disease

Good prognostic indicators
No volume overload
No gross valvular abnormalities
Limited area of regurgitant flow detected on pulsed-wave Doppler mapping

Poor prognostic indicators
Marked volume overload (LVDd > 14.5 cm, LAD > 15.5 cm)
Exaggerated IVS motion
Moderate diffuse or localised valvular thickening
Flail leaflet
Vegetative lesions of endocarditis
Dilated pulmonary artery
Large area of jet of regurgitant blood detected on pulsed-wave Doppler mapping
Pathological arrhythmias

Estimation of pressure gradients

Measurement of the velocity of a jet allows the pressure gradient between the two chambers between which the jet is flowing to be estimated. For this calculation a simplified version of the Bernoulli equation is used (Table 4.4). If the pressure within one chamber is known, the pressure within another can be estimated if a regurgitant jet of blood flows between them. From a practical standpoint, this is seldom helpful in the case of assessment of the severity of valvular regurgitation. However, it is very helpful in evaluating the haemodynamic effects of VSDs (see section 5.5.5).

Table 4.10   Summary: Echocardiographic features of tricuspid regurgitation

Aims of echocardiographic examination
Use 2DE to evaluate valvular structure:
  gain subjective impression of volume overload
Use pulsed-wave Doppler to detect and map area of jet

Technique
Right parasternal long-axis view for overall assessment of cardiac function
Right parasternal long- and short-axis and oblique views for assessment of degree of
  volume overload and degree of IVS flattening
Right parasternal long- and short-axis and oblique views to assess valve structure
Standard and tilted right parasternal long-, short- and oblique-axis views for pulsed-wave
  Doppler mapping

Common findings
No gross valvular abnormalities
No volume overload of right atrium or ventricle
Limited area of regurgitant flow detected on pulsed-wave Doppler mapping
Regurgitant jet positioned along right atrial wall where it borders the aorta

Other significant findings
Diffuse or localised valvular thickening
Valve prolapse
Flail leaflet
Arrhythmias
Other cardiac disease

Good prognostic indicators
No volume overload
No gross valvular abnormalities
Limited area of regurgitant flow detected on pulsed-wave Doppler mapping

Poor prognostic indicators
Marked volume overload
Flattening of the IVS
Paradoxical septal motion
Substantial diffuse or localised valvular thickening
Flail leaflet
Vegetative lesions of endocarditis
Large area of jet of regurgitant blood detected on pulsed-wave Doppler mapping
Pathological arrhythmias

4.2.8   Contrast echocardiography

Contrast echocardiography is a useful technique, particularly if Doppler is not available. Selective studies can be performed with the use of intra-cardiac catheters; however, non-selective echo-contrast studies are also useful and are simpler to perform. Non-selective investigations can be used to show movement of regurgitant blood across the tricuspid valve, or jets of blood flowing through congenital shunts. A video recording is very helpful for later replay and analysis.

A number of different contrast agents have been used, but a convenient medium which provides very good contrast is a plasma volume expander such as Haemaccel (Hoechst UK Ltd.). This must be agitated to produce microbubbles. This is easily achieved by repeatedly passing the solution from one syringe to another via a three-way tap. Around 10–15 ml of agitated solution are injected

Table 4.11 Summary: Echocardiographic features of aortic regurgitation

Aims of echocardiographic examination
Confirm diagnosis
Use 2DE to evaluate valvular structure
Use M-mode to detect vibration of aortic valve and septal mitral leaflet
Use pulsed-wave Doppler to detect and map area of jet
Assess significance
Use 2DE to gain subjective impression of volume overload
Use M-mode to measure left ventricular diameter at end-diastole and end-systole

Technique
Right parasternal long-axis view for overall assessment of cardiac function
Right parasternal long- and short-axis views for identification of lesions
Right parasternal short-axis view for positioning of cursor for measurement of LVD
Tilted left parasternal long-axis view for CW Doppler measurement of jet velocity
Tilted left parasternal long-axis view for pulsed-wave Doppler mapping

Common findings
Nodular thickening of the aortic valve (2DE)
High-frequency vibration of the aortic valve (M-mode)
High-frequency vibration of the septal mitral leaflet (M-mode)
Increased end-diastolic LV dimensions (M-mode)
Increased fractional shortening % (M-mode)
Detection of regurgitant blood flow (Doppler)
Filling throughout diastole (2DE or M-mode)

Other significant findings
High-frequency vibration of the IVS
Flail leaflet
Valve prolapse
Mitral valve abnormalities
Left atrial volume overload
Large vegetations
Pulmonary artery dilation
Ventricular septal defect
Pressure gradient estimated from velocity of jet using CW Doppler

Good prognostic indicators
LVDd < 15 cm
No vegetative lesions of endocarditis
Limited area of jet of AR
Velocity of jet measured using CW Doppler drops little during diastole

Poor prognostic indicators
Volume overload
Significant MR
Pathological arrhythmias
Rupture of the valve or sinus of Valsalva
Early closure of the mitral valve
Rapid decline in velocity of jet on CW Doppler
Vegetations indicating presence of endocarditis
Pulmonary artery dilation
VSD present

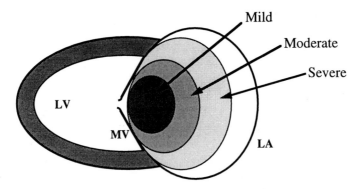

Fig. 4.30 Pulsed-wave Doppler mapping.
Pulsed-wave Doppler echocardiography can be used to 'map-out' the extent of a jet of regurgitation such as mitral regurgitation. As a rough approximation, the more widespread the area over which the jet can be detected in the left atrium, the more severe the MR. In fact, the area of origin of the jet at the valve is a more accurate approximation to severity, but it is more difficult to measure. Some jets run in a direction which makes it difficult to align the beam parallel with flow; others can be difficult to map because they cannot be detected in standard planes of view. However, if the limitations are recognised, mapping is a guide to severity. It can be useful to record diagrams of the jet for future reference. Mapping of tricuspid regurgitation is also helpful; however, some regurgitation is detected close to most valves, especially the tricuspid valve, even in normal horses.

rapidly through a catheter into the jugular vein. Contrast is seen filling the right side of the heart with a dense white cloud. It does not pass through the pulmonary capillaries and therefore does not opacify the left side of the heart unless a right-to-left shunt is present.

4.2.9 Echocardiographic heart score

Electrocardiographic measurement of the QRS duration and conversion into a figure known as 'heart score' was a technique popularised by Steel and co-workers in Australia (see section 4.1.5). In view of the practical and theoretic limitations of the electrocardiographic measurement of heart score, there has been some interest in the use of echocardiography to measure the size of the LV and predict the racing potential of an individual horse. The practice is based on the assumption that those horses with the large hearts are more likely to win races than those with smaller hearts. This assumption is unproved and may be flawed. Although the general principle that the best horses have large hearts may be correct, there is no evidence to show that this is why they win races. Evidence in human athletes indicates that athletes have bigger hearts than sedentary individuals and that elite athletes have particularly large hearts. However, the differences are only great enough to be significant when populations are compared rather than individuals. Furthermore, heart size changes in response to training so that those athletes that train harder develop larger hearts and this may be the reason that they win races, rather than any intrinsic differences in cardiac capacity.

4.3 Radiography

4.3.1 Plain radiography

Adults

Satisfactory radiography of the entire adult chest requires high output radiographic equipment which is not widely available in practice. Only lateral views are feasible in the adult; four separate radiographs are usually needed to show all the lung fields and even the cardiac silhouette cannot be included on one film. Radiographs may provide some useful information about pulmonary disease which may be relevant in animals with suspected cardiac disease, but thoracic radiographs must be of high quality to avoid over-interpretation and experience is required to distinguish the subtle indicators of disease from the wide range of normality. Pulmonary oedema may result in an interstitial pattern and in some cases an alveolar pattern; however, a number of other conditions have a similar radiographic appearance. Very limited information about heart chamber size can be obtained and radiography is therefore of very limited value in evaluation of animals with suspected cardiac disease.

Foals

Adequate quality radiographs of the thorax of foals can be taken with many portable X-ray machines. However, radiographs in foals are of limited value for assessment of cardiomegaly, which must be marked to result in a reliable, detectable degree of tracheal elevation and increased sternal contact. Severe cardiac disease may result in changes in the pulmonary vessels or cause pulmonary oedema. Radiographs are more valuable for identifying some pulmonary diseases. Conditions such as pneumonia may result in clinical signs which could be confused with those of cardiac insufficiency, or may complicate clinical signs in animals in which significant cardiac disease is present.

4.3.2 Angiography

Angiography has been used to identify congenital heart lesions and acquired conditions in foals and small (< 300 kg) adults. Expensive equipment is required, including a wide field-of-view image intensifier, a rapid film changer, cineangiography or video recording, a high output X-ray generator and a pressure injector capable of injecting up to 150 ml of contrast in under 4 seconds. Angiography has largely been replaced by 2DE and DE as the diagnostic method of choice for congenital heart disease in all species and is unlikely to be used in future clinical investigations. Selective echocardiographic contrast studies can also be performed and are more practicable than angiography. However, these studies are seldom required in order to reach a diagnosis.

4.4 Catheterisation

Until recently, catheterisation techniques were required in some cases, particularly in animals with congenital heart disease, in order to make a definitive diagnosis. Now, this technique has limited application in clinical cases, largely because 2DE and Doppler echocardiography are non-invasive and provide more diagnostic information. However, catheterisation is a very useful technique in some situations. Measurement of arterial blood pressure can be useful in assessing changes induced by drugs and is often performed during anaesthesia. It can also be used to illustrate the wide pulse pressure difference which can occur in horses with moderate or severe aortic regurgitation. In cardiovascular research, catheterisation is useful in the following situations.

(1) Placement of a balloon-tipped catheter such as a Swan–Ganz catheter in the PA for measuring pulmonary artery wedge pressures.
(2) Thermodilution or dye dilution measurement of cardiac output.
(3) Measurement of pressures in the chambers and great vessels.
(4) Measurement of blood gas levels in the chambers and great vessels.
(5) Injection of radiographic or echocardiographic contrast agents.

These techniques are unlikely to be performed outside a research institute and are therefore not discussed in detail. The reader is referred to the list of further reading for more detailed descriptions and normal catheterisation data.

4.4.1 Equipment

The type of equipment used depends on the study which is performed, the size of the animal, and whether it is under general anaesthesia. For injection of contrast media and measurement of blood gas concentrations, simple sterile polyurethane tubing can be used. Measurement of pressures can be performed through fluid filled systems; however, electronic catheter-tip transducers, such as the Millar catheter, are preferable. Dye dilution and thermodilution techniques require two catheters to be placed in the right side of the heart, one in the atrium and the other in the PA. Special balloon-tipped catheters such as a Swan–Ganz catheter are required for measurement of pulmonary wedge pressures. A length of approximately 150 cm is required for a catheter to reach from the cervical jugular vein, through the right side of the heart, to the PA. Pressure monitoring equipment, chart recorders, equipment for blood gas analysis and measurement of dye concentration, cardiac output computers, sensitive thermistors and pressure injectors may be required, depending on the type of study performed.

4.4.2 Technique

Catheters can be placed into the jugular vein and the carotid artery percutaneously. Catheterisation of the carotid artery is more easily performed with the animal anaesthetised; however, this may not be desirable, depending on the type of study which is being performed. Catheterisation of the jugular vein using the modified Seldinger technique is a relatively simple procedure. A needle or small catheter is placed in the vein, a small guide wire is passed through this and the needle or catheter is removed. A wide-bore dilator is then passed over the wire so that a much larger catheter can be inserted. The position of the catheter can be confirmed from the pressure trace, which has characteristic contours in the different chambers and great vessels, or by identification on fluoroscopy or echocardiography.

Pressure measurements are useful to identify the haemodynamic effects of disease. For example, raised pulmonary wedge pressures would be detected in an animal with severe MR and congestive heart failure; abnormally high right ventricular pressure might be detected in an animal with a large VSD or an outflow obstruction such as the pulmonary hypoplasia or valvular stenosis found in tetralogy of Fallot. However, the pressure changes are seldom specific for any one condition.

Oxygen tension measurements are useful in cases with shunts. With right to left shunts, there will be an abnormally low oxygen tension and high carbon dioxide level in the left side of the circulation at the level at which the shunt is occurring. With left to right shunts, there will be raised oxygen tension in the right side of the circulation. For example, an animal with significant flow through a VSD would have raised PO_2 in the RV. The extent of these changes is indicative of the severity of the shunt.

4.5 Indirect blood pressure monitoring

Peripheral arterial blood pressure can be measured using a simple manometer, a direct pressure recorder, or using indirect methods. The indirect methods are more easily applied and involve wrapping a cuff around an appendage such as the tail. The 'Dynamap' monitor is a commercial cuff system which is more accurate and convenient than the traditional mercury manometer. Measurement of blood pressure can be useful in conditions such as AR (see section 6.5.3); however, indirect measurements are subject to greater sources of error than direct techniques.

4.6 Phonocardiography

Phonocardiography is a useful technique for demonstrating the characteristics of murmurs. It is also applied in conjunction with other techniques such as echocardiography and pressure measurement to identify the timing of events during the cardiac cycle. The technique has many applications in an academic situation: however, it is seldom useful in clinical practice. The principal limitations are that it is difficult to obtain quality, artefact-free recordings and that equipment suitable for use in the horse is quite expensive. Good quality phonocardiography transducers are often bulky and are difficult to position in the axilla where the PMI of some murmurs is located.

4.7 Clinical pathology

Clinical pathology is helpful to distinguish cardiac and extracardiac disease and to investigate some cardiac conditions. It is discussed in detail in section 2.3.

Chapter 5

Congenital Heart Disease

The incidence of different types of congenital heart disease (CHD) varies markedly between species. Congenital heart disease is relatively uncommon in the horse compared with dogs or cattle. Many veterinary students will be exposed to a large number of dogs with CHD during their training and will be familiar with patent ductus arteriosus, aortic stenosis and pulmonary stenosis, the most common forms of CHD in the dog. These defects are, however, very rare in the horse. Some congenital abnormalities have been reported more often in certain breeds. Standardbred horses are reported to have an increased incidence of CHD compared with Thoroughbreds, and complex CHD has been reported most frequently in the Arabian breed, but CHD is uncommon in horses compared with other domestic species.

The severity of CHD varies enormously and may cause a range of clinical signs. CHD may be recognised at post-mortem examination following fetal or early neonatal death, but usually the condition is detected when the animal is presented to the veterinarian as a foal, or at the beginning of its athletic career if it results in poor athletic performance. In some animals the disease may not be noticed until well into adult life, or it may be an incidental finding in an apparently normal foal or a horse with normal athletic performance. An accurate diagnosis must be made to aid prognostication.

Some congenital cardiac malformations have been shown to be heritable in certain domestic species and in man, although not as yet in the horse. In other instances, CHD may result from teratogens, usually unknown, during early gestation. However, it must be assumed that CHD may be heritable and, once diagnosed, appropriate advice must be given with regard to breeding. The mare/ stallion pairing which is responsible should not be repeated and an animal affected by CHD should not be used for breeding.

In evaluating an animal with suspected CHD, it is important to:

- establish that the primary problem is cardiac.;
- distinguish congenital from acquired heart disease;
- make a specific diagnosis of the form of CHD;
- assess the cardiovascular effects of the condition and establish a prognosis for survival and athletic performance in that individual;
- investigate the animal for evidence of other conditions such as respiratory disease which may complicate treatment and management;
- advise about future breeding programmes.

5.1   The fetal circulation

In the fetus, the circulatory system develops from a single circuit into two circuits acting in parallel. The purpose of this pattern of distribution of blood is to deliver oxygenated blood to those parts of the body which have the highest requirements.

Blood returning from the placenta in the umbilical vein to the fetus is shunted through the liver via the ductus venosus and enters the heart via the caudal vena cava. The majority of it (approximately 80%) is directed through the foramen ovale by the shape of the structure of the junction of the vena cava and atrium. Oxygenated blood therefore enters the left atrium (LA) and is ejected into the aorta and the coronary and carotid arteries supplying the heart and brain. A small portion of the caudal vena caval blood flow is directed by the lower edge of the atrial septum secundum into the right atrium (RA) where it mixes with deoxygenated blood returning from the head and forelimbs and passes into the right ventricle (RV) and pulmonary artery (PA). However, the pulmonary circuit is the high resistance circuit in the fetus and this results in the majority of the deoxygenated blood being diverted through the ductus arteriosus into the aorta and thence to the systemic circulation (but not to the brain). Blood returns to the placenta via the umbilical arteries (Figure 5.1).

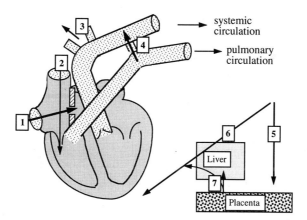

Fig. 5.1 Fetal circulation.
Key: **1.** Oxygenated blood from the placenta flows through the caudal vena cava and enters the right atrium, where it is funnelled through the foramen ovale into the left atrium. **2.** Deoxygenated blood returning from the cranial vena cava is guided through the right atrium into the right ventricle. **3.** Richly oxygenated blood is delivered to the heart and brain. **4.** Blood from the pulmonary artery is diverted through the ductus arteriosus into the aorta, bypassing the high pressure pulmonary circuit and supplying the low pressure systemic circulation (except the heart and brain). **5.** A large portion of aortic blood flow is directed towards the placenta through the umbilical artery. **6.** Some blood from the systemic circulation passes through the liver. **7.** Some placental blood supplies the liver but a large proportion of this richly oxygenated blood passes through the ductus venosus into the caudal vena cava.

5.2   Changes in the fetal circulation at birth

Since the source of oxygen in the fetus is the placenta, the system must necessarily undergo change to adjust to gaseous exchange in the lungs at the point of birth. At birth, the placental blood supply is removed and the pulmonary circuit changes from a high resistance circuit to a low resistance circuit when it is exposed to oxygen by breathing. The systemic circulation now becomes the high pressure circuit and there is no longer a pressure gradient to drive blood flow across the ductus arteriosus from the PA to the aorta. When exposed to oxygenated blood and prostaglandins released at birth, the ductus constricts and closes in the following 24–72 hours. This increases the amount of blood flowing through the lungs and results in an increase in left atrial pressure. This, in turn, pushes the atrial septum primum against the septum secundum, functionally closing the foramen ovale. The ductus venosus in the liver closes when placental flow stops. Thus, at birth the system changes from a pulmonary and systemic system in parallel to a double circulation in series.

5.3   Clinical diagnosis of congenital heart disease

Identifying CHD depends on classification of cardiac murmurs, palpation of the arterial pulse and detection of other clinical signs such as precordial thrills, jugular distension and/or pulsation, peripheral oedema, tachypnoea and cyanosis. Foals with significant CHD may be poorly grown. Clinical evaluation is performed as described in Chapter 3.

A complicating factor in evaluating foals with cardiac murmurs is that functional murmurs are particularly common in the neonate. They may also be relatively loud (up to grade 4/6). Often these are functional murmurs due to non-laminar flow in the great arteries, of the same nature as those commonly found in adults. A continuous waxing and waning murmur can also be associated with flow through the ductus arteriosus in neonates. The time period during which normal closure of the ductus arteriosus occurs is a matter of some debate and may depend on the technique used to document cessation of flow. The murmur usually disappears in the first 24 hours after birth; however, a systolic element may persist until there is complete closure of the ductus after three or four days.

Although cyanosis is uncommon in horses, it is an important finding in a small number of cases of CHD. It can be described as peripheral or central. Peripheral cyanosis is associated with poor local delivery of oxygenated blood and removal of deoxygenated blood. Central cyanosis indicates the presence of a right to left shunt resulting in deoxygenated blood reaching the systemic circulation, or severe pulmonary disease.

5.4   Investigative aids to diagnosis of CHD

Until recently, definitive diagnosis of CHD depended on the use of relatively difficult, invasive techniques such as catheterisation for angiography and measurement of chamber pressures and oxygen tension. Now, diagnosis is usually made on the basis of two-dimensional echocardiography (2DE). Doppler echo-cardiography (DE) and contrast echocardiography are also useful techniques in the diagnosis of CHD. DE is particularly useful for estimating pressure gradients, which may be directly related to the haemodynamic significance of a defect and the prognosis for that individual.

Echocardiography may also be useful to differentiate acquired heart disease from CHD. The distinction between acquired and congenital disease may affect the prognosis, influence future breeding programmes and may also be important in insured animals because many policies have an exclusion clause covering congenital disease. Acquired cardiac disease may be severe even in young animals. Endocarditis has an increased incidence in foals and may affect the atrioventricular (AV) valves more often in neonates than in adults. Ruptured chordae tendineae are also reported in young animals and may result in congestive heart failure (CHF).

Other acquired diseases, particularly respiratory disease, may result in clinical signs which are similar to those with CHD. For example, a foal with tachypnoea and tachycardia may have heart disease or may have pneumonia. A thorough investigation of all body systems is essential so that the relative significance of different problems can be evaluated.

The effect of a congenital lesion on future use as a breeding animal, resale value and insurance certification should also be considered when advising owners.

5.5 Ventricular septal defect

A ventricular septal defect (VSD) is the most common congenital cardiac lesion in the horse. The defect is usually situated at the base of the interventricular septum in the membranous or semi-membranous portion, just below the aortic root. Normally the septum fuses with the endocardial cushion at this point early in fetal development. Occasionally, defects are found in the septum just below the base of the pulmonary valve. These are due to abnormal development of the bulbus cordis. Defects in the muscular portion of the septum have also been reported. VSDs can also be found as a component of more severe complex CHD such as tetralogy of Fallot, tricuspid atresia and endocardial cushion defects.

5.5.1 Haemodynamic effects

The haemodynamic effect of a VSD depends on its size and the amount of blood shunting across it. The larger the defect, the greater the amount of blood that can flow from the high-pressure left ventricle (LV) to the low-pressure RV. If a substantial proportion of the LV stroke volume flows into the RV, there will be volume overload of the RV, pulmonary circulation, LA and LV. If the volume overload is large, this may also result in an increased pressure in the pulmonary circulation and a rise in RV pressure. Flow across the defect depends on the pressure gradient between the LV and RV. An increase in RV pressure will decrease the flow across the VSD because it reduces the pressure gradient. Some right to left (reverse) shunting may occur at some time during the cardiac cycle in animals with large VSDs, but very seldom does RV pressure increase to the point that a right to left shunt predominates (Eisenmenger's syndrome).

Pulmonary hypertension and volume overload are likely to result in systemic signs such as jugular distension and peripheral oedema. Small defects limit the amount of blood that can flow from the LV to the RV and are termed restrictive VSDs. They are associated with high velocity jets in just the same way that a high velocity jet is created by almost complete occlusion of the end of a hose by one's thumb.

5.5.2   Clinical signs

The clinical signs seen in animals with a VSD depend on the haemodynamic effects of the defect. Large defects will result in volume overload early in life and CHF may be the presenting sign. Tachypnoea and dyspnoea may be noted and may be directly due to pulmonary oedema, or to pneumonia developing as a complication of pulmonary oedema. Other animals with less severe disease may not be noticed to be abnormal until it is found that they have difficulty in keeping up with their dams at pasture, or that they have a reduced exercise tolerance compared with other foals. Often a murmur is detected in foals as an incidental finding when they are examined for other purposes. Some animals behave quite normally initially and a significant murmur is only detected later in life when the horse shows signs of reduced exercise tolerance or is examined for another reason. This usually occurs at the start of an animal's athletic career. However, VSDs have been detected well into adult life, particularly in horses which do not perform arduous athletic work.

5.5.3   Clinical diagnosis

VSDs in the semi-membranous part of the septum are usually associated with a characteristic loud plateau-type murmur. The point of maximal intensity (PMI) is on the right side of the chest, just above the sternum in the apex beat area (Figure 5.2). A palpable thrill is frequently present. The murmur may radiate to the left side of the chest. The murmur can be confused with that of tricuspid regurgitation, although it is usually much louder and harsher and the PMI is slightly more

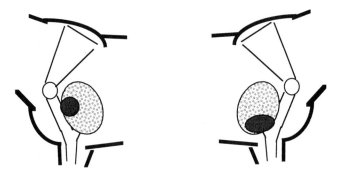

Fig. 5.2 PMI of murmurs associated with VSDs.

ventral. If a significant left to right shunt is present, there may also be a functional ejection-type murmur heard over the pulmonary valve area at the left base, related to the increased volume and velocity of blood flow into the PA. This is termed a murmur of 'relative' pulmonary stenosis.

Frequently, auscultation of the characteristic murmur will be the only significant clinical finding, but in some animals other abnormalities will be noted. The second heart sound may be markedly split due to the late closure of the pulmonary valve and early closure of the aortic valve which can result from the changes in effective stroke volume. A very loud second heart sound may be heard in animals with pulmonary hypertension, and a loud third heart sound may be related to volume overload of the LV. A brisk arterial pulse may be present in animals with moderate sized VSDs but without myocardial failure; a weak arterial pulse may be palpated in animals with more severe haemodynamic changes. CHF may develop in some cases. Sudden death has been reported in some animals with a VSD and is likely to be a result of rupture of the PA or malignant arrhythmias.

The murmur of a VSD may be less loud in animals in which there is pressure overload of the RV, thus the loudest murmurs are not necessarily the most significant. Sub-pulmonary VSDs have a PMI over the left base rather than the right apex. VSDs in the muscular septum have a variable PMI and radiation depending on their exact location. In some cases, a murmur of aortic regurgitation (AR) will also be associated with a VSD due to the effect of the defect on the aortic root. This results from prolapse of a cusp of the aortic valve, usually the non-coronary cusp, into the potential space created by the defect, resulting in regurgitant flow through the valve.

5.5.4 Further diagnostic aids

A definitive diagnosis of a VSD is best achieved using echocardiography, once a suspicious murmur is detected. Semi-membranous VSDs are usually identified in the long-axis view of the LV outflow-tract just below the right coronary cusp (RCC) of the aortic valve (Figure 5.3). It is important to rotate the transducer to

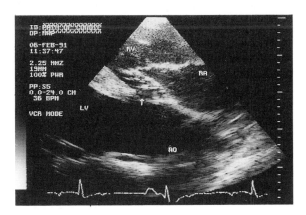

Fig. 5.3 An echocardiogram (right parasternal long-axis view) showing a ventricular septal defect just below the aortic valve at the base of the septum (arrow).

examine this area in the short-axis view. This ensures that the lesion will not be missed and also allows measurement of the size of the defect in two image planes. Often the septal leaflet of the tricuspid valve will be seen to have high-frequency vibrations during systole. Abnormal looking chordae may insert on this valve leaflet. Occasionally, the RCC of the aortic valve will be seen pro-lapsing into the defect, or the whole of the aortic root may appear to be displaced into the defect.

Contrast echocardiography is a useful technique to document the presence and location of a left to right shunt (see section 4.2.8). If a VSD is present, a jet of negative contrast (normal blood) will be seen entering the contrast-filled RV just below the tricuspid valve, adjacent to the aortic root. It is useful to record an ECG on the echocardiogram and to review these studies on video tape because echo-free blood from the caudal vena cava tends to flow down the atrial septum adjacent to the aortic root and can be mistaken for a jet of blood flowing through the VSD. To distinguish the two, the VSD shunt occurs during systole and the caudal vena cava flow is seen during diastole. The venous flow also enters the right side of the heart on the atrial side of the tricuspid valve, although this can be difficult to identify in the contrast-filled chamber. Selective contrast echocardiography is also possible but is much more invasive and is seldom required.

DE is a useful and sensitive technique for detecting the abnormal shunt flow. Pulsed-wave DE is used to detect blood flow by placing the sample volume on the RV side of the suspected defect. Echocardiography and DE should also be used to conduct a thorough examination to rule out the presence of other congenital anomalies which might complicate the clinical picture.

Catheterisation has been used to demonstrate an increased pressure and oxygen tension in the RV as a result of blood shunting from the LV. The extent of these changes will depend on the size of the shunt. Small shunts may be missed.

Angiography may demonstrate intracardiac shunting of blood. Selective angiography is ideal although non-selective angiography can also be performed along similar lines to non-selective contrast echocardiography; however, this requires a pressure injector in order to inject sufficient contrast to produce a diagnostic image. Angiography requires expensive equipment and has largely been replaced by echocardiography.

Electrocardiography is of little or no value in assessing heart chamber changes as a result of a VSD, but is of use in identifying arrhythmias which may com-plicate the condition. The most frequently occurring arrhythmia which is of clinical significance is atrial fibrillation. The presence of this arrhythmia in a foal with a VSD is suggestive of volume overload and indicates a poor prognosis.

5.5.5 Prognosis

Horses with a VSD are unlikely to perform at the very highest level; however, many animals are able to perform useful work on the racecourse or in less athletic pursuits. An echocardiographic examination is imperative for accurate prognostication in animals with a VSD, unless clinical signs are already suffi-ciently severe to suggest a grave prognosis.

Using 2DE, the size of the VSD should be measured in two different axes, usually the parasternal long and short axes. Occasionally, the largest dimension will be seen in an oblique axis some way between these two conventional views. As a general guide, defects under 2.0–2.5 cm in diameter are thought to be restrictive and carry a better prognosis for useful athletic function than larger defects. Sub-pulmonary VSDs and defects in the muscular septum appear to have a worse prognosis. Horses with VSDs associated with other congenital lesions also have a poor outlook. 2DE can also be used to assess the degree of volume overload which results from the shunt. Very similar guidelines apply in this instance to that in animals with mitral regurgitation (MR). In fact, the haemodynamic changes resulting from a VSD are in many ways similar to those associated with MR except that with a VSD there is also pulmonary overcirculation as a result of the left to right shunt. It is important to assess the PA dimension as a dilated PA may precede rupture of this artery and sudden death.

The presence of aortic incompetence due to prolapse of the non-coronary cusp of the aortic valve or the aortic root into the defect is associated with a worsened prognosis compared to animals with a VSD and no aortic incompetence.

The best way to assess the haemodynamic significance of a VSD is to estimate the pressure gradient across it using DE. If the defect is small and restrictive, only a small amount of blood will be able to flow between the high-pressure LV and the low-pressure RV during systole. Consequently, the pressure in the RV will be almost normal and the pressure gradient between the two chambers results in a high velocity jet of blood through the VSD. If the defect is large, a large quantity of blood may shunt from the LV to the RV, resulting in an increase in the RV pressure. There will also be significant volume overload of the left side, the RV and the pulmonary circulation which may result in pulmonary hypertension, also increasing RV pressure. With a lower-pressure gradient between the LV and the RV than normal, the velocity of the jet of blood will be reduced.

Pulsed-wave Doppler can be useful for detecting the presence of a jet; however, because the jet is high velocity, even in severe VSDs, aliasing may occur and continuous-wave Doppler is preferable. The pressure gradient is calculated from the estimated jet velocity using the Bernoulli equation (see section 4.2.7). For example, a jet of 4 m/sec would correspond with an estimated pressure gradient of 64 mm Hg. Since the LV systolic pressure is likely to be in the region of 120 mm Hg this means that the RV systolic pressure is 56 mm Hg. Normal RV systolic pressure is up to 40 mm Hg. It is important that the ultrasound beam is parallel with the jet so that the highest velocity is detected, otherwise the severity of the VSD may be exaggerated. If the velocity of the jet is 4.0–4.5 m/sec or more, the prognosis for future athletic use is good.

Clinical and historical evidence is also pertinent in giving advice on the use of horses with VSDs for athletic work. A recent, normal performance record is supportive evidence for the presence of a relatively insignificant lesion. Owners should be warned of the initial signs of deterioration (reduced exercise tolerance, cough, signs of CHF) and encouraged to allow repeated echocardiographic examination of their animals so that potentially important changes such as increased volume overload or PA dilation can be detected before they present an unacceptable risk to the rider.

5.5.6   *Treatment*

No specific treatment is available. Surgical repair is impracticable at present. CHF should be managed in the standard fashion (see section 6.9) if it develops.

The clinical, diagnostic and prognostic features of VSDs are summarised in Table 5.1.

Table 5.1   Summary: Ventricular septal defects

The most common congenital cardiac defect in the horse
Usually in membranous portion of the interventricular septum, just ventral to the aortic root
Typically pansystolic, harsh, grade 3–6, plateau-type murmur, PMI right apex

VSDs which may be compatible with athletic performance
No other clinical signs
Normal resting heart rate
Normal pulse quality
No abnormal arrhythmias
Normal intensity heart sounds
No volume overload
VSD < 2.5 cm diameter
Jet > 4.0–4.5 m/sec on CW Doppler
Normal PA diameter
No excessive tachycardia after exercise

Poor prognostic indicators
Other clinical signs including tachypnoea, jugular distension, jugular pulsation, ventral
  oedema
Raised resting heart rate
Brisk or weak arterial pulse quality
Abnormal arrhythmias such as AF or VPCs
Loud S2 or S3 heart sounds
Volume overload
VSD > 2.5 cm, subpulmonic or muscular
Jet < 4.0 m/sec
Dilated PA
Poor exercise tolerance

5.6   Tetralogy of Fallot

Tetralogy of Fallot is a complex defect which is uncommon in the horse. This anomaly has four elements: a VSD, an overriding aorta (the aortic root straddling the interventricular septum), RV outflow obstruction and RV hypertrophy. Sometimes the aorta is termed 'dextraposed' which means that the root is entirely within the RV. The cause of the RV hypertrophy may be pulmonary valve stenosis or PA hypoplasia. The latter is more common in the horse.

5.6.1   *Haemodynamic effects*

Tetralogy of Fallot is a severe defect with significant haemodynamic effects. RV outflow obstruction results in increased RV pressure and this is the cause of the hypertrophy. Infundibular hypertrophy may itself result in an element of outflow obstruction. The presence of a VSD means that there is a communication between the RV and the LV so that deoxygenated blood can pass into the systemic circulation. High RV pressure allows blood to flow into the LV. The presence of the overriding aorta means that some of this blood is ejected directly into the aorta.

5.6.2 Clinical signs

Owing to the presence of a right to left shunt, one of the cardinal signs of tetralogy of Fallot is central cyanosis. This may or may not be apparent on clinical examination, depending on the degree of shunting. Other signs include profound exercise intolerance, poor growth and CHF. Auscultation reveals loud (grade 4–6/6) murmurs on both sides of the chest, predominantly at the left base. A thrill is often present.

5.6.3 Diagnosis

Diagnosis is based on clinical signs (particularly if cyanosis is present) and echocardiography. 2DE shows a VSD (usually quite large), an overriding aorta and RV hypertrophy, with thick walls and marked trabeculation (Figure 5.4). Pulmonary stenosis may be identified if present; pulmonary hypoplasia is more difficult to see. Contrast studies are useful to demonstrate right to left flow. Injection of echo-contrast into the jugular vein results in opacification of the RA, RV and aorta. Hypoxaemia may be identified by blood gas analysis; a haematocrit may reveal polycythaemia.

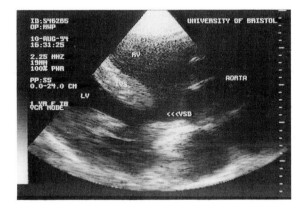

Fig. 5.4 An echocardiogram (right parasternal long-axis view) showing a VSD and an overriding aorta (the base of the valve is in the RV).
RV dilation and hypertrophy and pulmonary atresia was most easily seen in short-axis and olbique views. The diagnosis was therefore tetralogy of Fallot.

5.6.4 Prognosis

The prognosis for life with tetralogy of Fallot is poor. These horses will not become athletes. Euthanasia is usually warranted.

5.7   Atrial septal defect

Atrial septal defects (ASDs, communications between the RA and LA) are rare in horses. They can occur at a number of points in the atrial septum. Defects of the septum can take the form of:

- a sinus venosus ASD associated with a hole at the top of the septum at the junction of the LA and the pulmonary veins;
- a secundum defect in the mid-portion of the septum;
- a primum defect at the base of the septum (associated with an endocardial cushion defect);
- a patent foramen ovale (persistence of the normal fetal structure which allows blood to shunt from the right to the LA, see section 5.1).

Small ASDs may go unnoticed because they may not result in a cardiac murmur or any clinical abnormalities. Large ASDs occurring in the absence of other defects are very rare. Theoretically these defects would have a similar effect to a VSD except that there would be volume overload of the RA in addition to the other chambers. However, ASDs are usually associated with other cardiac defects, and may be essential for life in some defects such as tricuspid atresia (see section 5.8).

5.7.1   Haemodynamic effects

ASDs allow blood to be shunted from the high pressure LA to the low pressure RA, or from right to left if RA pressure is high. In fact, the left to right flow is seldom of great haemodynamic significance except if the defect is large. Blood flow through a large ASD increases flow through the pulmonary valve and may result in an ejection-type murmur of 'relative pulmonary stenosis', with a PMI at the left base. More often, the haemodynamic significance of ASDs is to allow right to left shunting in animals with a right-sided obstruction (e.g. tricuspid atresia). In some animals, the shunt may only open up during exercise, when right-sided pressures rise significantly.

5.7.2   Clinical signs

Clinical signs associated with an ASD vary from subclinical, undetected lesions to early neonatal death when they are part of a complex lesion.

5.7.3   Diagnosis

Diagnosis is based on echocardiography. The defect may go unnoticed without careful examination. If an ASD is identified, a thorough search for other cardiac anomalies is warranted. Contrast echocardiography and DE are useful aids. Care should be taken not to interpret artefactual drop-out of the atrial septum as a defect. A characteristic 'T sign' with apparent increased echogenicity of the septum either side of the hole is usually seen with real defects (Figure 5.5).

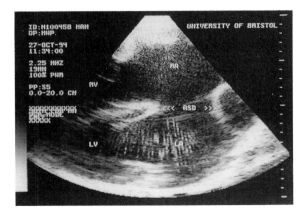

Fig. 5.5 An echocardiogram (right parasternal long-axis view) showing an absence of the interatrial septum.
This can be produced artefactually, but in this case was a consistent finding. The radiating lines in the left atrium are an artefact produced by electrical interference.

5.7.4 Prognosis

The prognosis for life and athletic performance with a small ASD, in the absence of other defects, is good. The presence of a complex defect, including an ASD, carries a very grave prognosis.

5.8 Tricuspid atresia

Tricuspid atresia is a rare defect in which the right AV (tricuspid) valve is poorly developed or imperforate. In the early fetus, this defect may not have severe consequences because blood can pass through the foramen ovale, left AV valve and the primary interventricular foramen to perfuse the lungs. For the fetus and neonate to survive, it is essential that this pathway remains patent, particularly after birth when blood flow to the lungs dramatically increases. An ASD and a VSD are therefore part of this complex anomaly.

5.8.1 Haemodynamic effects

The defect means that blood returning to the RA must pass into the LA and LV before returning to the RV. There is therefore marked volume overload of the left side which may result in CHF. In addition, deoxygenated blood flows into the LV and from there into the systemic circulation so cyanosis is likely.

5.8.2 Clinical signs

Affected foals may die in the immediate neonatal period or may survive for some months. They are usually stunted and severely exercise intolerant. They may show signs of CHF, tachypnoea and collapse. On examination, there will be a grade 4–6/6 pansystolic murmur with a PMI at the left base, also radiating to the right side. Tachycardia, weak pulses and cyanosis may be noted.

5.8.3 Diagnosis

A definitive diagnosis can be made using echocardiography. The tricuspid valve is replaced by an echogenic band of fibrous tissue. The ASD and VSD will be identified, along with a dilated LA, large mitral valve, volume overloaded LV and poorly developed RV. Polycythaemia may be evident on clinical pathology.

5.8.4 Prognosis

The prognosis for these foals is hopeless and euthanasia is the only humane course of action.

5.9 Pulmonary stenosis

Pulmonary stenosis is rare in the horse. When present, it is often associated with other congenital malformations such as tetralogy of Fallot.

5.9.1 Haemodynamic effects

The effect of pulmonary stenosis is to increase RV pressure and the work performed by the RV. This results in concentric hypertrophy. This may lead to RV failure, weakness or collapse, and signs of right-sided CHF. If an intracardiac communication with the left side such as an ASD or a VSD is present, it may result in right to left shunting of blood and cyanosis.

5.9.2 Clinical signs

A grade 3–6/6 crescendo–decrescendo ejection-type murmur will be heard at the left heart base. Clinical signs depend on the severity of the obstruction and the presence or absence of other defects. Exercise intolerance is the most likely clinical presentation to be seen with the more mild obstructions, but these are the minority.

5.9.3 Diagnosis

Diagnosis is made on the grounds of auscultatory findings and echocardiography. Cardiac catheterisation can be used to measure the pressure gradient across the valve and is a relatively simple technique for the investigation of right-sided heart lesions. A less invasive method is the use of DE to measure blood flow velocity and calculate the pressure gradient (see section 4.2.7).

5.9.4 Prognosis

The prognosis depends on the severity of the pressure gradient and presence or absence of other defects. Extrapolating from findings in other species, a gradient of more than approximately 50 mm Hg is likely to have a significant effect on exercise tolerance.

5.10 Patent ductus arteriosus

A patent ductus arteriosus (PDA) is a rare defect in foals over 4 days of age (see above). When present, it is often part of a complex anomaly.

5.10.1 Haemodynamic effects

A PDA allows blood to pass from the high pressure aorta to the relatively low pressure PA, i.e. in the opposite direction to blood flow in the fetus. This leads to overcirculation of the lungs. If the ductus is large it will lead to volume overload of the left side of the heart; a small PDA will be less significant. Frequently the ductus remains patent because other defects have resulted in abnormal pressures and oxygen concentrations within the circulatory system. For example, a PDA is essential for life in animals with severe pulmonary hypoplasia.

5.10.2 Clinical signs

Clinical signs will depend on the presence of other congenital lesions and the size of the ductus. Animals with a large shunt or complex defects are likely to present with CHF at an early age. Horses with small shunts may present with exercise intolerance later in life. On examination, a continuous waxing and waning 'machinery' murmur is heard, with a PMI over the left base. The murmur is continuous because a continuous pressure gradient exists between the high-pressure aorta and the relatively low-pressure PA. The murmur waxes and wanes in relation to the change in pressure gradient and volume of flow throughout systole and diastole. It may radiate widely, but the diastolic element may be heard over a localised region only. In some cases, if pulmonary hyper-tension develops, the murmur may may loose its diastolic element so that the continuous sound may be replaced by a predominantly systolic murmur. Bounding water-hammer arterial pulses may be palpated because of the large stroke volume which results from volume overload and the 'let-off valve' effect of the PDA.

5.10.3 Diagnosis

Diagnosis is made on the basis of the characteristic murmur. It is difficult to identify the vessel on 2DE, but turbulence may be detected in the PA using Doppler echocardiography. Catheterisation will show a raised oxygen tension in the PA.

If a murmur typical of a PDA is heard in an animal of more than a few days of age, a search for additional congenital cardiac lesions is warranted.

5.10.4 *Prognosis*

The prognosis for life with complex defects is grave. PDAs are theoretically amenable to surgery, although there are no reports of successful surgery with a return to normal athletic function as yet.

5.11 Endocardial cushion defect

Endocardial cushion defects cover a spectrum of abnormalities including ostium primum ASDs, VSDs, and malformed tricuspid and mitral valves. A cleft in the septal mitral leaflet may be present. The haemodynamic effects of the anomaly are variable but will include volume overload of the left side of the heart due to mitral regurgitation and the presence of the VSD. Cyanosis may be present. Affected foals are weak, stunted, and usually show signs of CHF. The diagnosis is made on echocardiography or post-mortem examination. The prognosis is hopeless.

5.12 Other defects

A large number of other congenital abnormalities have been reported including pulmonary atresia, cor trioculare biatrium (single ventricle with two atria or 'Frog heart'), truncus arteriosus (single large artery comprising of the fused PA and aorta), coarctation of the aorta (narrowing of the aorta, usually early in the descending portion), LV hypoplasia and double-outlet RV. Often the definition and terminology of some of the more complex lesions reported is not clear in papers describing these lesions. Complex lesions almost invariably carry a grave prognosis for life.

5.13 Arrhythmias in the neonate

Many arrhythmias, including ventricular premature complexes and atrial fibrillation, have been reported in foals immediately after birth. The majority of these abnormalities are short-lived and sinus rhythm usually returns after 24–72 hours without treatment. Persistent arrhythmias may be associated with underlying structural disease or systemic illness.

5.14 Detection of cardiovascular compromise in the fetus

Assessment of cardiac function is a useful technique for monitoring the well-being of the fetus. The technique is poorly developed at present but offers potential for future use. Transabdomenal ultrasonography can be used for monitoring fetal heart rate by placing the M-mode cursor through the fetal heart and calculating the rate from the M-mode trace. A persistent tachycardia (> 120 bpm in a near-term fetus) or bradycardia (< 70 bpm), a fixed heart rate, or arrhythmias, are suggestive of fetal distress. The advantage of the ultrasound technique is that the fetal fluids and fetal position can also be assessed.

Fetal electrocardiography can be used to monitor fetal heart rate and document the presence of a live fetus. A bipolar lead system is used, with the leads placed in either a ventro–dorsal configuration or from one flank to the other. Small complexes will be seen superimposed on the normal ECG of the dam. Good electrical contact must be maintained in order to avoid artefact obscuring the fetal trace.

Chapter 6

Acquired Cardiovascular Disease

Acquired cardiovascular disease is much more common than congenital disease. Usually it affects the valves, but the myocardium, the pericardium or the peripheral vasculature may also become diseased.

Optimal management of horses with cardiac disease requires the clinician to make a specific diagnosis, to assess the severity of the condition and to identify any underlying cardiac or systemic disease. Only after these factors have been addressed should treatment be considered. This may be corrective or palliative, depending on the disease process and the individual case. The most important considerations are usually the prognosis and advice about the future athletic use of the animal.

The majority of horses with cardiac disease do not benefit from any form of treatment. This is because most animals have signs which are limited to exercise intolerance, and in the case of valvular disease this is unlikely to improve with any treatment. However, selected individuals with arrhythmias, pericardial disease, bacterial endocarditis and congestive heart failure (CHF) may require specific treatment. Basic rules for the management of horses with cardiac disease are summarised in Table 6.1.

Table 6.1 Basic rules for management of horses with cardiac disease

1. Make a specific diagnosis.
2. Determine whether or not the disease is causing clinical signs at present. Consider whether it may deteriorate in the future.
3. Identify complicating factors such as systemic illness, endocarditis, management limitations.
4. Corrective treatment if appropriate.
5. Palliative treatment if appropriate.
6. Prognosis and advice for future use.

6.1 Valvular heart disease

6.1.1 Causes of valvular heart disease

Valvular disease may be caused by the following:

(1) Degenerative or myxomatous disease (common).
(2) Rupture or disease of the chordae tendineae supporting the atrioventricular (AV) valves (infrequent).

(3) Bacterial endocarditis (uncommon).
(4) Congenital valve malformation (rare).

Small nodular lesions which result from degenerative disease are quite commonly found on the mitral and aortic valves. It is unclear to what extent these constitute normal ageing changes similar to those seen on the valves of other species such as man and the dog; certainly they are not always associated with cardiac murmurs. However, in some animals these nodules, or more diffuse structural changes occurring in the valve, do result in valvular incompetence. Theoretically, valvular disease may also lead to stenosis and increased resistance to outflow of blood. However, true valvular stenosis as a result of degenerative change is exceptionally rare in the horse (compared with mitral stenosis in humans), and congenital stenosis is equally uncommon (compared with aortic stenosis in dogs).

The integrity of the atrioventricular (AV) valves depends on the supporting network of chordae tendineae, so rupture of these structures results in a billowing of the valve leaflet into the atrium during systole. This usually has a serious effect on valvular competence. Bacterial infection of heart valves is termed endocarditis, and represents a life-threatening disease because it usually causes severe damage to valvular integrity and because it acts as a nidus of infection. Congenital valvular malformations are much less common in the horse than in other species, although cardiac murmurs may result from structural defects which are congenital and may be confused with those which result from acquired cardiac disease.

6.1.2 Clinical findings in horses with valvular heart disease

The clinical finding most commonly associated with valvular heart disease is that of a cardiac murmur; however, a murmur may be found in the absence of valvular disease because functional murmurs are common in horses (see section 3.5.2). In addition, AV valve incompetence can result from dilation of the ventricles and the valve annulus. Rarely, significant valvular disease can also be present without causing turbulent blood flow. For example, the absence of a murmur does not always exclude a diagnosis of endocarditis. A variety of clinical signs may result from reduced cardiac reserve caused by the haemodynamic effects of valvular disease.

Two important steps must be made in the clinical examination of horses with heart murmurs:

1. *To identify the source of the murmur.* It is very important that functional murmurs are distinguished from those which result from disease. The characteristics of murmurs determined from clinical examination are normally sufficient for this distinction to be made (see section 3.5).
2. *To make a judgement regarding the significance of the murmur.* Functional murmurs have no deleterious effect on cardiac function, although some physiological murmurs are present as a result of systemic disease which alters cardiac output. Once a murmur has been determined to result from a pathological process, its likely effect on athletic performance and future health can be

evaluated. Appropriate use of further diagnostic aids is prompted by these findings and helps the clinician to direct treatment (where appropriate) and to give a prognosis for the animal. These techniques have been discussed in Chapter 4.

Murmurs typical of MR and functional murmurs may also be detected in horses during episodes of colic. The reason for this is not clear; however, it seems likely that it is related to altered fluid balance rather than to myocardial depression or primary valvular disease. In some cases, the murmur may have been present but undetected for some time. It is wise to re-examine animals in which murmurs are detected in these circumstances, after other clinical problems have resolved, before any judgement is made as to their significance.

6.2 Mitral valve disease

Mitral valve (MV) disease is the most important valvular condition affecting athletic performance. Degenerative myxomatous change is the most common cause; however, the exact aetiology of this disease is poorly understood. Anecdotal reports link the occurrence of the condition with previous viral or bacterial respiratory infections, but there is little clear evidence of this. Recently, there has been interest in the possibility of a valvulitis associated with streptococcal respiratory infections which may affect the mitral or other valves. However, although the concept is attractive, there is little evidence for such a link at present. It may be that murmurs are more commonly detected in these animals because they are more likely to be auscultated. If the degenerative change is sufficient the valve may become incompetent. This may be due to a change in the collagenous structure of the valve resulting in a billowing of the valve leaflet, rather than due to the nodules on the margin of the valve. Horses of all ages can be affected, but chronic degenerative disease is most frequently seen in middle-aged or older horses. MV disease may also be caused by bacterial endocarditis, but this is relatively rare (endocarditis is discussed in section 6.6).

6.2.1 Clinical signs

Murmurs typical of mitral regurgitation (MR) are frequently found in horses with no history of poor performance or other signs of cardiac disease. However, even in these animals, the detection of a murmur compatible with MR is a significant finding because it may be progressive and may lead to reduced athletic performance or even to cardiac failure later in life. The initial approach to such an animal is therefore to determine the effects of MR on cardiac function at the time of examination, in particular the effect it may have on exercise tolerance. Where the condition is deemed to be clinically insignificant at the time of examination, periodic re-examination should be recommended to follow the progression of the disease so that any deterioration is detected.

The clinical signs associated with MR are commonly insidious in onset. Often excessive tiring and increased respiratory effort after work are noted first. Owners may not associate these signs with cardiac disease, particularly in animals that may be unfit or in which the expectations of athletic performance are low. A useful diagnostic feature is that if excess expiratory effort is due to lack of fitness it usually resolves after exercise in a matter of minutes, but it may persist for a prolonged period (e.g. 10–30 minutes) in animals with significant cardiac disease. However, other conditions such as respiratory disease can lead to similar signs and should also be considered.

When MR is sudden in onset, such as when a major chorda tendinea ruptures, pulmonary oedema may develop, resulting in severe respiratory distress, frothy fluid appearing at the nostrils, coughing at rest and weak arterial pulses. In these situations, the left atrium (LA) and pulmonary veins do not have the capacity to cope with the sudden increase in pressure and volume. Hydrostatic pressure overcomes colloid pressure and lymphatic drainage so that the interstitial spaces and then the alveolae fill with fluid (see section 2.2.2). Initially, this may only happen during times of high demand such as exercise, particularly in athletic animals. Frequently this stage of left-sided congestive heart failure (CHF) is not observed by the owners. The LA and pulmonary veins adapt to the load but the increased pulmonary wedge pressure, and possibly pulmonary arteriolar constriction, result in pulmonary arterial hypertension. The exact pathophysiological mechanism of the development of pulmonary hypertension is unclear and local hypoxaemia may also play a role.

MR which is sufficiently severe to cause pulmonary hypertension will result in signs of right-sided heart failure. Signs include distension of the jugular veins, oedema of the ventral abdomen and brisket area, filling of the sheath in males and oedema of the distal limbs. These signs are often more readily recognised by owners than signs of left-sided CHF such as pulmonary oedema, which are frequently short-lived. It is important that other causes of peripheral oedema formation are considered when these signs develop, even when a cardiac murmur is detected. The differential diagnoses for ventral oedema were summarised in Table 3.3.

6.2.2 Clinical examination

Auscultation

The murmur associated with MR is typically holo- or pansystolic. This is because regurgitation starts as soon as the pressure of the left ventricle (LV) rises above that of the LA and lasts until the end of systole. The character of the murmur is usually described as plateau or band-shaped (see section 3.5.1). This is due to the fact that a relatively constant pressure gradient exists between the left ventricle and the LA throughout systole. In some animals, particularly those with MV prolapse, the murmur may be restricted to a limited period of systole. Murmurs associated with valve prolapse are typically loudest in late systole, are crescendo in character, and may have a musical or honking quality.

Typically, the point of maximal intensity of a murmur (PMI) associated with MR is over the apex beat area of the heart, but it may radiate dorsally and cranially up towards the base, or sometimes in a dorsal and caudal direction (Figure 6.1). The pattern of radiation of the murmur will depend on the position of the regurgitant jet within the LA. Some very loud murmurs of MR are loudest over

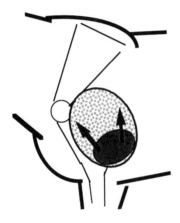

Fig. 6.1 The point of maximal intensity and radiation of a murmur typical of mitral regurgitation.

the cardiac base in the region of the aortic valve. This may lead to some confusion as to their origin. The pansystolic plateau-type characteristics remain, and the localisation of the PMI to this area is likely to be because of a cranially and dorsally directed jet running up the aortic aspect of the LA.

The intensity of murmurs which result from MR may be relatively quiet or very loud. They are usually at least grade 2/6, are most often grade 3 or 4, but may be associated with a precordial thrill and murmurs of grades 5 or 6/6.

Some cardiologists have described diastolic murmurs which they have attributed to mitral stenosis. There is, however, no documented evidence of a true stenosis seen on M-mode, two-dimensional or Doppler echocardiographic (DE) examination of these animals. Volume overload of the LV and LA, which may result from significant MR, can cause an increase in the intensity of S3 due to the increased volume of blood flowing through the MV. This finding can be a useful clinical observation, although S3 may also be loud in animals with LV eccentric hypertrophy caused by exercise training.

Additional characteristics of the murmur associated with MR can be identified in some animals. Quiet musical murmurs are heard in some horses, often in younger animals with no other signs of cardiac disease. The significance of these murmurs is often particularly hard to define. They are unlikely to be of any clinical significance at the time of examination, but it is unclear whether they progress to cause significant valvular incompetence later in life. In animals with rupture of the chordae tendineae the murmur may have a vibrant, rasping quality and may be associated with a precordial thrill.

6.2.3 Other clinical findings

A thorough clinical examination is required in all animals in which a murmur compatible with a diagnosis of MR is found. Mucous membrane colour is likely to be normal in all but the most severe cases, and capillary refill time is usually within normal limits except in animals with CHF. The facial pulse quality should be assessed, but this is also unlikely to be abnormal except in animals in heart failure. The pulse rate is measured once the horse is at rest. The relationship between the pulse and the heart sounds should be examined in animals with an arrhythmia or a tachycardia. The nostrils should be examined for evidence of pulmonary oedema. The jugular veins are inspected for evidence of distension or pulsation. The lung fields should be auscultated, and a re-breathing test should be performed in selected cases. The abdomen and distal limbs should be examined for signs of dependant oedema (see section 3.3.7).

6.2.4 Diagnosis

Diagnosis of MR depends in the first instance on accurate auscultation. Usually the diagnosis can be made with reasonable certainty on these grounds alone. In some cases, DE is useful to confirm the presence of a jet of blood flowing into the LA during systole. Frequently, no evidence of gross valvular change is seen using two-dimensional echocardiography (2DE), although this does not exclude the possibility that MR is present.

   Once MR has been diagnosed, it is important to consider other conditions which may cause similar clinical signs to MR. If signs such as tachypnoea and dyspnoea are present, the respiratory system should be examined further to establish whether any other disease processes are contributing to the signs. It is often particularly relevant to rule out the presence of allergic respiratory conditions in adults and respiratory infections in foals. Radiography, endoscopy, cytological examination of tracheal or bronchio–alveolar lavage samples and clinical pathological investigations may be appropriate if respiratory disease is considered to be a differential diagnosis or a complicating factor. If inflammatory small airway disease (COPD) is present, appropriate managemental changes should be instituted so that it does not compromise athletic performance or allow clinical signs, attributable to this condition, to become confused with signs of a deterioration in the severity of the MR at a later date.

6.2.5 Clinical guides to prognosis

Judgement of the significance of MR on clinical grounds alone can be difficult. The intensity of a murmur is not an accurate guide to the severity of MR. However, in general, loud murmurs are more often associated with significant disease than quiet murmurs. It can be helpful to note the radiation of the murmur; if the regurgitation is moderate or severe, the murmur is likely to radiate widely. In cases in which a thrill is palpated, significant regurgitation of blood is likely to be present. The position of the apex beat and the area over which heart sounds are heard may be more caudal than usual in cases with severe MR and cardiomegaly. Percussion may also reveal an enlarged cardiac silhouette in these cases. Pulse quality is seldom affected in animals with MR, except in those cases with CHF. The pulse rate is a more useful guide to the response of the heart in compensation for the haemodynamic effects of MR. In order to maintain cardiac output in the face of a significant regurgitant fraction, heart rate will be increased. It is very difficult to judge the appropriate heart rate for horses after exercise, particularly in animals other than racehorses. However, measurement of resting heart rate is very useful, as a persistently raised heart rate often accompanies severe MR. In the author's opinion, any heart rate above 45 bpm, when the animal is genuinely at rest, requires investigation to rule out non-cardiac causes. However, MR can be significant in horses with a resting heart rate below this level.

Arrhythmias may be found in animals with MR and should be characterised, using electrocardiography if necessary. Physiological arrhythmias (see section 7.7) are less likely to be found in animals with significant valvular disease than in normal horses because vagal tone is usually less marked. The presence of abnormal rhythms, particularly atrial and ventricular premature beats and atrial fibrillation, in animals with MR, is significant. These findings suggest that the valvular disease has caused, or is associated with, myocardial dysfunction or chamber dilation. Although the effects of exercise on the intensity of cardiac murmurs is an overvalued part of the clinical examination (see section 3.8.2), in some cases where valvular disease is present, arrhythmias may only be present during exercise. Auscultation after exercise and, ideally, radiotelemetry during exercise is helpful in order that these abnormalities are detected.

Sequential examinations can help to give a more accurate prognosis in horses with MR than a single examination because the rate of progression of the condition can be monitored. It is seldom possible to know the rate at which MV disease will progress, but it must be assumed that the degenerative change will continue, resulting in an increased regurgitant fraction over a period of months or years. Sudden deterioration of the condition, which may precipitate more severe clinical signs, may be associated with rupture of chordae tendineae as a result of the degenerative change, the development of an arrhythmia such as atrial fibrillation, or non-cardiac disease which results in a further load on the heart.

Many horses can still perform useful work with mild or moderate MR; however, few horses will do well in athletic competition with moderate MR. If poor athletic performance develops, it may be appropriate to reduce the level of activity. The principle danger is that the animal will tire easily and then become more likely to fall. Owners should be made aware of this possibility and it may affect the suitability of the horse for different riders. Collapse is very uncommon except in animals which are showing signs of cardiovascular compromise (e.g. tachycardia, jugular distension) at rest. These individuals should not be ridden. As a rule, problems are most likely to be encountered when athletic activity is increased beyond the level at which it has been established that the horse can manage satisfactorily. The most difficult situation is in young animals with mild MR and little performance history. In some cases, after echocardiographic appraisal and a discussion of the signs of exercise intolerance with the owners, it may be appropriate to continue to increase the level of work in order to establish what sort of performance the horse is capable of providing. The progression of MR should be monitored regularly. A follow-up examination approximately three months after the problem is first identified, and then at six-month intervals, is justified in moderate cases of MR.

6.2.6 Diagnostic and prognostic aids

Echocardiography

Echocardiography can be helpful to identify gross valvular lesions, generalised valve thickening, valve prolapse, or abnormal motion such as flail leaflet. However, in most horses with MR, little gross valvular change is visible on echocardiography. The main purpose of the examination is to identify any volume overload of the LA and LV in an animal in which MR has already been diagnosed from auscultation. In animals with no volume overload, it is likely that the MR is of limited clinical significance at the time of examination (although it does not mean that the condition will not deteriorate to this point at some time in the future). Animals with marked volume overload are likely to have clinical signs of decreased cardiac reserve or even CHF. Echocardiography is most helpful in enabling the clinician to make an objective assessment of the significance of MR in those cases where mild volume overload may have resulted in clinical signs such as decreased athletic performance.

Echocardiographic evaluation of MR combines examination of the structure and motion of the MV, and subjective and quantitative assessment of the consequences of the regurgitation in terms of the degree of volume overload and the effect on cardiac function. In order to evaluate MV structure fully, it is essential that long- and short-axis views are obtained from the right and left parasternal positions. The long-axis views are particularly helpful and may allow detection of localised or nodular thickening of the valve, or abnormal motion of the valve such as prolapse or flail of a leaflet. Both the right and left parasternal views are required because they transect the valve along different axes. For example, the right commissural leaflet is best seen from the left parasternal view because this view tends to be along a left cranial to right caudal axis, which takes it through this leaflet.

Quantitative measurements can also be made from both sides of the chest. Usually, LV diameter is measured from the right parasternal short-axis view at the level of the chordae tendineae, using 2DE to guide the position of the M-mode cursor. Measurement of LAD is made from a left parasternal long-axis view with the dimension of the atrium maximised (see section 4.2.4). Although LAD cannot be measured as accurately as LVD, it is a very useful measurement because it is a good guide to the significance of MR. A range of measurements from normal Thoroughbred horses was given in Table 4.7. As a very rough guide, adult Thoroughbred horses with MR resulting in LVD measurements at end-diastole (LVDd) > 14.5 cm and LAD > 15 cm are unlikely to perform well in competition, those with LVDd > 15.5 cm, LAD > 16 cm should not be ridden at all. However, these figures are only approximate and should be considered in combination with other clinical information, and after due consideration of the circumstances of each individual owner and horse. Measurements for other breeds are not available. Generally speaking, large horses have larger cardiac dimensions than smaller animals, and fit, athletic horses have larger chambers than those which have little exercise training. Severe MR may result in pulmonary hypertension, leading to dilation of the pulmonary artery (PA). Since sudden death due to rupture of the PA has been reported, these horses should not be ridden (see below).

In addition to assessment with two-dimensional echocardiography and measurement with 2DE and M-mode echocardiography, DE can be used to show the extent of the jet of MR within the LA. This is performed by mapping out the area of the LA over which the regurgitant jet can be detected (see section 4.2.7).

Quantitative echocardiography is the most objective method of assessing the severity of MR in clinical practice and is an exceptionally helpful technique. The echocardiographic features of MR were summarised in Table 4.9.

Electrocardiography

Electrocardiography is a useful technique in cases in which arrhythmias are detected at rest, during or after exercise. These may be caused by atrial dilation and may complicate the prognosis in horses with MR. However, ECGs are not useful in a clinical setting for the detection of either atrial or ventricular enlargement.

Clinical pathology

Clinical pathology is rarely of any value in the evaluation of MV disease except in animals in which endocarditis is suspected. There is no clear evidence of any association between MV disease and raised cardiac isoenzymes. Clinical pathology may be helpful in order to evaluate the presence of other diseases which may be related to MR, or which may result in similar clinical signs. The evaluation of horses with MR is summarised in Table 6.2.

6.2.7   Treatment

Treatment of horses with MV is inappropriate except in valuable animals in which the condition is sufficiently severe to have resulted in CHF or is caused by endocarditis (see section 6.6). It is seldom more than palliative in either case.

6.3   Tricuspid valve disease

Abnormalities of the tricuspid valve (TV) are an uncommon finding at post-mortem (PM) in the horse, but tricuspid regurgitation (TR) can be found in animals with no gross valvular lesions. Although TR is not well documented in the literature, it is not as uncommon as some reports would suggest. TR can result from pulmonary hypertension due to pulmonary disease such as severe inflammatory small airway disease (COPD). Pulmonary hypertension may also result from left-sided CHF. The TV may be particularly likely to leak as a result of dilation of the valve annulus because of the three leaflet structure. It is also possible that dilation of the right side occurs as a result of the normal eccentric hypertrophy which results from exercise training and may lead to TR. TR detected by DE is more common in human athletes than in sedentary individuals and a similar situation may occur in trained racehorses.

6.3.1   Clinical signs

A murmur compatible with a diagnosis of TR is a common finding in Thoroughbred racehorses which show no signs of clinical abnormality and in which athletic performance is normal. In horses presented for poor performance, TR should only be considered to be the likely cause after a thorough examination to

Table 6.2   Summary: Clinical evaluation of horses with mitral regurgitation

History
Variable signs noted by owners depending on the severity of the condition:
   incidental finding
   poor exercise tolerance (stopping, fading, prolonged recovery, EIPH)
   left- and/or right-sided congestive heart failure
Sudden onset or progressive over days to years

Clinical findings
Mucous membrane colour usually normal
CRT normal to slow
Arterial pulse normal to weak
Pulse rate normal (24–45) to rapid (> 45), regular or irregular
Grade 2–6/6 plateau-type pan or holosystolic murmur with a PMI over the left apical area or
   just dorsal to this
Murmur may radiate dorsally and cranially or caudally
Murmur may radiate to right side of the chest
Late systolic murmurs may also be heard, suggestive of valve prolapse
Endocarditis seldom affects this valve in adults

Evaluation of significance
Most likely to be significant if:
   associated with poor athletic performance
   slow CRT
   weak or variable pulse quality
   resting heart rate > 45 bpm
   intensity grade 4/6 or greater
   widespread radiation
   associated with abnormal arrhythmia, especially atrial fibrillation, APCs
   associated with signs of left-sided congestive heart failure (pulmonary oedema evident
     by white froth at nares, tachypnoea, weakness, exercise intolerance)
   associated with signs of right-sided congestive heart failure (dependent oedema, jugular
     filling)

Note: The progression of MR is seldom predictable, so detection of MR may be a significant
finding, for future athletic use, even if no clinical signs are attributed to the condition at the
time of examination.

Helpful diagnostic tests
Echocardiography
Electrocardiography, if arrhythmia present

rule out other possible conditions and, ideally, an echocardiographic examination, unless it is obviously severe.

Moderate and severe TR may result in a reduction in athletic performance. Severe TR can lead to right-sided failure, with prominent jugular pulsation. The pulsation results from the force of ventricular systole ejecting blood in a retrograde direction into the right atrium (RA) and great veins. If the RA becomes dilated as a result of the volume overload, it may predispose to the development of atrial fibrillation.

Degenerative disease of the TV is uncommon. Occasionally rupture of the chordae tendineae of the valve is seen. TR is most often accompanied by prolapse of the valve leaflets which may be seen on echocardiography. Prolapse of the TV is often regarded as clinically insignificant by the author and may apparently resolve on later examinations; however, it does lead to significant TR in some cases. The TV is seldom affected by endocarditis.

6.3.2 Diagnosis

Auscultation

Diagnosis of TR is based on the finding of the typical pan or holosystolic plateau-type murmur with a PMI over the TV region, on the right side of the chest (Figure 6.2). These murmurs often have a soft blowing quality. When they are harsh they are more likely to be related to primary TV disease. In some animals with TR, the murmur can also be heard on the left side of the chest cranial to the MV region, usually low down in the second intercostal space.

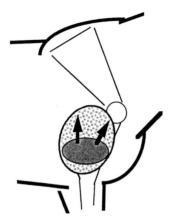

Fig. 6.2 The point of maximal intensity and radiation of a murmur typical of tricuspid regurgitation.

An important differential diagnosis in the case of a loud pan or holosystolic plateau-type murmur over the TV region is a ventricular septal defect. Typically, the murmur associated with this congenital defect is lower on the chest wall, just above the sternum, has a harsh quality and an associated palpable precordial thrill. These characteristics are, however, dependent on the exact location and size of the defect and on secondary changes (see section 5.5.3).

6.3.3 Further diagnostic aids

Echocardiography

Although mild–moderate TR may not be associated with any clinical signs, it can be significant in some individuals and therefore further investigation may be justified. Echocardiography is the best method to assess whether TR is resulting in significant volume overload. Unfortunately, accurate measurement of the RV or RA size from either M-mode echocardiography or 2DE is difficult because of the absence of good landmarks and the trabeculations of the RV surface. However, a subjective assessment of the size of the structures is useful. The RA and RV should be examined from the right parasternal location in long-axis and short-axis views, and at angles between the two. Familiarity with these views will allow a subjective assessment of the size of the atrium and ventricle. The aorta acts as a reference point. A thick chest wall can give the appearance of a large RV because more of the free-wall is visible. Prolapse of the TV is most often seen in the long-axis view. Using pulsed-wave Doppler, a jet of regurgitant blood is most frequently detected in the long-axis view running along the side of the atrium where it borders the aorta. Jets which can be detected over a much wider area of the RA are more likely to be associated with clinically significant disease. If RV volume and pressure are particularly high, the interventricular septum (IVS) will be flattened, i.e. it is pushed towards the LV, and in extreme cases, the motion of the IVS will be paradoxical (see section 4.2.6).

Contrast echocardiography can be a useful technique in animals with loud pansystolic murmurs on the right side of the chest, particularly when Doppler equipment is not available. Contrast may be seen regurgitating back into the RA in cases of TR. Some animals with TR may have increased amounts of spontaneous contrast within the RA and RV. When TR is present this may be seen moving back into the RA during systole. The echocardiographic features of TR were summarised in Table 4.10.

Electrocardiography
Electrocardiography is indicated in horses with arrhythmias, but is not helpful for assessing the degree of volume overload in individual animals with TR.

Clinical pathology
Clinical pathology may be helpful in animals with suspected endocarditis; however, this is very uncommon.

6.3.4 Treatment

Treatment of horses with TR is valid in some valuable animals when it is caused by endocarditis (see later in this chapter). Treatment of CHF using diuretics is seldom worthwhile in the long term.

Clinical evaluation of horses with TR is summarised in Table 6.3.

6.4 Ruptured chordae tendineae

Rupture of the chordae tendineae is a condition which has been reported relatively infrequently, but it is an important complicating factor in a significant proportion of cases with MR and some animals with TR. Rupture of MV chordae tendineae is much more common and more significant than TV chordae tendineae rupture and may be immediately life-threatening. Rupture of the chordae tendineae is likely to result from degenerative disease affecting the whole of the valve, rather than being a primary problem. Frequently, however, animals have been known to have pre-existing cardiac disease. In the author's experience, the right commissural cusp of the MV is most frequently affected, although other leaflets can be involved. Ruptured chordae tendineae are recognised with greater frequency since the advent of echocardiography.

Table 6.3 Summary: Clinical evaluation of horses with tricuspid regurgitation

History
Variable signs noted by owners depending on the severity of the condition:
  incidental finding (usually)
  poor exercise tolerance (uncommon)
  right-sided congestive heart failure (very uncommon)

Clinical findings
Clinical signs are rarely noted
Most commonly found in racehorses presented for poor athletic performance, but
  frequently an incidental finding even in these animals
Grade 2–6/6 plateau-type pan or holosystolic murmur with a PMI over the right apex area
Murmur may radiate to left side of the chest in the 2nd ics
Endocarditis rarely affects this valve

Evaluation of significance
Most likely to be significant if:
  associated with poor athletic performance
  weak or variable pulse quality
  resting heart rate > 45 bpm
  intensity grade 4/6 or greater
  widespread radiation
  associated with more significant valvular disease such as MR
  associated with abnormal arrhythmia, especially atrial fibrillation (uncommon), APCs
  associated with signs of right-sided congestive heart failure (dependant oedema, jugular
    filling)
  jugular pulsation is present

Helpful diagnostic tests
Echocardiography
Electrocardiography if arrhythmia present
Evaluation of other body systems is indicated in investigation of poor athletic performance
  using diagnostic tools such as endoscopy

6.4.1 Clinical signs

The clinical signs associated with a ruptured chorda tendinea depend on whether the MV or TV is affected, and the contribution of the affected chorda to support of the valve. The larger the chorda involved, the more severe the clinical signs are likely to be. The rupture may or may not occur at a time of strenuous exercise.

Rupture of a major chorda to the MV usually results in signs of acute left-sided CHF. Because the pressure within the LA increases rapidly, the atrium and pulmonary veins do not have an opportunity to adapt to the increased pressure and the pulmonary venous pressure increases sufficiently to cause pulmonary oedema. This may result in a rapid deterioration with tachypnoea and coughing. Exercise intolerance, weakness and even syncope may occur during this period. Often this initial crisis is followed by a period during which signs of pure left-sided CHF decrease in severity.

In the long-term, pulmonary hypertension, right-sided pressure overload, TR and signs of right-sided CHF such as distended jugular veins and dependant oedema develop. In some horses, clinical signs may not be observed immediately and these animals may be presented only later as a result of poor exercise tolerance, or right-sided CHF. Arrhythmias such as atrial fibrillation may result from distension of the atria. Rupture of the MV chordae tendineae may result in sudden death in some animals, although this is uncommon. However, a murmur of AV regurgitation due to ruptured chordae tendineae may be an incidental finding in animals which do not perform strenuous work.

6.4.2 Diagnosis

Auscultation
Ruptured chordae tendineae result in moderate to severe valvular incompetence. Diagnosis is first based on auscultation of the characteristic murmur of MR or TR. Signs which may alert the clinician to the specific diagnosis of ruptured chordae tendineae include a history of a sudden deterioration of clinical signs, or the acute onset of clinical signs of heart disease in animals with no previously known disease. In some cases the murmur is particularly harsh, with a coarse vibrant quality. Musical murmurs are sometimes present and may have a honking quality. Frequently the murmur radiates a long way dorsally from the left apex, and may even appear to have a PMI over the base of the heart. This may be because of the vibration of the left atrial wall in association with the regurgitant jet of blood.

6.4.3 Further diagnostic aids

Echocardiographic examination is required to confirm the presence of ruptured chordae tendineae ante-mortem. The affected valve leaflet may be seen to flail into the atrium. If the plane of the beam is in the long axis of the affected valve, this appears as a curve of the leaflet into the atrium during systole (Figure 4.23). If the plane of the beam is not aligned with the valve, a flash of an echogenic dot may be seen in the atrium, just behind the valve. Often, careful examination from the right and left parasternal positions is required in order to identify the abnormal motion. Flail due to rupture of the right commissural cusp chordae tendineae is usually best seen in a left parasternal long-axis view.

At PM, a ruptured chorda may be difficult to find without careful inspection (Figure 2.2). Usually a tag will be present where the chorda originates on the papillary muscle, while a curled-up piece of tissue is found on the ventricular side of the leaflet where it inserts. Jet lesions may be seen in the atrium (Figure 2.1).

6.4.4 Prognosis

Most ruptured chordae tendineae lead to significant volume overload and carry a poor prognosis. The fact that a ruptured chorda tendinea is the cause of valvular incompetence has no direct bearing on the prognosis, except that the signs may be particularly severe immediately after the rupture, before compensation occurs. When a murmur of MR or TR develops in a short period and is associated with clinical signs, a period of box rest during which the animal is given a chance to compensate may be justified in animals which are not expected to perform at an arduous athletic level. However, very few animals will return to work, even if they are only required for hacking, although some may have an adequate quality of life to be kept as a pet. In these circumstances, monitoring the resting heart rate and close observation for signs of tachypnoea and ventral oedema are advisable, so that the horse is not ridden when unsafe and for the welfare of the animal. Ideally, echocardiographic examinations should be repeated at three- to six-month intervals to monitor for signs of deterioration such as increased volume overload or PA dilation which may precede rupture of this vessel.

6.5   Aortic valve disease

Small nodules and fenestrations of the aortic valve cusps are common findings in normal horses. Fenestrations are usually found on the leading edge of the valve and may even be found in the fetus. Small nodules are more often found in older animals and become most common in horses over approximately seven years of age. These nodules are due to degenerative change, but frequently appear to have no effect on valve function. In some animals band-type lesions are found, and these are more often associated with signs of abnormal valve function. Nodules and bands are most frequently found on the right coronary cusp of the valve, although the left coronary cusp and the non-coronary cusp are also affected. Lesions, particularly those of a band-type, may result in valvular incompetence; however, there is no evidence that they ever result in sufficient obstruction to outflow to merit the term 'stenosis' (see section 6.5.4). Aortic regurgitation (AR) is quite common in older horses, but is occasionally found in younger animals.

6.5.1   Auscultation

The murmur associated with AR is usually characteristic. It is a decrescendo holodiastolic murmur, with a PMI over the aortic valve region at the heart base, radiating down to the apex (Figure 6.3). The murmur may also be heard on the right side of the chest at a lower intensity. AR can be difficult to hear in mild cases, where it may be a faint, sighing grade 1/6 murmur. However, in other

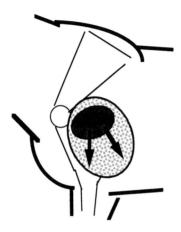

Fig. 6.3 The point of maximal intensity and radiation of a murmur typical of aortic regurgitation.

cases it can be musical, or harsh and rasping and in some animals it is extremely loud, up to grade 6/6 in intensity. It is important to listen carefully with both the diaphragm and the bell of the stethoscope so that sounds of high and low pitch can be heard. It is often helpful to try to ignore systolic sounds and concentrate on diastolic sounds of different pitch over a period of a few minutes.

In some animals, a relatively loud (grade 2–3/6) functional ejection-type murmur is also heard. This may be present because of the large stroke volume of the LV and high velocity of blood flow through the aortic valve which results from severe AR.

6.5.2   Clinical signs and prognosis

In mild cases, the athletic performance of the horse is usually unaffected, and the finding of a murmur of AR is not sufficient alone to warrant a reduction in the level of exercise. The condition is likely to deteriorate with time, but usually AR is not the reason for the eventual retirement or death of the animal. If the condition is more severe, the arterial pulse may become bounding, or 'water hammer' in character, due to the volume overload and rapid diastolic run-off in pressure. The pulse quality has been shown to be a very useful clinical guide to the severity of the disease. The resting heart rate can also be a useful guide to significance, as with other conditions. Resting heart rates in excess of 45 per minute are a cause for concern and would indicate the need for further investigation.

The intensity of the murmur of AR is of very little value as a guide to severity. Some animals with very loud murmurs of AR (grades 5 or 6/6) may have relatively little volume overload, while animals with quieter murmurs may have sufficient volume overload to result in clinical signs of poor athletic performance or even CHF. Identification of coexisting disease is another important consideration. For example, if the condition is found in conjunction with MR, the prognosis is much worse.

Endocarditis, although relatively uncommon, most commonly affects the aortic valve in adult horses. Identification of a murmur of AR in a sick animal should therefore lead to consideration of the possibility of an infectious cause for valvular incompetence. Many more animals will coincidentally have a murmur of AR and an illness other than endocarditis; however, the condition carries a grave prognosis if not diagnosed and treated early. Therefore, unless there are other obvious reasons for an illness in an animal with a murmur of AR, further investigative tests are warranted (see below).

6.5.3   Further diagnostic aids

Echocardiography
Echocardiography can be very helpful in the confirmation of a presumptive diagnosis of AR and in evaluating the significance of the condition, particularly because the intensity of the murmur is often of little value in determining the severity of the disease. A number of characteristic echocardiographic features may be seen in horses with AR. These were summarised in Table 4.11. Abnormal valve motion which results from regurgitant flow of blood is sufficiently

common for the examination to be a useful method of confirming the diagnosis; however, the most important consideration is to evaluate the effect of the condition in terms of the volume overload which may accompany it. This can be very substantial. It is the best guide to the severity of the condition and is very useful in making a suitable judgement regarding the future athletic use of the animal.

Examination of the aortic valve is best performed from the right parasternal long- and short-axis views at the level of the valve. In the long-axis view the dilation of the aorta at the level of the sinuses of Valsalva is easily seen. The left coronary cusp and sinus are most clearly seen because the beam bisects these structures. The right coronary cusp or non-coronary cusp are seen in the near field. In the short-axis view the valve is said to have a 'Mercedes–Benz' appearance, with the coronary arteries clearly seen (Figure 4.15). Echogenic lesions may be seen on the valve cusps in either of these views (Figure 4.21), and these may be the cause of AR or may be incidental findings in animals with no murmur. The valve structure appears more echogenic if it lies perpendicular to the line of the beam; this may artefactually give the appearance of thickening of the valve. For example, the tip of the left coronary cusp always appears to be thickened in the long-axis view. Real lesions may be missed in the long-axis view but are more easily identified in the short-axis view. In some animals with AR detected on auscultation, no clear echogenic lesion will be seen.

High-frequency vibration of the aortic valve cusps may be identified during diastole and is best seen using M-mode echocardiography. Flailing of the tip of a valve leaflet is found occasionally. In this situation, the murmur is often very loud and musical. A small piece of valve will be seen fluttering on the ventricular side of the valve like a flag in the wind. On rare occasions, the valve ruptures and a whole cusp can flail into the LV. Often the septal mitral leaflet is seen to vibrate; it may even fail to open fully as a result of the action of the jet. This has been termed 'relative mitral stenosis'. However, the flow of blood through the valve is more likely to be affected by changes in diastolic LV pressure than a jet impinging on the valve. In some animals, the IVS will vibrate if the jet is directed towards it.

In addition to confirming a diagnosis of AR and assessing its effects on cardiac function, it is also important to investigate the presence and the significance of other conditions which may have a bearing on treatment and prognosis. The most important complicating conditions are endocarditis and MR. Large valvular vegetations alert the clinician to the presence of endocarditis (Figure 4.20). If MR is present in addition to AR, the prognosis for future athletic use and eventually for life are diminished. It is therefore important to evaluate aortic and MV structure and to assess LAD, in addition to measuring LVD. AR may be detected in some cases of congenital heart disease. It may complicate a ventricular septal defect if the aortic root prolapses into the defect resulting in distortion of the valve. This would reduce the prognosis for athletic use in a horse with a VSD.

Having confirmed the diagnosis of AR, the most important part of the examination is to assess the severity of the condition. This can be judged on a number of features. Measurement of LVD is the most helpful guide to the severity of the disease. However, in horses with AR, the same amount of volume overload is less likely to be clinically significant than in animals with MR. Opinions differ as to the dimensions at which volume overload is sufficient to warrant advising against continued use of the animal. This advice, as always, is a matter of judgement, depending on the athletic demands and individual circumstances. As a rough guide, the author would not recommend the use of animals with a LVDd > 15 cm for hard athletic use and one with a LVDd > 16 cm under any circumstances (in an adult Thoroughbred horse). However, these are only arbitrary guidelines; there are anecdotal reports of Thoroughbred horses with LVDd measurements in excess of 16cm competing successfully, but others have poor exercise tolerance with LVDd measurements of < 15 cm. Other criteria such as the presence of myocardial disease or arrhythmias also have to be taken into account.

In animals with severe AR, there will be exaggerated motion of the IVS, which may give the appearance of continuous motion towards the RV throughout diastole. If the LV diastolic pressure rises to very high levels as a result of the volume of blood regurgitating through the aortic valve, the MV may close in mid–late diastole instead of remaining open throughout the conduit phase of diastasis. In these situations the prognosis is likely to be poor.

Doppler echocardiography
Doppler echocardiography is helpful for identifying the retrograde flow of blood through the aortic valve during diastole, and for assessing the severity of the disease. The extent of the jet of AR, mapped using pulsed-wave DE, is a semi-quantitative measure of severity. Very extensive jets suggest a significant degree of regurgitant flow. However, this guideline is not as useful with AR as with MR. The area of the origin of the jet of blood is another indication of the severity, with a large area of origin at the valve being associated with a larger quantity of regurgitant blood flow. A small amount of regurgitant flow is found in many apparently normal animals. The velocity of the regurgitant jet is related to the pressure gradient across the valve during diastole.

Blood pressure measurement
Arterial blood pressure measured either directly, or more commonly indirectly using a pressure-cuff system such as a 'Dynamap', allows the pulse profile to be quantified (see section 4.5). In severe AR, there is an increase in the difference between the systolic and diastolic pressures, which is why the arterial pulse feels strong. This is largely due to the increase in the systolic pressure in main arteries, which is a consequence of the large stroke volume which results from severe regurgitation, and run-off of pressure as blood regurgitates back into the LV. If myocardial failure occurs, the systolic pressures may drop and the arterial pulses may feel weaker; however, this is usually an end-stage event. Blood pressure measurement is thus a relatively simple way of assessing the severity of AR.

Clinical evaluation of horses with AR is summarised in Table 6.4.

6.5.4   Aortic 'stenosis'

Some confusion arises over the term aortic 'stenosis'. This description is used by some authors to describe the degenerative nodular change which commonly affects the aortic valve. While it is possible that these nodules could result in turbulent flow, generating a murmur, it appears to be very rare that they are

Table 6.4 Summary: Clinical evaluation of horses with aortic regurgitation

History
Variable signs noted by owners depending on the severity of the condition:
   incidental finding (common)
   poor exercise tolerance (uncommon)
   left- and/or right-sided congestive heart failure (uncommon)
Sudden onset or progressive over days to years

Clinical findings
Mucous membrane colour usually normal
CRT normal to slow
Arterial pulse may be normal, strong and bounding, or weak
Pulse rate normal to rapid, regular or irregular
Grade 1–6/6 descrescendo holodiastolic murmur with a PMI at the left base
Murmur may radiate ventrally
Murmur may radiate to right side of the chest
Look for signs of endocarditis (very uncommon, but aortic valve is commonest site)

Evaluation of significance
Most likely to be significant if:
   associated with poor athletic performance
   slow CRT
   strong, bounding pulse
   weak or variable pulse quality (usually only when in CHF)
   resting heart rate > 45 bpm
   widespread radiation
   associated with MR
   associated with abnormal arrthythmia, especially AF
   associated with signs of left-sided or right-sided congestive heart failure
   valve affected by endocarditis

Note: The murmur of AR may be very loud in animals with relatively little volume overload

Helpful diagnostic tests
Echocardiography
Electrocardiography if arrhythmia present
Blood pressure measurement (wide pulse pressure)
Clinical pathology if endocarditis suspected

sufficiently large to produce a significant functional narrowing of the valve. Murmurs associated with these nodules would sound like flow murmurs, but there is no evidence that they have any significant deleterious effect on cardiac function; in fact they may be found in animals with no murmurs at all.

6.6   Endocarditis

Endocarditis is a very uncommon disease in the horse. It is caused by bacterial infection of the endocardium resulting in damage to the valves, although vegetations may also be found on the chordae tendineae or on the surface of the ventricular lumen.

Endocarditis can result from poor aseptic technique with intravenous injections, but there is usually no apparent predisposing factor and the source of the infection is seldom established. Horses of any age may be affected, although it is most commonly found in foals, or in middle-aged or older horses. The condition most commonly affects the aortic valve and MV, with the TV and pulmonary valve being affected rarely. The aortic valve is affected more often in adult horses, suggesting that underlying valvular degeneration may predispose to the condition. However, because endocarditis is so uncommon, it is difficult to make valid statements about predisposing factors.

6.6.1 Clinical signs

Horses with endocarditis are usually systemically ill. The signs can relate to the direct effect on the heart as a result of valvular incompetence. Additional signs are due to the effect of infection or sepsis, or emboli from the infected thrombus, and sometimes associated immune-mediated disease. The horse may be depressed and inappetant. Pyrexia, tachycardia and weight loss are common findings and signs of heart failure may be apparent. The mucous membranes may be injected and the capillary refill time increased or reduced as a result of toxaemia. Auscultation usually reveals the murmur of regurgitation through the affected valve. Uncommonly, in severe cases, the lesion may cause a functional stenosis of the valve. Rarely, endocarditis is present in the absence of a cardiac murmur and the animal may be presented with signs of systemic disease only. The facial pulse quality should be assessed as a guide to severity of aortic regurgitation if this valve is affected. Dysrhythmias, particularly premature ventricular beats, are not uncommon and may be caused by emboli in the coronary vasculature.

6.6.2 Diagnostic aids

In any animal in which endocarditis is suspected a thorough investigation is indicated in order to allow early diagnosis for there to be any chance of successful treatment. It is a good principle to perform clinical pathological tests in any horse which is unwell and in which a murmur of AR is detected, although other differential diagnoses need to be considered.

Clinical pathology

Haematology and biochemistry Haematological examination may show a neutrophilia, with or without a left shift. Toxic signs in the neutrophils are sometimes seen. These changes can be very variable. More consistent findings are a hypergammaglobulinaemia and a high plasma fibrinogen level. The latter is particularly useful; a fibrinogen assay should be requested in any animal in which endocarditis is considered a differential diagnosis. Very high fibrinogen levels of 8–13 g/l are often found in animals with endocarditis. However, fibrinogen levels may be raised due to an inflammatory and/or infectious process in other organs and further diagnostic tests pertinent to these organs may be indicated. For example, animals with cardiogenic pulmonary oedema and secondary pneumonia may have high fibrinogen levels. Although the prognosis in the long-term is likely to be poor in these animals also, the pneumonia is more likely to respond to treatment than endocarditis.

Blood culture   A wide variety of bacteria have been isolated from endocarditis lesions so the identity of the causative organism is unlikely to be known without successful blood culture. Scrupulous aseptic technique is needed to avoid contamination; nonetheless, the results of bacterial isolation and antibiotic sensitivity should be interpreted in the light of potential contaminants. If fever spikes are identified, it is theoretically advantageous to take a sample on a rising peak, although this is seldom practicable. At least three samples should be taken directly into blood culture media and cultured for aerobic and anaerobic organisms. Although bacteria can usually be isolated from the lesion itself at PM, blood cultures are often negative. The best results are obtained when large quantities of culture medium and blood are used and when the samples are taken before any antibiotic treatment is given.

Echocardiography

Ideally, echocardiography should be performed in any animal in which endocarditis is suspected, particularly those with a high plasma fibrinogen. It may also be helpful in any animal with a fever of unknown origin, whether a murmur is present or not. The purpose of the echocardiographic examination is to attempt to make a definitive diagnosis and to evaluate the effects of the valvular disease on cardiac function.

In order to make a definitive diagnosis of endocarditis, the location of the infective focus should be isolated to the heart valves or the walls of the ventricles. The lesions caused by endocarditis are usually large, florid and echogenic and are easily identified by echocardiography (Figure 4.20). Occasionally lesions are small and may be attributed to degenerative valvular disease. Serial echocardiographic examinations are likely to show a change in the size or number of lesions with endocarditis. Measurement of any consequent volume overload may help to indicate the severity of valvular regurgitation. If severe, the prognosis is grave even if treatment of the infectious process is successful. It is therefore essential to judge the severity of volume overload before embarking on treatment.

In some animals, systemic disease related to an infectious process other than endocarditis may result in increased demands for cardiac output and may precipitate heart failure in animals with underlying degenerative valvular heart disease.

Clinical evaluation of horses with endocarditis is summarised in Table 6.5.

6.6.3   Treatment

The prognosis for most animals with endocarditis is grave. Frequently the systemic disease is advanced and the damage to the affected valve is extensive; however, on some occasions treatment can be successful. If the horse has sufficient breeding potential or sentimental value, aggressive antibiotic treatment may be justified. Some animals have returned to athletic performance after successful treatment of endocarditis; however, this is uncommon and depends on the degree of valvular compromise.

The aim of treatment is to achieve a bacteriological cure, to reduce systemic embolisation of infected thrombi, and to reduce valve damage and subsequent

Table 6.5 Summary: Clinical evaluation of horses with endocarditis

History
Very uncommon
Usually chronic history of malaise
Weight loss

Clinical findings
+/– cardiac murmur
+/– signs of cardiac disease
+/– pyrexia
signs of systemic illness

Evaluation of significance
All cases are significant
Most cases are fatal
Prognosis depends on degree of damage to valve and resultant valvular insufficiency
Identify arrhythmias which may affect treatment and prognosis
Early diagnosis and intensive treatment with appropriate antibiotic regime required to have
    any hope of successful treatment

Helpful diagnostic tests
Echocardiography
Plasma fibrinogen (usually very high)
Haematology (often a neutrophilia and left shift)
Blood culture and antibiotic sensitivity of isolates
ECG if arrhythmia present

incompetence. Echocardiographic examination is important not only to help to confirm the diagnosis, but also because it allows the degree of valvular damage and resultant volume overload to be assessed. If there is substantial volume overload associated with the damage to the valve structure, the long-term prognosis is poor even if a bacteriological cure is achieved.

Successful treatment depends on early diagnosis and treatment with appropriate antibiotics. High doses of bactericidal drugs, to which the organism is sensitive, are required for prolonged periods. Ideally the drug should also have good properties for penetration of the mass of fibrin which accumulates around an infected valve. Additional considerations are the potential side-effects of long-term antibiosis and the cost of treatment.

Initially, the agent involved and its drug sensitivity are seldom known. A wide variety of bacteria have been reported to cause endocarditis; no one species appears to be particularly prevalent. Treatment with broad-spectrum antibiotics is therefore indicated, while the results of culture and sensitivity tests on multiple blood culture samples are awaited. Two antibiotic regimes are widely used. Potentiated sulphonamide preparations should be used intravenously initially (15 mg/kg bid). Oral treatment at a dose of 15 mg/kg bid can be instituted once the initial systemic illness has resolved. Long-term use of potentiated sulphonamides has been associated with development of diarrhoea. Another option is to use a combination of penicillin and gentamycin. This must be administered parenterally, ideally four times daily initially, and is much more expensive. In addition, the potential nephrotoxicity of gentamycin should be considered if treatment is long-term. It is helpful to monitor plasma fibrinogen levels, which are a good guide to the presence of an inflammatory process. It is usually advisable to maintain antibiosis until fibrinogen levels have been normal for approximately two weeks. It is wise to repeat the fibrinogen assay periodically thereafter, to ensure that the infection has completely resolved.

Non-steroidal anti-inflammatory drugs (NSAIDs) have also been recommended as part of treatment. They may reduce the pyrexia and improve the horse's demeanour, and are particularly valuable in animals with gram-negative bacteraemias and endotoxaemia. In addition, NSAIDs may decrease further platelet aggregation on the vegetative lesion. Phenylbutazone or flunixine meglumine can be used, although low doses are advisable in the light of possible toxicity associated with long-term use, particularly if renal function is compromised.

6.7 Myocardial disease

Myocardial disease can affect cardiac function because the normal electrical activation processes are disturbed, or because of abnormal contraction or relaxation of cardiac muscle. The incidence of myocardial disease in the horse is a matter of some debate. Certainly, few animals develop myocardial failure without severe underlying valvular heart disease. However, lower grade disease leading to the development of arrhythmias or to sufficiently poor myocardial function to result in poor athletic performance may be more common than has been recognised previously. The use of echocardiography, in conjunction with exercise and 24-hour ECGs and clinical pathology where appropriate, may lead to an improvement in the understanding of myocardial disease in the horse.

The aetiology of myocardial disease in horses is poorly understood, although there are a number of situations in which myocardial disease may be identified. The most common is myocarditis which may occur in animals which have suffered from viral or bacterial respiratory infection. Myocardial fibrosis and/or necrosis have also been recorded. In addition, myocardial function may be affected by systemic disease such as septicaemia. Drugs, toxins and electrolyte disturbances may also result in arrhythmias and/or poor myocardial function. Idiopathic cardiomyopathy, which is common in other domestic species such as the dog and cat, is seldom recognised in the horse. This may be partly because of a failure to recognise the disease. However, the difficulty in making a specific, definitive diagnosis of myocardial disease may also lead to over-diagnosis of these conditions.

6.7.1 Diagnosis of myocardial disease

Clinical examination
The clinical signs associated with myocardial disease vary from sub-clinical to fatal. Myocardial disease is most often a consideration in horses presented for poor athletic performance, but it can be difficult to diagnose with any degree of certainty. In horses with CHF it is important to distinguish primary myocardial disease from valvular heart disease. Some animals with CHF due to myocardial disease will recover, and may, in some instances, return to athletic use, but the

prognosis is usually hopeless with CHF due to valvular heart disease. Myocardial failure may also occur secondary to severe valvular heart disease. In addition, horses with systemic disease may have myocardial dysfunction as a secondary complication. This is particularly common in foals with septicaemia, and in exhausted animals with profound electrolyte imbalance.

A thorough clinical examination is required in the evaluation of animals with suspected myocardial disease. Other causes of poor athletic performance may need to be investigated (see section 8.2). Examination of the cardiovascular system is performed along the lines previously described (Chapter 3). In animals with mild myocardial disease there may be no abnormal findings on clinical examination at rest. The disease may only be suspected after arrhythmias are detected during exercise. In other animals, arrhythmias at rest may be the only significant finding. This is most often the case with myocarditis. A raised pulse rate and poor pulse quality are common findings in animals with more severe myocardial disease. In cases in which there is a marked reduction in myocardial contractility, a weak apex beat and quiet heart sounds may be detected. Signs of CHF should also be noted if present. Abnormal heart murmurs should be classified and evaluated to determine whether they indicate the presence of primary valvular disease, and whether they alone are sufficient to account for the clinical signs. Animals with myocardial disease may develop cardiac murmurs, particularly MR, as a result of dilatation of the valve annulus. Further diagnostic tests are usually required to determine the primary problem.

Echocardiography
Echocardiography is a very important tool in the diagnosis of myocardial disease. It may allow a diagnosis to be made in those animals which have no abnormalities detected on clinical examination. In horses which have obvious clinical signs, it is a helpful guide to the severity of the disease and is a useful prognostic indicator. Echocardiography may also allow the clinician to determine whether the primary problem is valvular or myocardial.

The heart should be carefully examined for evidence of valvular and myocardial abnormalities. In myocardial fibrosis, a diffuse or localised increase in echogenicity of the myocardium may be noted. Care should be taken not to over-interpret artefactual changes in density which are very dependent on the gain settings and the angle of incidence of the ultrasound beam. The size of the cardiac chambers should be assessed.

Echocardiography is particularly useful for assessment of myocardial contractility. An impression of the effectiveness of myocardial contraction can be made from subjective assessment of the 2DE and M-mode image. A more quantitative method is to measure fractional shortening (FS%) of the LV from the M-mode image (see section 4.2.6). A marked reduction in contractility will result in a reduced FS%. A measurement of less than 26% can be regarded as abnormal (Figure 6.4). However, as with all echocardiographic measurements, this is a guideline rather than an absolute value and may be affected by measurement errors and the level of excitement of the animal. When there is dyskinesis of the ventricles, FS% may be of little value and a subjective assessment of contractility may be sufficient. Sedation affects FS% and should not be used in horses in which myocardial disease is suspected. In some animals, such as those

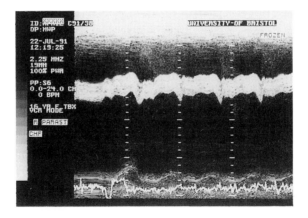

Fig. 6.4 M-mode trace showing poor myocardial contractility. The limited motion of the IVS and LV free-wall suggest poor myocardial contractility. The RV is also dilated.

with extensive myocardial fibrosis, diastolic dysfunction is the primary problem. This may be evident echocardiographically as a slow rate of filling and abnormal mitral valve motion on the M-mode trace (Figure 4.14), and may result in an increase in the relative size of the A wave compared with the E wave.

It is impossible to perform an echocardiographic investigation in the actively exercising horse; however, useful recordings can be made immediately after exercise. The examination is complicated by respiratory motion and is not easily performed. Animals with myocardial disease may show a reduction in FS% during this period which was not evident at rest. The consequences of other physiological changes which occur after exercise, such as the effects of dehydration and cutaneous vasodilatation for thermoregulation, need to be considered, but post-exercise echocardiograms may prove to be useful in selected cases.

Electrocardiography

Myocardial disease often causes arrhythmias. Detection of an abnormal arrhythmia may therefore indicate the presence of myocardial disease. Reduced athletic performance may result directly from the effect of the arrhythmia on ventricular filling and cardiac efficiency, or result from poor myocardial contractility.

ECGs recorded at rest may show arrhythmias which are likely to result in poor athletic performance, or other signs of heart disease. Ideally, echocardiography and clinical pathological tests should be performed if frequent atrial premature beats (APCs), ventricular premature beats (VPCs), atrial or ventricular tachycardia, or other abnormal rhythms are detected at rest. In many animals, the significance of arrhythmias detected at rest is unclear. It is helpful to assess their incidence during exercise in order to evaluate their likely effect on performance. ECGs recorded during exercise, either with the horse on a treadmill, or on the gallops if radiotelemetry is available, are therefore extremely useful in these cases. Some animals with poor athletic performance, but no evidence of cardiac disease at rest, will be shown to have significant arrhythmias during exercise which may explain the clinical signs. In other animals, arrhythmias such as APCs and VPCs, which were present at rest, may be abolished once the sinus rate is increased. 24-hour resting ECGs are also useful for assessment of the significance of arrhythmias detected intermittently at rest (Chapter 7).

In addition to identification of arrhythmias from the ECG, abnormalities in the morphology of the complexes and the intervals between them can result from myocardial damage. However, the changes are very non-specific and, because complexes may vary between different normal animals, these changes are difficult to interpret.

Clinical pathology

A variety of clinico-pathological tests are helpful in evaluating myocardial disease. Details of each test are described in Chapter 2.

Haematology is helpful in assessing the possibility of viral infection, but is not helpful in specifically identifying the presence or absence of myocardial disease. Both haematology, viral antibody titres and virus isolation may be helpful if a viral cause for myocarditis is suspected; however, the clinical pathological evidence for viral infection is most likely to be found in the active infection phase, and myocardial disease is seldom suspected or present until weeks or months later.

Abnormal electrolyte levels may be responsible for arrhythmias, and may be found following muscle damage. However, changes are seldom specific, and electrolyte measurements are of more help in ruling out other causes of arrhythmias than in evaluating the presence or absence of myocardial disease.

Isoenzymes of creatinine kinase (CPK) and lactate dehydrogenase (LDH) have been suggested as useful indicators of myocardial damage. However, a number of problems exist with the assays and in the author's opinion they should be interpreted with caution (see section 2.3).

6.7.2 Specific myocardial conditions

Myocarditis

Myocarditis is a poorly defined condition characterised by reduced myocardial contractility and arrhythmias. Clinical signs include exercise intolerance, dyspnoea and sometimes episodic collapse or CHF. Myocarditis may follow a recent history of fever, anorexia, depression and respiratory disease that apparently responded to treatment. Pre- and post-exercise echocardiography, resting, 24-hour and exercise ECGs, and possibly isoenzyme assays are worthwhile investigative procedures in animals with poor exercise tolerance following a bout of respiratory disease. However, it is important that all body systems are examined thoroughly. Long-term respiratory dysfunction resulting in poor gaseous exchange is a much more common sequel to respiratory disease and may result in similar clinical signs.

Myocardial fibrosis

Myocardial fibrosis is thought to caused by ischaemia resulting from emboli, such as fibrin from vascular intima damaged by strongyles. These areas could act as ectopic foci and can be responsible for arrhythmias, but are more commonly seen as incidental findings at PM. More widespread fibrosis may follow myocardial necrosis.

Myocardial degeneration/necrosis

Conditions causing myocardial degeneration or necrosis are very uncommon. However, they have been reported to occur in outbreaks and may therefore have profound economic implications. The clinical significance of the conditions in an individual animal vary from sudden death to subclinical disease. The mechanisms of the diseases are poorly understood. The most well-known condition resulting in myocardial degeneration and necrosis is ingestion of ionophore antibiotics, such as monensin or salinomycin.

Monensin toxicity

This drug is used as a growth promoter in cattle feed and as a coccidiostat in poultry feed, but it is highly toxic to horses. A number of outbreaks of monensin poisoning associated with the accidental feeding of cattle feed to horses or contamination of horse feed at a feed mill have been reported in recent years. Monensin causes acute cellular necrosis, leading to fibrosis. In addition, hepatic, renal and skeletal muscle necrosis may result. When monensin toxicity is suspected, specialist analysis of the feed is required.

Clinical signs   Clinical signs of monensin toxicity can vary from sudden death due to per-acute hypovolaemic shock, to mild inappetance. Anorexia, ataxia, sweating, increased urination, jugular pulses, tachycardia and dysrhythmias have been documented. CHF is a common feature. In some horses, the clinical signs may be delayed for weeks before the myocardial damage leads to the development of dysrhythmias. In animals which have been exposed to low doses, exercise intolerance may be the only abnormality observed.

Prognosis   Echocardiography may show LV volume overload, and regional dyskinesis is common. Monitoring progress with ultrasound appears to be the best prognostic indicator. The outcome is largely dependent on the dose ingested. Some horses with mild disease may recover and return to normal athletic performance.

Treatment   There is no specific treatment. Fluid therapy is indicated in the acute case; supportive treatment and strict rest is helpful. Vitamin E may have a cardio-protective effect because it scavenges free radicals produced by cellular necrosis and may be helpful in the treatment of monensin toxicity. Digoxin is contraindicated because it exacerbates the effect of monensin on ionic transport at the cellular level.

Nutritional causes of myocardial disease

Rarely, vitamin E and selenium deficiency can lead to myocardial degeneration in horses. This is very unlikely to be a problem in the UK, except in the most bizarre diets, and would most commonly be found in foals whose dams are malnourished. The condition has been reported in other parts of the world where local soil conditions result in a mineral inbalance. It is usually seen in association with skeletal muscle weakness.

Vitamin D toxicity due to over supplementation has been reported to produce a myopathy leading to valvular insufficiencies, in addition to tachycardia, anorexia, weight loss, polyuria and polydipsia, and muscular stiffness. In some parts of the world, ingestion of toxic plants can result in hypervitaminosis D. Treatment involves removal of the offending feed and fluid therapy. The prognosis is dependent on the degree of irreversible renal and cardiac damage, but recovery has been reported.

Idiopathic cardiomyopathy

Cardiomyopathy can be described as idiopathic if no other predisposing factor, such as viral infection, can be found. It is rare in the horse compared with small animals. However, it may be more common than has been thought; with the increasing use of echocardiography it may become a more common diagnosis. Cardiomyopathy should be considered in cases where murmurs and CHF develop fairly acutely and there are no signs of obvious valvular disease. Arrhythmias are frequently found in other species with cardiomyopathy and are likely to be common in horses with the condition also. Diagnosis is made on echocardiographic findings of poor myocardial contractility. Supportive treatment involves the use of diuretics, such as frusemide, and positive inotropes, such as digoxin. However, the prognosis is likely to be poor.

6.7.3 Treatment of myocardial disease

There are limited options for treatment of myocardial disease. Most of these are palliative rather than aimed at correcting the underlying disease.

Rest

The most important treatment for myocardial disease is rest. Animals which show more severe clinical signs should be box rested, but pasture rest is sufficient in most cases. A rest period of two months prior to re-evaluation is a guide in most cases.

Other treatments

A number of treatments have been used in myocardial disease, most of which are largely empirical. Corticosteroids have been used, and appear to reduce the incidence or severity of arrhythmias in some cases of post-viral myocarditis. There is always a risk of inducing a recrudescence of the viral disease, but a gradually reducing dose of corticosteroid may be appropriate. There is little rationale for the use of antibiotics in myocardial disease. Vitamin E and selenium supplements have been used with apparent success, but rest may have been a more significant part of treatment. Digoxin and frusemide are indicated in animals with CHF and may allow time for the animal to recover. Some animals have recovered from severe myocardial disease and returned to previous racing form. However, the prognosis for animals with CHF and volume overload resulting from myocardial disease is usually poor. Anti-arrhythmic drugs such as quinidine may be helpful in some instances in which arrhythmias are life-threatening.

Vasodilators may be beneficial, although little is known about the pharmacology of these drugs in the horse and they would be extremely expensive.

As a general rule, rest alone should be the first line of treatment except in cases where the myocardial disease is life-threatening, or there is great pressure to return the animal to work as soon as possible.

Clinical features of myocardial disease are summarised in Table 6.6.

Table 6.6 Summary: Clinical evaluation of horses with myocardial disease

Equine myocardial disease is poorly understood

History
Uncommon
Variable signs noted by owners depending on the severity of the condition:
  sub-clinical
  poor exercise tolerance
  left- and/or right-sided congestive heart failure
  sudden death (rare?)
Usually associated with recent viral respiratory infection (myocarditis)
May be a problem in a group of animals if associated with toxic origin

Clinical findings
Arrhythmias
Apex beat may be weak
Murmurs may or may not be present
Heart sounds quiet in some cases
Left- or right-sided congestive heart failure

Evaluation of significance
Most likely to be significant if:
  associated with poor athletic performance
  slow CRT
  weak or variable pulse quality
  resting heart rate > 45 bpm
  murmurs present of grade 3–4/6 or greater
  associated with abnormal arrhythmias, e.g. APCs, VPCs, AF
  associated with signs of left- or right-sided congestive heart failure

Helpful diagnostic tests
Echocardiography (pre- and in some cases post-exercise)
Electrocardiography (resting, 24-hour, exercising)
? CPK MB fraction isoenzymes
?? LDH isoenzyme 2 fraction
Serial viral titres and haematological evaluation

6.8 Pericardial disease

Congenital pericardial disease is exceptionally rare in horses. Acquired pericardial disease is a very uncommon problem in this species, but is an important cause of cardiac disease because it can be difficult to diagnose and treat. It can be a life-threatening condition, although in some cases it may be asymptomatic. The more widespread use of echocardiography may result in the identification of pericardial disease when it would previously have gone unrecognised.

Pericardial disease usually results from inflammation of the pericardial sac around the heart, i.e. pericarditis. The condition is divided into two forms, effusive and constrictive. In effusive pericarditis, a transudate, modified transudate, exudate or blood fill the pericardium and may compress the low-pressure right side of the heart, leading to poor venous return (tamponade). In constrictive pericarditis, the pericardium loses its elasticity and restricts filling of the ventricles. In practice, the two conditions may be present in the same animal to varying degrees.

6.8.1   *Pericardial effusions*

Aetiology
Pericarditis can be bacterial in origin, but most commonly it is idiopathic. It is sometimes found in association with an infectious disease such as viral respiratory infections. Traumatic pericarditis resulting from penetrating wounds has also been recorded. Neoplastic causes are very rare. Pericarditis appears to be much less common in the UK than in the USA. This may be because pericarditis is sometimes associated with pleuro-pneumonia, which is more common in animals transported long distances overland between two climatic extremes.

Effusive pericarditis results in right-sided CHF when the pressure within the pericardium rises so that it exceeds that within the heart, restricting diastolic filling of the cardiac chambers. The low-pressure RA is the first chamber to collapse under the pressure of the intra-pericardial fluid. This limits venous return. The increase in filling pressure leads to venous congestion and the limited preload means that cardiac output cannot be raised to meet any increased demands. The greater the pressure within the pericardium, the higher the pressure required to fill the RA and ventricle. The rate at which the effusion develops also affects the severity of the condition, because the pericardium can stretch to accommodate larger volumes of fluid if it accumulates slowly. If an acute effusive episode occurs, the fibrous sac will have little time to dilate and intra-pericardial pressure will be high.

Clinical signs
A spectrum of clinical signs may be attributable to a pericardial effusion, depending on the quantity of fluid, the rate of accumulation and the aetiology of the condition. Pericarditis may go unrecognised or may result in relatively minor clinical signs if the volume of the effusion is small. In the athletic horse, a reduction in performance may be noted. In more severe cases, clinical signs of right-sided CHF are evident, indicating cardiac tamponade. In other animals, signs of systemic disease such as fever, anorexia, weight loss, dyspnoea, tachypnoea and tachycardia are seen. Horses with a pericardial effusion may appear to be in pain and discomfort.

Diagnosis

Clinical examination   If the pericardium is inflamed and only a small quantity of pericardial fluid is present, a pericardial friction rub may be heard on auscultation. This is a harsh sound which may be confused for a murmur. It is usually triphasic, in time with atrial systole, ventricular systole and ventricular diastole. Occasionally one or more of these sounds will be absent; however, the sound can be distinguished from a pleural rub because it is in time with the cardiac cycle. The sound of a pericardial friction rub is similar to that of a creaking branch or door. Heart sounds are muffled if a significant effusion is present and the friction rub may be lost. If anaerobic bacteria are present, gas formed by these organisms may result in splashing sounds being heard, although this is unusual.

Further diagnostic aids

Electrocardiography   Small complexes and electrical alternans (variable size complexes which are alternately large and small) may be seen on an ECG, although these findings are not specific for a pericardial effusion.

Echocardiography   The technique of choice for diagnosis of pericardial disease is echocardiography. The effusion may be sufficiently clear to be seen with linear-array transducers or sector scanners of up to 5 MHz. The main echo-cardiographic feature is the presence of an anechoic space (fluid) between the echogenic pericardium and the myocardium (Figure 4.29). In some animals with septic pericarditis, fibrin tags forming echogenic fronds within the fluid, or thickening of the pericardial or epicardial surface will be seen. Pleural fluid may also be present, either as a result of right-sided CHF or due to the effects of systemic disease which also involves the pleura. It is important that pleural fluid is not confused with fluid within the pericardium.

The volume of pericardial fluid and its effect on cardiac function should be assessed; this will dictate whether immediate drainage is required. If cardiac tamponade is present, the RA will be seen to collapse during diastole. If the condition is more severe, restriction of RV filling may be observed. An M-mode image is useful to identify paradoxical septal motion, which occurs when RV pressure is high. The heart may be seen to swing from side to side in the fluid and this may make septal motion appear unusual.

Radiography   Radiography may be a helpful diagnostic technique in animals with large pericardial effusions if equipment of a suitable output is available. A globular or pumpkin-shaped cardiac outline may be seen. A gas cap may be present if anaerobic organisms are involved.

Clinical pathology   Clinical pathological tests are useful in animals which show signs of systemic disease. A plasma fibrinogen assay and haematology should be performed to investigate the likelihood of active inflammation of the pericardium. Cytological, biochemical and bacteriological examinations of pericardial fluid are indicated if pericardiocentesis is performed (see below).

Treatment
Effusive pericarditis which results in cardiac tamponade is a life-threatening condition which requires immediate, aggressive treatment. Pericarditis may also occur without compromising venous return, in which case the need for treatment

depends on whether there are systemic signs of infectious disease. It is essential that the horse receives box rest during the course of treatment and convalescence. Although pericardial effusions carry a relatively poor prognosis, recent reports show that treatment can be rewarding, with a successful long-term outcome.

Where pericarditis is suspected, echocardiographic examination is invaluable in order to identify the severity of the condition. It is important to identify fibrin tags or echogenic particles within the pericardial fluid which may suggest that an inflammatory or infectious process is occurring. In anaerobic infections, very echogenic particles may be seen indicating the presence of gas-forming organisms, and suitable antibiotics (e.g. metronidazole) must be used (ideally based on the results of bacterial culture and antibiotic sensitivity tests). The cause of the effusion may also be determined from cytological examination of pericardial fluid. Thus for both accurate diagnosis and treatment, placement of a catheter into the pericardium is desirable. However, many horses with CHF, or effusions in other body cavities, have a small amount of pericardial fluid which may be seen echocardiographically but which does not result in tamponade. In these instances, drainage is unwarranted and should be avoided.

Drainage/sampling technique   The optimal site for pericardiocentesis can be selected from echocardiographic examination. Alternatively, an area over the left or right fifth intercostal space between the level of the costo–chondral junctions and the shoulder can be selected. The region should be aseptically prepared. A bleb of local anaesthetic is placed under the skin and is infiltrated into the underlying muscle. The skin can be moved slightly so that the puncture site does not directly overlie the muscular puncture site. A stab incision can be made with a No.11 scalpel blade. A $3\frac{1}{2}$ in or longer 10–12 gauge catheter or a chest drain is advanced into the chest until a slight 'pop' is felt and fluid is aspirated. If a large-bore catheter is used for the puncture, a longer, finer catheter such as a dog urinary catheter can be advanced through it and left in place. If a pleural effusion is also present it may be difficult to distinguish whether the fluid has been aspirated from the pleural or pericardial space. Echocardiographic guidance is particularly helpful in this situation.

An indwelling drain can be left in place, secured with a purse string suture, if drainage or lavage and infusion of drugs is required. Isotonic fluids can be used for lavage. Flushing of the pericardial space with one litre of isotonic fluid, followed by instillation of drugs in a similar volume, has been reported to be successful.

Drainage of pericardial fluid is not without risk. The most worrying complications are laceration of major thoracic or coronary vessels and resultant haemorrhage, or induction of ventricular arrhythmias. The equine epicardium is reported to be particularly sensitive to stimulation. VPCs are not uncommon and could precipitate ventricular fibrillation. An ECG should therefore be recorded during the procedure so that arrhythmias can be recognised early and treatment given if necessary. It is advisable to have lignocaine or quinidine gluconate on hand for treatment of arrhythmias; however, the arrhythmia will usually resolve when the catheter is withdrawn. An indwelling intravenous catheter should be placed prior to the procedure to allow rapid administration of drugs if necessary.

Long-term complications of the condition and of pericardiocentesis include constrictive pericarditis.

Drug treatment   Bacterial pericarditis should be treated with systemic antibiotics but, in addition, broad spectrum antibiotics such as a combination of penicillin and gentamycin, can be infused into the pericardial sac two to four times daily. Idiopathic pericarditis carries a better prognosis than bacterial pericarditis. Animals with idiopathic effusions have been treated with corticosteroids, systemically and by local infusion, with success (see Appendix). Corticosteroids are only advisable if an infectious cause has been ruled out and the fluid collects repeatedly following drainage.

Non-steroidal anti-inflammatory drugs such as flunixine meglumine may also be useful in pericardial disease as analgesic and anti-inflammatory agents. If CHF is present, drainage of the effusion is the only suitable form of treatment. Diuresis is unlikely to result in any significant improvement of clinical signs. Vasodilators are contraindicated. Digoxin will have no beneficial effect and should not be used unless atrial tachycardia is present.

6.8.2   Constrictive pericarditis

Constrictive pericarditis may develop following resolution of effusive pericarditis as a result of an inflammatory response to the accumulation of fluid, or may occur without a known previous effusive episode. Frequently the epicardium is also involved, resulting in a limitation of diastolic filling. Constrictive pericarditis can be more difficult to recognise on clinical grounds than a pericardial effusion because there may be no abnormal auscultatory findings. However, clinical signs are very similar to those in effusive pericarditis. If constrictive pericarditis is suspected, echocardiography is very useful to confirm the diagnosis. A thick, echogenic pericardium is seen and in some cases tamponade is present despite there being a relatively small volume of effusion. Diastolic filling and wall motion may halt abruptly when the elastic limit of the pericardium is reached. Steroid treatment may be worthwhile, but the prognosis is grave.

Clinical features of pericardial disease are summarised in Table 6.7.

6.9   Treatment of congestive heart failure in horses

The prognosis for horses with congestive heart failure (CHF) is poor. They very seldom recover to a point where they are able to perform useful work except when the CHF is due to an arrhythmia, pericardial disease or in some cases, myocardial disease. Where, much more commonly, valvular heart disease is the underlying cause, treatment is at best short-term and palliative. However, long-term treatment may be justified if the horse has great sentimental or breeding value. Thus, in selected individuals, it may be valid to control the clinical signs using drugs.

The principal categories of drugs used to control signs of CHF in small animals and humans are diuretics, positive inotropes, and vasodilators. However, the choice of these drugs for the equine clinician is very limited. To appreciate the

Table 6.7 Summary: Clinical evaluation of horses with pericardial disease

History
Variable signs noted by owners depending on the severity of the condition:
  sub-clinical
  poor exercise tolerance
  associated with systemic illness or thoracic disease, e.g. pleuro-pneumonia
  right-sided congestive heart failure
Sudden onset or progressive over days

Clinical findings
Mucous membrane colour usually normal
CRT normal to slow
Arterial pulse normal to weak, apex beat may be weak
Pulse rate normal to rapid
+/– juguar distension
+/– quiet heart sounds
Weakness, lethargy

Evaluation of significance
Most likely to be significant if:
  associated with poor athletic performance
  slow CRT
  heart rate > 45 bpm
  associated with signs of right-sided congestive heart failure
  associated with other diseases such as pleuro-pneumonia
  bacterial, traumatic or neoplastic aetiology

Helpful diagnostic tests
Echocardiography
Electrocardiography
Clinical pathology, especially examination of perciardial fluid

rationale of the use of these drugs it is important to understand the pathophysiology of CHF (Chapter 2). Horses with CHF should be rested. Box rest with some daily walking in hand is ideal.

6.9.1 Diuretics

Diuretics alleviate the congestive signs seen in heart failure by reducing preload. They may also improve oxygenation of peripheral tissues by removing excess interstitial fluid. A reduction in preload reduces the hydrostatic pressure which is driving fluid out into the extracellular spaces, reducing oedema. It also reduces the dilutional effects of excessive water retention which is found in animals with CHF. This benefits the animal because the main clinical signs of CHF are due to oedema formation. Diuretics can be life-saving in animals with acute pulmonary oedema and dyspnoea as a result of flooding of alveoli (left-sided CHF). They are less effective in reducing oedema which has formed through the effects of increased hydrostatic pressure in the systemic capillaries (right-sided CHF).

A significant side-effect of reducing preload by the use of diuretics is that, if the fall in preload exceeds compensatory mechanisms, cardiac output can be decreased. Preload reserve is lost in CHF and as a result of diuresis, so a delicate balance must be struck. Box rest ensures that demands for increased cardiac output are kept to a minimum.

The choice of diuretics which are suitable for use is the horse is limited. Frusemide is the only diuretic which has been widely used and there seems little to be gained by trying other drugs. The dosage can be varied according to individual requirements (see Appendix). Intravenous use is required to relieve acute pulmonary oedema; intramuscular and oral preparations can be used for maintenance.

6.9.2 Positive inotropes

Digoxin was the only positive inotrope used in long-term management of cardiac disease in humans and small animals for many years. Recently, new positive inotropes have been developed, although none have been as successful as was hoped. The long-term use of positive inotropes in humans and small animals is controversial, because there is little evidence that they increase longevity or quality of life. Their use in primary valvular disease is particularly controversial; many cardiologists believe that they are of no value in these conditions. There is no role for the use of digoxin in management of cardiac disease in the horse except when there is evidence of CHF or if a supraventricular tachycardia is present and requires treatment (see Appendix).

The pharmacology of digoxin in the horse is poorly understood and may be quite variable in animals with heart disease. Side-effects include inappetance and diarrhoea. The drug can actually increase the frequency of arrhythmias, particularly ventricular arrhythmias. It must therefore be used with great care and only when absolutely necessary. There is a narrow margin between the therapeutic and toxic ranges. Blood digoxin assays can therefore be useful to monitor treatment. The therapeutic range is thought to be 1.0–2.0 µg/l. Other factors may also affect the pharmacology of the drug. Because of interactions, the dose should be reduced by approximately 50% when used in conjunction with quinidine. Digoxin is cleared from the body by the kidney and should therefore be used at a reduced rate in horses with renal failure.

Dopamine and dobutamine are catecholamines which increase myocardial contractility. This may be helpful in selected animals with low output heart failure. They must be used as an intravenous infusion (see Appendix). Unfortunately, both drugs also result in selective vasoconstriction. This may increase blood pressure, but it also increases afterload and therefore raises myocardial oxygen consumption. Dobutamine is potentially arrhythmogenic and should not be used in the presence of ventricular arrhythmias.

6.9.3 Vasodilators

Vasodilators are now an important part of the treatment of heart disease, including CHF, in humans and small animals. They act by reducing afterload and preload. A variety of drugs are available which affect arterial or venous tone to differing degrees. Vasodilators can reduce the work of the heart and allow an increase in cardiac output and muscle perfusion, which may reduce signs of weakness. Angiotensin converting enzyme (ACE) inhibitors also reduce sodium and water retention. There is some evidence that ACE inhibitors improve both longevity and quality of life in humans and small animal patients with valvular and/or myocardial disease.

Unfortunately, there are very limited pharmacological data on vasodilators in horses. Drugs which could be used include arteriolar vasodilators such as hydralazine; mixed arteriolar and venodilators including acepromazine and ACE inhibitors (e.g. captopril and enalapril), and venodilators such as nitroprusside and nitroglycerine. Prolonged treatment would be very expensive in adult horses. Enalapril (an ACE inhibitor) has recently been licensed for use in dogs in the UK and, although it would be very expensive if it was used at the same dose, might find some use in horses, particularly if pharmacological studies were performed.

Without the benefit of experience of the action of these drugs in a substantial number of animals, treatment is fraught with potential danger. All these drugs are potentially hypotensive and need to be titrated in order that they have beneficial effects without precipitating profound hypotension. However, there could be circumstances in which, with informed owner consent, their use could be justified. Doses are empirical (see Appendix).

6.10 Peripheral cardiovascular disease and conditions affecting the great vessels

6.10.1 Rupture of the aortic root

Rupture of the aortic root is a rare condition which is reported most frequently in aged stallions. It is thought to result from necrosis and degeneration of connective tissue in the aortic wall. Blood penetrates the myocardium surrounding the base of the aorta 'dissecting' the tissue. Usually the dissection runs into the basal part of the IVS from the right coronary sinus. Animals may die suddenly or may present with acute cardiac decompensation. Distress and signs of pain can be seen. A sinus tachycardia is likely to be present, although junctional or ventricular tachycardias have been reported with dissection of IVS. These arrhythmias may be life threatening and may require immediate treatment (see section 7.8.9).

Diagnosis

Diagnosis of a rupture of the aortic root is made on echocardiographic examination or at PM. On echocardiography, an area of hypoechogenicity may be seen in the IVS if the dissection has taken this route. The area around the aortic root may appear abnormal; however, changes may not be very dramatic. Frequently other abnormalities such as aortic valve disease or MV disease may be present and murmurs associated with these conditions may be noted on clinical examination.

Prognosis

The prognosis for animal with a rupture of the aortic root is very poor and, although they may recover from the initial period of distress and tachycardia, a recurrence of signs or sudden death are likely at a later date.

6.10.2 Sinus of Valsalva aneurysm

An aneurysm of the sinus of Valsalva is an uncommon condition which may be found in association with a murmur of aortic regurgitation or may be identified incidentally on echocardiography or PM. The aetiology of the aneurysm is unclear. Usually the right coronary sinus is involved and, on echocardiography, this may appear as a defect in the junction between the aortic root at the base of the IVS and the junction of the RV and RA. This may at first resemble a VSD; however, the defect is more dorsally situated and there is no flow through it unless rupture has occurred.

The lesion is a very significant finding because it is possible that the aneurysm may rupture at any time, usually resulting in sudden death. Horses with this condition should be regarded as unsafe to ride for this reason.

6.10.3 Rupture of the pulmonary artery

Rupture of the PA is an event which usually results in sudden death and may occur in animals with pulmonary hypertension. Usually the degree of pulmonary hypertension required to result in rupture is caused by severe left-sided cardiac disease. Animals with severe MR are most at risk.

Clinical signs
No clinical signs may be attributed to the dilation of the PA which precedes rupture; however, clinical evidence of the primary disease is likely to be present. However, the PA can be dangerously dilated in some horses in which cardiac disease has not been recognised by the owners. Usually animals will be showing signs of CHF such as dependent oedema, but this may not be evident in all animals in which the artery is dilated.

Diagnosis
Diagnosis of rupture of the PA is usually made at PM, although it may be missed because the condition does not figure prominently in the literature. Occasionally animals will survive long enough to be presented for echocardiographic examination, in which case, flailing of the pulmonary valve and dissection of blood into the surrounding tissue may be seen. Prior to rupture, dilation of the PA will be seen on echocardiography. Although measurement of the PA diameter cannot be made with absolute precision, adult Thoroughbred horses with PA diameters >8 cm at the valve base should be considered to be at risk of rupture if accompanying signs of severe left-sided heart disease are present. In general terms the PA diameter should not exceed the aortic diameter.

Owners of animals with moderate to severe MR should be encouraged to present them for periodic repeat echocardiographic examinations (approximately every 3–12 months), so that signs of dilation of the artery can be detected before the risk of rupture becomes too great to allow the animal to be ridden.

Prognosis
The prognosis for animals with dilated pulmonary arteries is poor and they are unsafe to ride. The prognosis for animals with a rupture of the artery which has

not resulted in sudden death is hopeless and euthanasia is the only course of action.

6.10.4 *Jugular vein thrombosis*

Occlusion or partial occlusion of the jugular vein by a thrombus is a relatively common complication of long-term catheterisation (> 24 hours). Usually the thrombus is small and does not present a clinical problem other than complicating the administration of intravenous fluids or drugs. However, in some cases the situation becomes more serious. The vein may become inflamed (thrombophlebitis) or even infected. This may occur following intravenous injection of irritant drugs, poor aseptic technique, or simply due to the presence of foreign material such as a catheter. It is most commonly a problem in animals recovering from colic surgery and in those with septicaemia, endotoxaemia or bacteraemias (particularly salmonellosis). This is because these animals are frequently in a hypercoagulable state and are usually catheterised for prolonged periods. In severe cases, the condition can be life threatening and complications such as pulmonary thrombo-embolism and endocarditis can occur. Long-term scarring of the vein may result in reduced venous return, although recanalisation usually results in resolution and a collateral circulation may develop over time.

Clinical signs

Palpation of the affected vein reveals a firm cylindrical mass within the lumen. Distension of the vein above the thrombus will be present to varying degrees depending on how much of the lumen is occluded. Oedema and venous distension of the head may be visible if the vein is severely occluded, particularly if both left and right jugular veins are affected. Swelling can become marked and is usually worse after exercise. Athletic performance can be reduced due to pressure on the pharynx. Pain, heat and swelling around the site may be present with thrombophlebitis; if the site is infected a discharge may break out at the skin surface.

Diagnosis

Diagnosis can be made on clinical grounds. In addition, ultrasonography is a valuable technique which allows the clinician to detect the build up of thrombus within the lumen before it becomes clinically apparent. It will show a moderately echogenic mass within anechoic blood filling the vein and allows the size of the thrombus to be measured. Slow flowing blood may appear to contain echogenic particles similar to the smoke occasionally seen in the heart (see section 4.2.6). Pockets of fluid may be seen within the thrombus and hyperechoic areas suggestive of gas may be found in thrombi which are infected. Recanalisation may become visible as the thrombus matures and the condition resolves.

Haematology and plasma fibrinogen analysis are useful aids if infection is considered possible, but interpretation is frequently complicated by the primary problem for which the animal was under treatment.

Treatment

If a substantial thrombus is detected, indwelling catheters should be removed. Further catheterisation or intravenous injections in the affected vein should be avoided if possible. However, if the thrombosis is small and uninfected, it may be better to place catheters in the same vein lower down rather than risk losing both jugular veins. Alternative sites should be used if possible for taking blood sample or administering intravenous injections. The lateral thoracic, cephalic and saphenous veins are suitable. If sepsis is suspected, the contents of catheters should be submitted for bacteriological culture and isolates should be tested for antibiotic sensitivity. Broad spectrum antibiotic treatment is indicated until the results are available. Local poulticing may help to bring an abscess to a head. NSAIDs may reduce the inflammatory response and prevent further aggregation of thrombus.

Most cases of jugular thrombosis resolve without complication. However, the prognosis is not so good if marked thrombophlebitis is present, or if infection develops. Long-term antibiosis may be required for infected thrombi. In intractable, severe cases, surgical resection of the affected vein is required.

6.10.5 Aorto–iliac thrombosis

Thrombosis of the terminal section of the aorta, internal iliac arteries, external iliac arteries, or combinations of these vessels, has been reported to result in an ischaemic myopathy of the hind limbs. The aetiology of the condition is unclear, although it may be associated with larval *Strongylus vulgaris* migration.

Clinical signs

One or both hind limbs may be affected, depending on the extent of the occlusion of the vessel(s) by thrombus. The typical history is of a hind-limb lameness which is induced or exacerbated by exercise. The condition is usually insidious in onset. Clinical examination may reveal a weak greater metatarsal arterial pulse and slow filling of the saphenous vein. These signs may be more marked following exercise. Tachypnoea and sweating may be observed during exercise, possibly due to pain.

Diagnosis

Rectal examination is usually diagnostic. Thrombus may be palpated in any of the arteries at the terminal aorta, although they are most commonly recognised in the terminal aorta itself. The pulse quality may be reduced. A thorough examination of the aorta and both branches of the iliac arteries on the left and right side is required.

A more definitive method of diagnosis is ultrasonography of the affected vessel. This has been diagnostic in some cases where clinical examination did not pinpoint the source of the lameness. A 5 or 7.5 MHz linear array real-time scanner is recommended, although some sector scanners are suitable for examinations per rectum. A mass of variable heterogeneous echogenicity may be seen on either the dorsal or ventral wall of the aorta, or in its branches (Figure 6.5). The degree of occlusion can be estimated.

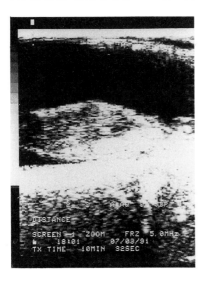

Fig. 6.5 Aorta–iliac thrombosis.
An oval mass of heterogeneous echogenicity is visible on the ventral surface of the artery, which is otherwise filled with hypoechoic blood. (Courtesy of Dr Alistair Barr)

Treatment
Treatment consists of box rest, NSAIDs such as phenylbutazone, and larvicidal doses of anthelmintics such as ivermectin. Resolution of the thrombus may occur in some cases, however the outcome is seldom favourable. Ultrasound is a useful method of assessing progress.

Chapter 7

Cardiac Arrhythmias

Disturbances of cardiac rhythm are called arrhythmias or dysrhythmias. The term arrhythmia means a lack of rhythm, while a dysrhythmia is a disorder of rhythm. However, in practice they are often used synonymously. In the normal heart, rhythm is dependant on the discharge of the sinus node and is therefore known as sinus rhythm. In normal horses, disturbances from sinus rhythm are common due to high parasympathetic (vagal) tone. However, other arrhythmias may be associated with pathological processes such as myocardial disease, electrolyte imbalance, or toxaemia. Some arrhythmias have no identifiable cause.

Even if arrhythmias are associated with pathological change, they may not be sufficiently severe to result in clinical signs. However, they can reduce cardiac output directly, or they can be symptomatic of cardiac disease which itself is affecting cardiac function. A normal cardiac rhythm ensures that the filling and contraction of the heart is co-ordinated. An irregularity may reduce stroke volume by reducing the time available for ventricular filling during a short diastolic interval. In addition, cardiac arrhythmias may affect overall heart rate. In normal animals, the ability to alter heart rate is essential to maintain blood pressure at rest and to allow animals to respond to increased demands, for example during exercise. An abnormally high rate may prevent complete ventricular filling, so that stroke volume falls, in turn reducing cardiac output. An abnormally slow heart rate may reduce cardiac output sufficiently for clinical signs to be apparent. Usually this will be mediated by a drop in blood pressure, so the clinical signs seen are those of weakness or syncope, but it is very uncommon in horses.

7.1 Clinical examination of horses with arrhythmias

Clinical examination of horses with arrhythmias may reveal a number of different findings depending on the type of arrhythmia and its severity and the presence or absence of underlying heart disease. Arrhythmias may be continuous or intermittent; some are present only at rest, or during or after exercise. Presenting signs vary from poor athletic performance to congestive heart failure, syncope, collapse and sudden death, or the arrhythmia may be an incidental finding. The arterial pulse may be normal, rapid or slow in rate; normal, weak or strong in quality; regular or irregular. A pulse deficit occurs when the stroke volume of a contraction is too small to produce a palpable change in arterial pressure and when ventricular contraction takes place, systolic sounds are heard, but a weak or absent pulse is palpated. The heart sounds may be abnormally loud, quiet or absent. Auscultation is particularly useful for rhythm analysis in the horse compared with small animals and humans because the sound associated with atrial contraction (S4 or *A* sound) can be heard in most normal animals. It is therefore possible to identify whether atrial depolarisation has occurred. During auscultation, some time should be spent specifically assessing cardiac rhythm before concentrating on murmurs. However, some arrhythmias can only be detected electrocardiographically.

7.2 Identification of arrhythmias

When an arrhythmia is suspected from clinical examination or historical findings, it is helpful to document the rhythm disturbance using an ECG. In certain situations it may be important to record the ECG over a prolonged period with a Holter monitor, or to examine the effect of exercise on rhythm using radio-telemetry. These techniques of recording ECGs and the principles of interpretation of the ECG were described in section 4.1.

In order to assess the significance of an arrhythmia, a specific diagnosis must be made. The important steps when an abnormal rhythm is detected are to:

(1) Classify the arrhythmia. This requires a good knowledge of the normal anatomy and electrophysiology of the heart (see section 1.5), a clear ECG recording and a logical approach to the interpretation of the ECG (see section 4.1.4).
(2) Identify underlying cardiac or systemic disease.
(3) Direct management and treatment of the horse, if it is appropriate.

The clinical approach to horses with arrhythmia is shown in Table 7.1, and a summary of the main features of each arrhythmia is shown in Table 7.2.

7.3 Classification of arrhythmias

Rhythm disturbances can be classified according to:

(1) *Rate:* The normal range of heart rate in a quiet, relaxed horse, at rest is 24–40 bpm. Dysrhythmias may be faster than normal (tachydysrhythmias), or slower than normal (bradydysrhythmias). Bradydysrhythmias may result in clinical signs such as weakness or syncope when they result in an abnormally low cardiac output, but they seldom cause signs of congestive heart failure (CHF). Tachydysrhythmias are often due to severe cardiac disease and may result in, or be associated with, signs of CHF. Measurement of the heart rate and assessment of rhythm, are important parts of the interpretation of an ECG (see section 4.1.4).
(2) *Origin and conduction:* Dysrhythmias are further defined as supraventricular (originating from the SA node, atria, or AV node and junctional

Table 7.1 Summary: The clinical approach to horses with arrhythmias

Identify the arrhythmia by:
1. Careful auscultation to identify the regularity of heart sounds and heart sound intensity. Identify the A sound if possible
2. Simultaneous palpation of arterial pulse and auscultation of heart sounds
3. Resting ECG
4. Exercising ECG such as radiotelemetry
5. Identifying how often the arrhythmia is occurring (persistent or intermittent)
6. Establishing whether the arrhythmia is induced or abolished by changes in heart rate, vagal manoeuvres, excitement or exercise

Evaluate the clinical status of the patient:
1. Can the signs be attributed to the arrhythmia?
2. Is the animal sufficiently compromised that it requires urgent treatment?
3. Is there any evidence of underlying cardiac or systemic disease (clinical examination, echocardiography, clinical pathology, known side-effects of drugs)?

Treatment of the arrhythmia
1. What, if any, treatment is required?
2. What are the possible side-effects of the drug, what is its cost?
3. How does the pharmacology of the drug dictate its use?

tissues) or ventricular in origin. The origin of an arrhythmia can usually be determined by careful interpretation of the waveforms and their relationships on the ECG. The origin of the arrhythmia makes up the essential part of the terminology of arrhythmias.

(3) *Timing:* When isolated, abnormal depolarisations are seen, they can be determined to be premature (they occur before the normal timing for the P wave or QRS complex) or escape complexes (they occur late, to rescue the ventricles from asystole).

(4) *Frequency:* Abnormal complexes may occur as intermittent single complexes, in groups, or may be persistent.

(5) *Cause:* Arrhythmias can be roughly divided into physiological or pathological types. Physiological arrhythmias may result from alterations in autonomic tone. Pathological arrhythmias may be related to abnormalities such as valvular or myocardial disease, or electrolyte disturbances. In addition, arrhythmias are often categorised as being caused by abnormal impulse formation, or by abnormal conduction. In fact, this classification is a gross simplification, because the pathogenesis of arrhythmias is incompletely understood and is extremely complex. Some arrhythmias may be induced or abolished by exercise or other procedures such as eyeball pressure (a vagal manoeuvre).

7.4 The pathophysiology of conduction abnormalities and arrhythmias

Myocardial cell damage affects the electrophysiological features of the cell membrane and can result in the development of arrhythmias. This is principally

Table 7.2 Summary: Recognition of arrhythmias

Arrhythmia	Clinical examination	ECG findings
Supraventricular arrhythmias		
Sinus arrest/block Fairly common, usually physiological	slow/normal rate regular underlying rhythm with pauses	regular underlying rhythm with intermittent pauses >/ = 2 P–P intervals with no P wave
Sinus bradycardia Rare, usually pathological	slow regular rhythm	long R–R interval, normal P–QRS–T
Sinus arrhythmia Uncommon at rest, common after light exercise, physiological	slow/normal rate variable S1–S1 interval	variable R–R interval +/– wandering pacemaker (variable P wave morphology)
First degree AV block Fairly common, usually physiological	slow/normal rate long A sound – S1 interval	prolonged R–R interval (> 0.5 sec)
Second degree AV block Nearly always physiological, abolished by increased sympathetic/decreased vagal tone, very common	slow/normal rate regularly irregular rhythm or occasional pauses (dropped beats) A sound not followed by S1 + S2 pulse deficit isolated jugular A wave may be palpable	P wave blocked and not followed by QRS double R–R interval at block Mobitz type 1 = variable P–R interval prior to block Mobitz type 2 = constant P–R interval
Third degree AV block Pathological, may cause collapse or death, rare	slow rate regular rhythm A sounds have no relation to S1 + S2	no relationship between P waves and QRS regular junctional or ventricular escapes
Atrial premature complexes (APCs) Fairly common, abnormal, variable significance, may be associated with poor performance	normal/fast rate irregular rhythm premature beat usually followed by non- compensatory pause +/– pulse deficit	premature P wave P' wave may be different configuration P–R interval may change P' wave may be buried in previous T wave

Table 7.2 Continued

Arrhythmia	Clinical examination	ECG findings
Atrial tachycardia Uncommon, pathological, significant, may need treatment, box rest advisable	fast rate regular or irregular may be abolished by vagal manoeuvre +/– signs of cardiovascular compromise	irregular if short bursts regular if sustained P waves often obscured P waves may be abnormal normal QRS
Junctional tachycardia Uncommon, pathological, significant, may need treatment, box rest advisable	fast rate regular or irregular +/– signs of cardiovascular compromise +/– signs of systemic disease	irregular if short bursts regular if sustained P waves unrelated to QRS but can be retrograde normal QRS
Atrial fibrillation (AF) Most common arrhythmia affecting athletic performance. Careful case selection essential prior to treatment	normal or fast rate irregularly irregular rhythm may have long diastolic intervals followed by a flurry of beats no A sound variable intensity heart sounds variable pulse quality +/– signs of underlying heart disease	irregular R–R interval no P waves f waves usually seen normal QRS occasionally slight variation in QRS amplitude
Atrial flutter Rare, definitions vary, can be thought of as a similar condition to AF	fast rate irregular or regular rhythm no A sound	sawtooth f waves +/– fixed F–QRS relationship
Pre-excitation syndromes Rare, may or may not be significant, can be a mechanism for re-entry supraventricular tachydysrhythmias	normal or fast rate regular rhythm may sound normal +/– clinical signs	short P–R interval delta wave at beginning of QRS complex
Accelerated idiojunctional rhythm Sometimes found in very sick animals, e.g. those recovering from colic surgery Antidysrhythmic treatment not required Treat underlying condition	slightly raised rate (40–50) regular rhythm A sounds may not be heard, but if detected have no relationship to S1 + S2	normal QRS no relationship between QRS and P waves junctional rate slightly faster than sinus rate

Table 7.2 Continued

Arrhythmia	Clinical examination	ECG findings
Ventricular rhythms		
Premature ventricular complexes (VPCs) Variable significance Investigation for underlying myocardial or systemic disease required May be induced or abolished by exercise	premature S1 + S2 loud S1, quiet S2 usually followed by compensatory pause +/– pulse deficit	premature QRS not preceded by P wave QRS morphology differs cf normal QRS may be wide (>0.14 sec), but can be normal T wave orientation opposite to QRS
Ventricular tachycardia Uncommon, significant Box rest required, +/– antidysrhythmic drugs Treat underlying disease	fast regular rhythm may have burst of rapid beats usually signs of CV compromise +/– signs of underlying disease	More than four consecutive VPCs sustained or paroxysmal QRS different morphology cf normal P waves may be seen occasionally and bear no relationship to QRS Capture +/– fusion beats may be seen
Accelerated idioventricular rhythm Uncommon, similar mechanism to idiojunctional rhythm Antidysrhythmic treatment not required, treat underlying condition	slightly raised rate (40–50) regular rhythm A sounds may not be heard, if detected have no relationship to S1 + S2	abnormal QRS (may be wide, different morphology) no relationship between QRS and P waves ventricular rate slightly faster than sinus rate capture and fusion beats may be seen
Ventricular fibrillation Almost invariably fatal Institute emergency treatment	no pulse no clear heart sounds no palapable cardiac impulse	no clear complexes bizarre undulating baseline

caused by damage to the ion pumps and channels which determine the shape of the action potential (*see* section 1.5.2). The exact type of arrhythmia depends on the location of the damaged tissue and the extent of the damage. Autonomic factors, electrolyte levels and drugs may also affect the membrane potential and influence the genesis of arrhythmias. In general, myocardial cell damage results in a decreased resting membrane potential, slowed depolarisation (phase 0), and a shortened action potential plateau (phase 2).

Some arrhythmias result from conduction block, which can affect rhythm directly or which can lead to the development of re-entrant arrhythmias. Other arrhythmias result from abnormal impulse formation.

7.4.1 Abnormal impulse conduction

Conduction blocks at the sinoatrial and atrioventricular nodes may result in a bradycardia. These arrhythmias are common in horses and are usually physiological in origin. They reflect the large resting cardiac reserve in this species and are abolished by increased sympathetic and decreased parasympathetic tone. Abnormal conduction blocks can result from cell damage and lead to failure of the normal pathway to initiate ventricular contraction. In order to avoid asystole, a secondary pacemaker takes over. These are often seen as escape beats.

Re-entry arrhythmias are relatively common and can result in single or multiple premature beats or persistent arrhythmias. The most common of these in the horse is atrial fibrillation (AF). In a re-entry arrhythmia, an area of damaged tissue develops very slow conduction properties or a unidirectional block. This means that the impulse takes a long time to reach some areas of cardiac tissue in order to depolarise them. By the time that these areas are depolarised, adjacent areas, which would normally be refractory to further stimulus, have returned to their resting potentials and can be depolarised. This allows a loop to form so that the impulse can pass in a circuit and result in a premature depolarisation. The principle is demonstrated in Figure 7.1.

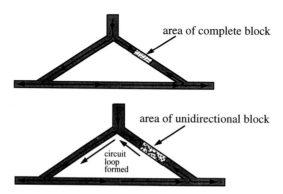

Fig. 7.1 Re-entry arrhythmias.
An area of complete block prevents a circuit loop developing. If a portion of myocardium has slow conduction it can be refractory to an initial stimulus, but has become able to be depolarised by the time an impulse is conducted to it via another route, allowing a re-entry circuit to develop.

7.4.2 Abnormal impulse formation

The most common mechanism of abnormal impulse formation is increased automaticity. This is often responsible for the generation of atrial or ventricular premature beats. Automaticity develops when an abnormal focus within the atria or ventricles becomes a pacemaker site which fires at a higher rate than the usually dominant sinus node. The enhanced impulse initiation results from fast phase 4 depolarisation. The other form of abnormal impulse formation is triggered activity. This form of ectopic focus requires an initiating depolarisation with an afterdepolarisation.

Mechanisms of arrhythmogenesis are important in order to understand the pathophysiology of arrhythmias and the potential effects of disease. More detailed discussions are contained in articles in the reading list. However, as yet, identification of the mechanisms of arrhythmias has had little practical influence on their treatment.

7.5 Principles of the treatment of arrhythmias

A limited range of antidysrhythmic drugs is licensed for use in animals. In small animal medicine, the pharmacology of a range of drugs, designed for use in humans, is understood. However, little is known about the pharmacology of most of these drugs in the horse. The number of drugs which can be safely used in horses is therefore very limited. Some have to be used on the presumption that their pharmacology and action is similar to that in other species. It is advisable first to obtain informed consent from owners prior to treatment because these drugs are unlicensed for use in horses in the UK.

Fortunately, the incidence of arrhythmias which require treatment in the horse is relatively low compared with small animals and humans. Atrial fibrillation (AF) is the most common arrhythmia which requires treatment. Although other arrhythmias are quite common, they are often intermittent and do not require treatment. Severe bradydysrhythmias are rare and tachydysrhythmias are relatively uncommon, perhaps as a result of the relatively low incidence of myocardial disease. An additional problem is that drugs are not always as effective at reducing the deleterious effects of arrhythmias as might be hoped. Even in human and small animal medicine, it is increasingly recognised that antidysrhythmic drugs may themselves cause arrhythmias and that they may not be as beneficial as was once thought. They may also have side-effects. As a general rule, therefore, drugs should be avoided except in cases where underlying disease cannot be controlled and the condition is life threatening, or when an arrhythmia is persistent and limits athletic performance.

The most important principles of treatment of arrhythmias are to:

- Identify the arrhythmia and determine whether it is physiological or abnormal.
- Identify any underlying heart disease.
- Identify any underlying systemic disease.
- Decide on the significance of the arrhythmia and perform any further diagnostic tests which may be required.
- Decide what treatment, if any, is required.

7.6 Normal cardiac rhythms

7.6.1 Normal sinus rhythm

The normal resting heart rhythm is called sinus rhythm because the sinoatrial node acts as the pacemaker governing rhythm (see section 1.5.3). The pulse rhythm is regular and pulse quality is consistent. On auscultation, clear A, S1, S2 and S3 sounds may be heard, with a regular rhythm. The ECG will show that each QRS complex is preceded by a P wave, and that a QRS complex follows each P wave. The R–R and P–P intervals are consistent (Figure 4.2).

7.6.2 Sinus tachycardia

Sinus tachycardia occurs when sympathetic discharge increases and parasympathetic tone decreases. A rate above 60 bpm would be considered a tachycardia. The SA node is the pacemaker. Sinus tachycardia is a normal response in order to increase cardiac output. This often results from pain, fear, excitement or exercise. At rest, it can be seen in animals with heart failure, haemorrhage, shock, pyrexia, or anaemia.

Auscultation reveals a regular, rapid rhythm. The intensity of the heart sounds may be greater than normal. An ECG demonstrates normal P and QRS complexes, with a regular R–R interval. At high heart rates, the P wave may be lost in the preceding T wave (Figure 7.2). The T wave is extremely labile and is profoundly affected by heart rate. At high heart rates it may be large and of a different configuration from normal. Before deciding that a tachycardia is due to heart failure, it is very important to be sure that the horse is truly at rest, preferably in its own environment, having become used to the presence of the examiner.

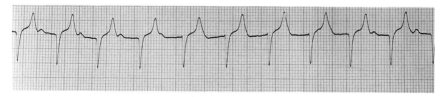

Fig. 7.2 Sinus tachycardia.
Some P waves are lost in previous T wave.

7.7 Arrhythmias which are frequently associated with high vagal tone

7.7.1 First degree atrioventricular block

First degree AV block (1°AVB) is caused by delayed conduction of the sinus impulse through the AV node resulting in prolongation of the P–R interval. Auscultation may reveal a prolonged A–S1 interval. The condition is difficult to define in the horse because of the wide variation of normality, but an interval of > 0.5 sec should be considered abnormal. In the horse it is usually due to high vagal tone, but it can also be caused by drugs such as xylazine, detomidine, and digoxin. It is rarely caused by AV nodal disease. 1°AVB is primarily an ECG diagnosis of little practical relevance in horses.

7.7.2 Second degree atrioventricular block

Second degree heart block (2°AVB), also called partial atrioventricular block (PAVB), or a missed, dropped or blocked beat, is the most common arrhythmia found in horses and may be found in up to 30% of fit horses at rest. It is associated with a slow or normal heart rate and high vagal tone. The percentage of animals with the arrhythmia is probably higher than recorded because horses are naturally wary of auscultation or the use of an ECG. 2°AVB is nearly always a normal homeostatic mechanism which is involved in the control of blood pressure, detected by baroreceptors and mediated by the cardiovascular centre in the medulla. Rather than reducing the sinus rate, which might predispose to atrial arrhythmias, the heart rate and therefore cardiac output can be reduced by blocking conduction of sinus beats. Blood pressure measurements will show a slight stepwise increase in the arterial blood pressure until a sinus beat is blocked. This allows the pressure to fall back to a basal level before the process is repeated. However, as soon as there is demand for increased cardiac output, the sinus beats are all conducted, immediately increasing the number of stroke volumes pumped per minute (see section 1.4.3).

Auscultation will reveal an A sound without subsequent S1 and S2 sounds. The A sound is sometimes heard best on the right side of the chest. An A wave may also be seen or palpated in the jugular vein. It is important to try and identify the A sound, but it cannot be heard in all cases. In addition, the arrhythmia is often noticeably 'regularly irregular', i.e. the blocked beats occur at regular intervals. Frequently, every third, fourth or fifth beat will be blocked. This may be a useful feature in distinguishing this physiological arrhythmia from AF (see section 7.8.5). It may be helpful to use one's foot or hand as a metronome, tapping in time with the cardiac rhythm. Often, the metronome will tap once in the middle of the long diastolic interval, and then again in time with the next conducted sinus beat.

The ECG will show a P wave which is not followed by a QRS complex. Most commonly, Mobitz type 1 or Wenckebach phenomenon is seen in the horse. If it is this form of block, there is variation in the P–R interval, often with gradual prolongation before an impulse is blocked (Figure 7.3). This is often recognisable on auscultation. In Mobitz type 2 2°AVB, the P–R interval is fixed. In small animals this can indicate the initial stages of AV node disease leading to 3°AVB, but there is no evidence that this is the case in the horse. Although usually only one sinus impulse is blocked, on occasions, double-blocked beats can occur. These are very seldom pathological.

If high vagal tone is abolished by excitement or exercise, normal sinus rhythm will return. This is the reason for the use of a trot-up as a way of assessing whether an arrhythmia is physiological or not. Many pathological arrhythmias will become more irregular with exercise, so the abolition of the arrhythmia at higher heart rates is a useful presumptive indicator of a vagal arrhythmia. Exciting an animal in its box has the same effect. However, 2°AVB can also

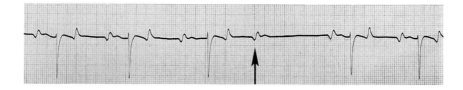

Fig. 7.3 Mobitz type 1 (Wenkebach) second-degree atrioventricular block.
The P–R interval gradually increases until the fourth P wave (arrow), which is not followed
by a QRS complex, was blocked at the AV node.

occur at higher heart rates under some circumstances. Sometimes it is noted while the heart rate is slowing during the phase of 'autonomic imbalance' (Figure 7.4). In these situations it is usually regarded as normal. It is has a similar mechanism to that of post-exercise transient sinus arrhythmia.

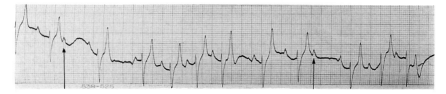

Fig. 7.4 Second-degree atrioventricular block at a high heart rate.
Some P waves are unconducted (*arrows*) despite an elevated heart rate (approximately 75 bpm). This ECG was recorded immediately after exercise in an apparently normal horse. It is a manifestation of the period of 'autonomic imbalance'.

2°AVB can also occur when atrial premature beats reach the AV node while it is still refractory. These APCs can be difficult to identify without careful examination of the ECG. On rare occasions, 2°AVB can be so profound that it can be considered an abnormal arrhythmia (see section 7.8.15). However, it must be emphasised that this is extremely uncommon.

7.7.3 Sinus arrhythmia

Sinus arrhythmia is the periodic waxing and waning of heart rate associated with changes in vagal tone. It occurs infrequently in resting horses with a high vagal tone and may be related to respiration. However, it is much less common at rest than in dogs or humans. More commonly, sinus arrhythmia occurs during the recovery period following exercise, particularly after light exercise. Usually, when the heart rate slows further, the rhythm becomes regular once more. In this circumstance it is known as post-exercise transient sinus arrhythmia.

Auscultation reveals a cyclical irregularity of rhythm which is frequently a source of confusion in assessment of animals during the post-exercise period. If sinus arrhythmia disappears after further rest or with more vigorous exercise it is a normal finding. The ECG will show cyclical changes in the R–R interval (Figure 7.5). The QRS complexes will be normal, but the P waves often vary in

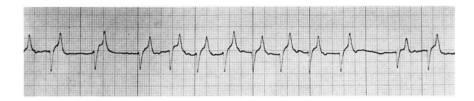

Fig. 7.5 Sinus arrhythmia.
The R–R interval gradually reduces and then increases in this example. It is difficult to see the P waves in this example recorded during exercise on a treadmill in an apparently normal horse, but it appears that there is also a gradual change in the P–R interval. Second-degree AV block can also occur during this vagally mediated arrhythmia, e.g. between the third and second last complexes. (Courtesy of Dr Jeremy Naylor)

configuration due to changes in the site of impulse origin within the SA node or in its propagation through the atria (a 'wandering pacemaker'). The condition usually disappears with decreasing parasympathetic or increasing sympathetic tone. A radiotelemetric ECG is very useful to demonstrate that the arrhythmia is not present during exercise. Commonly, during a pre-purchase examination, this arrhythmia will be heard after the first stage of the exercise phase, causing concern on behalf of the examiner (see section 8.1.5). If it is not possible to record an ECG at the time of the examination, increasing the level of exercise will often result in abolition of the arrhythmia, because the horse loses parasympathetic reserve. No treatment is required.

7.7.4 *Sinus block or arrest*

Sinus block or arrest are manifestations of high vagal tone which are much less frequent than AV block (see below), but which are not uncommon. Horses with these arrhythmias have a slow heart rate with pauses less than or equal to or greater than two normal R–R intervals. During these pauses no A sound will be heard and no P wave is seen on the ECG (Figure 7.6). Sinus block or arrest are very seldom pathological. In extreme cases, junctional or ventricular escape beats may be seen (see below). However, if syncopal episodes which can be attributed to the presence of these arrhythmias do occur, treatment with atropine is indicated in the short-term. In the long-term, implantation of an artificial pacemaker could be required if the syncope can be directly related to the dysrhythmia. It is very rare that any treatment is required.

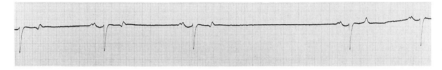

Fig. 7.6 Sinus block.
The third QRS complex is followed by a pause with no P wave which is approximately double the normal R–R interval.

7.8 'Pathological' arrhythmias

7.8.1 Sinus bradycardia

Sinus bradycardia is an abnormally slow heart rate (< 24 bpm) caused by infrequent but regular sinus discharge. It can be associated with high vagal tone, myocardial depression, electrolyte disturbances, or high cerebrospinal fluid pressure. Auscultation will identify a slow regular rhythm. The ECG shows regular R–R intervals and normal QRS complexes. If the condition is physiological, it will be abolished by excitement or exercise. However, it is usually pathological and may be associated with poor athletic performance. It is a rare condition. It is important to identify any underlying predisposing factors and treat these conditions rather than use atropine to try to increase the heart rate.

7.8.2 Atrial standstill

Atrial standstill is an uncommon arrhythmia, which is usually caused by hyperkalaemia. In atrial standstill, P waves are absent but there is apparent conduction of the sinus impulse to the ventricles. A slow sino-ventricular rhythm is present because the cells of the sinus node and internodal tracts are more resistant to hyperkalaemia than the atrial myocardiocytes. The effects of hyperkalaemia on the electrocardiogram are less predictable than are often reported; however, flattening of the P waves and pronounced or inverted T waves may be seen once the potassium levels approach 8–10 mEq/l. This may occur in animals with renal failure or a ruptured bladder. In these instances, treatment is aimed at reversal of the initiating disease process if possible, and administration of large quantities of intravenous normal saline to reverse the electrolyte imbalance. Sodium bicarbonate can also be given if required to encourage potassium to move into cells (0.25–0.5 mEq/kg).

7.8.3 Atrial premature complexes

APCs (or premature atrial systoles, PASs) are a relatively common supraventricular arrhythmia. Occasional APCs are sometimes found in otherwise apparently normal horses and do not appear to limit athletic performance. Frequent APCs can be a sign of myocardial disease, electrolyte inbalance, toxaemia, septicaemia, hypoxia or chronic valvular disease. They can be associated with previous episodes of respiratory disease and subsequent myocarditis. APCs may be a significant finding in animals with poor athletic performance. It is often unclear whether the effect on performance is directly due to the abnormal rhythm or is related to cardiac disease which is the underlying cause of the arrhythmia. When APCs occur, further investigation to establish the underlying cause is advisable. However, even after a thorough investigation it can be difficult to be certain of the effect of the arrhythmia on exercise tolerance.

Clinical examination

APCs occur due to abnormal impulse formation in the atrial myocardium. As the name implies, they occur earlier than a normal sinus impulse, causing a shortened P–P′ and R–R interval. They originate from outside the SA node (ectopic), may be of a different configuration from the normal P wave (P′) and may have a different P′-R interval. At high heart rates they may be lost in the preceding T wave. They often reset the SA node so that the subsequent P wave follows after a normal P–P interval (Figure 7.7). This is called a non-compensatory pause. It is a useful method of differentiating APCs from ventricular premature complexes (VPCs), which are usually followed by a full compensatory pause (see below), although this distinction is not reliable because there are exceptions to the rule. On auscultation, therefore, most APCs can be recognised because they are preceded by a short diastolic interval and are followed by a normal diastolic interval. With a compensatory pause there is a long diastolic interval following the premature beat. The first and second heart sounds (S1 and S2) are often normal in intensity unless the APC is very early. However, very premature APCs may have a relatively loud S1 and quiet S2, and result in a marked reduction in stroke volume which may be palpated as a weak pulse or a pulse deficit.

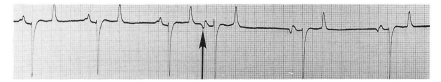

Fig. 7.7 A supraventricular premature beat (APC).
The fourth P wave (*arrow*) has a different conformation from the preceding P waves and occurs prematurely. (Subsequent P waves and R–R intervals vary slightly.)

Investigation of horses with APCs

When APCs are suspected on auscultation, it is helpful to document their presence and frequency by recording an ECG. APCs may be more frequent during exercise than at rest, or may be detected during exercise in animals in which they were absent at rest. Radiotelemetric recording of the ECG at exercise or in the immediate post-exercise period is therefore invaluable. In horses with poor athletic performance associated with APCs, ECGs recorded during exercise may be the only way in which a diagnosis can be reached. Radiotelemetry is very helpful in determining whether APCs are occurring sufficiently frequently during exercise to limit performance. In some horses, APCs are present at rest or during the recovery period, but do not occur during exercise. In these cases, APCs are less likely to be associated with poor athletic performance.

APCs may be detected periodically during the period of heart rate slowing after exercise, particularly after sub-maximal exercise. In some cases it can be difficult to determine whether these early beats with a slightly different shape P wave are APCs or are a normal variation as part of sinus arrhythmia and a wandering pacemaker. Sometimes the atrial complexes are found to have been blocked at the AV node, resulting in an irregular rhythm. This may be as a result of the return of vagal tone during the period of autonomic imbalance and is a normal finding in some cases. As a general guide, if the APCs are single and occur in a cyclical fashion every four or five sinus beats for a limited period during heart rate slowing, they are unlikely to be associated with atrial disease or poor athletic performance. If, however, they occur in groups, at irregular intervals, or are present in animals with suspected atrial disease, they are more likely to be significant.

24-hour Holter monitoring can be a useful aid in horses with APCs because periods of paroxysmal atrial tachycardia or multiple APCs may occur at times other than those in which the animals is being examined or during a standard ECG recording.

When more frequent APCs occur (e.g. 1–5 per minute), it is more likely that underlying atrial disease is present. A thorough clinical examination should be performed, with particular note to evidence of AV regurgitation, even if no clinical signs appear to be associated with the APCs. Echocardiography should be used to assess the severity of valvular and myocardial disease. If significant mitral regurgitation (MR) is present, the prognosis is guarded. If tricuspid regurgitation (TR) is detected, it is possible that the valvular insufficiency is coincidental; echocardiography will help to indicate the severity of the condition. In a few cases, fractional shortening will be reduced suggesting poor myocardial function. In most cases, no obvious underlying pathology is found, and it is usually assumed that the arrhythmia is caused by atrial myocarditis. Often there is a history of a previous respiratory infection (see section 6.7.2). Haematology, and viral antibody serology may therefore be useful aids in some cases, and biochemistry should be performed to investigate the possibility of underlying systemic disease or electrolyte imbalance.

Management and treatment

When APCs are very infrequent and are asymptomatic, no treatment or change in management is warranted. When APCs are more frequent and are thought to be related to poor exercise tolerance, it is important that the horse is rested for approximately two to eight weeks to allow the problem to resolve. Pasture rest is usually sufficient. The animal should then be re-examined, preferably with the use of 24-hour ECG recordings and radiotelemetry, before being returned to training. A premature return to full work may result in further incapacity. However, on occasions rest alone may not be sufficient and other steps need to be taken. There may also be pressure from trainers to get the horse back to work in a shorter time period. Corticosteroids have been used for their anti-inflammatory action in these circumstances, although their use is somewhat controversial. Dexamethasone can be used at a dose of 0.02–0.15 mg/kg twice daily by mouth (see Appendix). The dose should be decreased over a 2–4 week period, initially reducing the frequency to daily and then every other day treatment. Prednisolone can also be used (0.02–1.0 mg/kg). Corticosteroids are contraindicated if an active viral infection is present. In addition, when these drugs are used, care should be taken to note any signs of laminitis. This is a recognised problem with the use of corticosteroids in horses, but is unlikely to occur with low doses in the short-term. Although there is a rationale for the use of steroids as soon as frequent APCs are detected, the author prefers a more conservative approach and uses them only if the horse fails to respond to rest, except in exceptional cases.

If the APCs are sufficiently frequent to cause obvious clinical signs at rest or at low levels of exercise, then treatment should include box rest. Usually an atrial tachycardia will be present; treatment is as described below.

7.8.4 Atrial tachycardia

Atrial tachycardia is a supraventricular tachycardia with a rapid, regular rhythm and a rate which is often 120–220 bpm. It may be paroxysmal (short bursts) or sustained. Four or more consecutive APCs constitute an atrial tachycardia. The ECG will show normal QRS complexes, with regular R–R intervals, but the P′ wave may be a different configuration from normal. Often the P′ wave is lost in the preceding T wave and cannot be identified. In some cases, intermittent 2°AV block is also present and the rhythm may be fast and irregular.

It is important to distinguish atrial tachycardia from sinus tachycardia and ventricular tachycardia. Diagnosis is usually straightforward if a paroxysm of tachycardia starts during the ECG recording. This shows the normal sinus rate and the normal QRS complex configuration, followed by a different configuration P′ wave and a shorter P′–P′ and R–R interval. However, if the rhythm is persistent the distinction is more difficult. An atrial tachycardia can be distinguished from sinus tachycardia because the heart rate is inappropriately high, i.e. there are no other apparent causes for the high rate such as excitement, pyrexia, pain, etc. Ventricular tachycardia can be more difficult to distinguish from atrial tachycardia in horses than in small animals because the QRS complexes of ventricular origin may not be abnormally wide. However, if a normal QRS complex is seen, comparison allows complexes of ventricular origin to be identified. In addition, in ventricular tachycardia, P waves may be identified and bear no relationship to the QRS complexes.

The presence of atrial tachycardia may indicate underlying atrial myocardial disease. A thorough clinical examination and laboratory evaluation including haematology, plasma fibrinogen and serum biochemistry should be performed in order to try to identify any underlying systemic disease. If the clinical signs at rest are sufficiently severe, antidysrhythmic treatment should be used. However, underlying conditions such as electrolyte imbalance should be corrected before antidysrhythmic treatment is initiated. If clinical signs are severe, digoxin can be used to control the ventricular rate by slowing conduction through the AV node, or quinidine can be used to suppress the ectopic focus. However, quinidine is negatively inotropic, vagolytic and hypotensive, which may all exacerbate the clinical condition, so the drug must be used with caution. Digoxin should also be used with caution (see section 6.9.2).

Atrial tachycardia is occasionally seen during quinidine conversion of AF (see below).

7.8.5 Atrial fibrillation

Atrial fibrillation is the most common dysrhythmia affecting exercise tolerance. It is important to learn to recognise this dysrhythmia from clinical examination. It is particularly important to be able to distinguish AF from 2°AVB because long diastolic pauses can occur in both arrhythmias. With careful auscultation this should not be difficult; however, mistakes are sometimes made.

Poor athletic performance is the most common presenting sign in horses with AF. Less frequently, epistaxis, prolonged recovery following exercise and tachypnoea are seen and occasionally CHF, collapse, ataxia, myopathies and colic are associated with AF. In a significant number of cases, particularly in non-athletic horses, AF is an incidental finding.

In the USA, AF has been reported most often in Standardbred horses and is more common in animals of racing age. In the UK, it has been reported to affect heavy-hunter type animals and draught horses more frequently than other breeds, and is most often seen in horses aged 5–15 years. These reports may reflect the hospital populations at different institutions. In the author's experience, there are three general categories of animal which are most frequently affected by the condition. The first are young and middle aged racehorses (2–10 years) with no evidence of underlying heart disease that present with a sudden deterioration in performance. The second are middle-aged (8–15 years) large Thoroughbred or Thoroughbred-cross horses with no evidence of underlying heart disease which have a more vague history of exercise intolerance. The third group is animals with underlying heart disease, particularly MR. AF is rarely found in ponies.

The pathophysiology of atrial fibrillation

In most species, AF is associated with significant underlying heart disease which results in atrial enlargement, usually left atrial enlargement. For example, in dogs it is most commonly seen in animals with dilated cardiomyopathy or severe MR; in humans it is often associated with mitral stenosis. AF is usually initiated by an APC which may or may not be related to myocardial disease. Experimentally, rapid atrial stimulation can set up AF. The arrhythmia will only be maintained if there is inhomogeneity of the state of refractoriness of the atrial myocardium. The premature beat starts a circus movement of depolarisation around the atria spreading from one area of excitable tissue to another. This requires a large mass of atrial tissue and suitable refractory and excitable cells. Surface mapping of atrial electrical activity in the presence of AF demonstrates a number of wavefronts, with some areas of the atria being depolarised, some in a refractory state and others in an excitable state. The impulse can pass from the depolarising area to adjoining excitable areas, but cannot depolarise refractory areas. However, these refractory areas then become excitable, allowing the wavefront to come back and cause depolarisation. In sinus rhythm, once a wavefront has been conducted, it is surrounded by refractory tissue and the impulse cannot continue, but in AF, the wavefront always has an adjacent excitable area which can be stimulated so the wavefront is perpetuated. Marked atrial enlargement increases the chances of circus movement of wavefronts developing because the activation pathways are increased in length.

AF is particularly common in horses for two reasons. In normal horses, of approximately 15 hands or more in size, the atria are sufficiently large for AF to persist once it has been set up. In animals with atrial enlargement it is even more likely that the condition will persist rather than revert to sinus rhythm. An additional factor which is responsible for the persistence of AF in horses is the high vagal tone found in this species. The release of acetylcholine shortens the refractory period to differing degrees in different cells within the atria, resulting in an increased inhomogeneity of refractoriness. The inhomogeneity increases the chance of circus movements being set up. The effects of increased vagal tone are demonstrated in other species, for example, cattle with intestinal conditions which result in increased vagal tone may develop AF, but is abolished if the primary problem is reversed. Experimentally, dog atria have been maintained in AF by bathing them in acetylcholine (the neurotransmitter released by the vagus) once AF has been induced by rapid electrical pacing.

The cardiovascular effects of atrial fibrillation

Effective atrial contraction is important in animals with cardiac disease, because a stiff ventricle may not fill normally during the passive phase of early diastolic filling. Atrial contraction is required to force blood into the ventricles in this situation, so if AF develops, there may be a deterioration in clinical signs. However, in the absence of underlying heart disease, at normal resting heart rates, co-ordinated atrial contraction has little effect on ventricular filling. Consequently, many animals with AF show no clinical signs at rest.

Atrial contraction is of much greater importance during exercise when, at higher heart rates, it contributes a significant volume of blood to ventricular filling. AF may therefore limit ventricular filling during exercise, reducing stroke volume and affecting athletic performance. In addition, the priming effect of atrial contraction, which increases the force of ventricular contraction via the Frank–Starling mechanism, is lost when AF is present. AF results in higher heart rates during exercise at a lower level of work than would be found in the same animal if it was in sinus rhythm. Maximal heart rates may reach 240–260 bpm in these animals rather than 220–240 bpm. Cardiac output at peak exercise is reduced compared with normal animals because stroke volume falls. Horses with AF are unlikely to perform with success in athletic pursuits such as racing, three-day eventing, long distance riding, carriage riding, hunting or polo, although there are some exceptions to this rule. However, some animals, which are used for less arduous work such as show-jumping or dressage, may perform satisfactorily while in AF, at least in the short- to medium-term.

Clinical examination and electrocardiography

Clinical examination will reveal an irregular heart rhythm. The heart rate may be normal (as low as 24 bpm) or elevated. This contrasts with dogs, where AF is almost always accompanied by a tachycardia. There may be long pauses of up to 8 seconds or so, sometimes followed by flurries of beats. Sometimes the flurries will come in a cyclical fashion. The S1 and S2 sounds may vary in intensity due to the variable position of the atrioventricular valves at the beginning of systole. The most characteristic finding is the absence of the A sound (S4). This corresponds to the ECG finding of an absence of P waves in any lead, due to the lack of any co-ordinated atrial activity. The P waves are replaced by f (fibrillation) waves. The R–R interval will be irregular; this may be more obvious at normal heart rates than in tachycardias (Figures 7.8 and 7.9). The pulse quality will depend on the diastolic interval, and on the presence of any underlying heart disease. Pulse deficits are common with very short diastolic intervals.

As a general principle, when a long diastolic interval is heard, it is important to try and identify an A sound because if A sounds are present then the cause of the

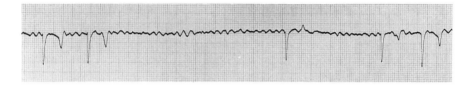

Fig. 7.8 Atrial fibrillation.
AF is easily recognised when it occurs at a normal heart rate as in this case. f waves are clearly visible and the R–R interval is completely irregular.

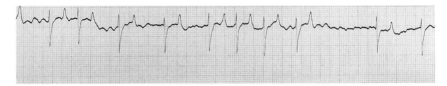

Fig. 7.9 Atrial fibrillation.
At high heart rates f waves are often less clear, but there are no P waves and the rhythm is irregularly irregular, giving the diagnosis.

arrhythmia is not AF. In 2°AVB the pauses are usually multiples of the normal R–R interval and the arrhythmia has a regularly irregular, predictable nature. It may be helpful to use one's foot as a metronome to get used to the underlying rhythm. With careful auscultation, if 2°AVB block is present, an A sound is likely to be heard during the pause. In AF, the rhythm can be described as irregularly irregular. Two relatively uncommon situations may confuse the issue. Long diastolic intervals with no atrial contraction may be due to SA block rather than AF. In this case, SA block is usually found intermittently, with normal sinus rhythm being the predominant rhythm. A second condition which is rarely encountered is a split S1, which can be confused for an A sound and S1. In this situation AF is suspected on the grounds of the irregularly irregular rhythm and the absence of an A sound during the longer diastolic intervals. Where AF is suspected, it is wise to perform an ECG to confirm the diagnosis and to be able to detect any QRS complexes which are ventricular rather than junctional in origin.

Diagnostic features of AF are summarised in Table 7.3.

Management of horses with atrial fibrillation
An essential part of the management of cases with AF is a careful examination for underlying heart disease which might predispose to the condition, and an assessment of historical details. Horses with valvular or myocardial disease and those with a long-standing AF (typically more than 4 months) are less likely to be successfully treated than those without evidence of underlying disease or a recent onset of the arrhythmia. These horses are also more likely to suffer a recurrence of the condition at a later date even if treatment is initially successful.

A thorough clinical evaluation should always be made prior to treatment. Pathological murmurs should be identified (Chapters 3 and 6). Measurement of an accurate resting heart rate is also helpful. An elevated heart rate is more common in horses with underlying heart disease. Electrolyte abnormalities,

Table 7.3 Summary: Clinical features of atrial fibrillation

Most common arrhythmia affecting athletic performance
Horses are predisposed to AF because they have high vagal tone and large atria
Horses often develop AF without underlying heart disease
May be paroxysmal or sustained
Paroxysmal AF may be difficult to identify
AF may develop in some animals with congestive heart failure but underlying heart disease
is the cause of the CHF

Presenting signs
Common
Poor athletic performance
Incidental finding
Uncommon
Ataxia
Epistaxis
Collapse (usually at exercise)
Myopathy
Weight loss

Clinical recognition
Irregularly irregular rhythm
Absence of atrial contraction sound ('A' sound)
Pulse quality may be variable
Heart rate normal or raised

ECG
No P waves
f waves
Irregular R–R interval
QRS complex normal (although may vary fractionally)

If CHF is present, do not treat with quinidine. The prognosis is poor

particularly hypokalaemia, may predispose to AF and therefore it may be beneficial to measure plasma levels in selected cases. Further tests such as a fractional excretion test can also be helpful (see section 2.3.6).

If echocardiography is available, it is the best method of assessing the severity of valvular or myocardial disease. The most common predisposing factor to AF is MR. Structural mitral valve abnormalities may not be seen echocardiographically, but measurement of left atrial size is very helpful. Pulsed-wave or colour-flow Doppler echocardiography can be used to map the area of the regurgitant jet and its origin, in order to provide a semi-quantitative measurement of the severity of MR. Myocardial contractility can also be assessed, (although fractional shortening should be measured over several cardiac cycles because widely differing R–R intervals affect measurements) (see sections 4.2.6 and 6.7.1). Aortic regurgitation is less commonly associated with AF, but if significant AR is detected on clinical examination or echocardiography, the prognosis for return to sinus rhythm is reduced. MR is usually present as well as AR in these cases. TR may result in dilation of the right atrium and predispose to AF. However, it should be remembered that TR is a frequent incidental finding in fit, large racehorses and may be an incidental finding in animals with AF also (see section 6.3). Echocardiography is a very useful aid to assessment of severity of

TR. In each case, particularly with MR, if echocardiography shows atrial or ventricular dilation the prognosis for conversion to sinus rhythm is worsened in comparison to animals with no volume overload. If severe myocardial disease is present, treatment should not be undertaken. In horses with a recent respiratory infection and reduced fractional shortening on echocardiography, treatment should be postponed for approximately 1–2 months, before re-evaluation.

In horses in which valvular disease is significant, or in which the arrhythmia may have been present for more than approximately four months, the risks of failure of treatment, potential complications during treatment or a reversion to AF later, and financial considerations, need careful discussion with the owner or trainer. These horses may not return to previous performance levels even if treatment is successful. In animals which have high financial or sentimental value, treatment can be pursued, but both the veterinary surgeon and the owner should be aware of these increased risks.

Horses with AF may have a better long-term prognosis if they are successfully treated rather than left untreated so, even in pet animals, treatment is usually beneficial in suitable cases. However, there are some circumstances when the prognosis for successful treatment is thought to be poor because of a prolonged history, or because treatment has been unsuccessful, or because AF has recurred, when the horses can continue in work despite the presence of AF. When AF is likely to have been present for some time and the horse is performing satisfactorily, with a normal resting heart rate and no signs of significant underlying heart disease, the potential risks of treatment may not be justified. Treatment is not risk free, and if the horse's performance is normal it may not be essential. In the author's opinion, AF does not in itself increase the risk of collapse at lower levels of exercise; it is when the condition is accompanied by significant heart disease and the horse is asked to work hard when it is tired that a risk to the rider develops. The first sign of compromise due to the condition and/or the underlying disease is likely to be tiring or prolonged recovery following exercise. Owners should be made aware of this and advised to pull up horses once they feel them beginning to tire. The horse may be unsuitable for riders who are too inexperienced to detect this or when the individual horse is the type which 'soldiers' on regardless.

Breeding animals with AF usually benefit from treatment to convert them to sinus rhythm unless there are signs of marked underlying heart disease. However, both mares and stallions may continue to perform satisfactorily when AF is refractory to treatment. If signs of CHF failure develop, these are best managed with diuretics and digoxin.

As a general rule, *animals with AF should not be used for arduous competition* and the level of work for which they are used should not be increased from that of which they were previously known to be capable without tiring, unless treatment is successful.

Horses with AF and CHF have a grave prognosis. Usually volume overload has resulted in dilation of the left atrium and myocardial changes which make a return of sinus rhythm unlikely.

Treatment of horses with atrial fibrillation
The most important consideration in treatment of AF is selecting suitable cases.

Animals with evidence of CHF or a resting heart rate of > 55–60 bpm are not suitable for treatment. However, treatment of cases without evidence of underlying heart disease frequently results in a permanent return to sinus rhythm and subsequent normal athletic performance. Some animals can be treated repeatedly and perform well during the periods in which they are in sinus rhythm.

Quinidine sulphate is the drug of choice for treatment of AF. This is insoluble and must be given orally in a suspension. There have been some reports of its use intravenously, but side-effects were common and this route of administration is not recommended under any circumstances. Quinidine gluconate is the soluble form of the drug, and has been used intravenously for treatment of AF with success. However, oral treatment is more reliable, particularly in cases which have been in AF for more than a few days. Quinidine gluconate is not available in the UK at the present time. Other drugs such as procainamide have been used for treatment of AF but do not appear to be as reliable as quinidine.

Oral treatment with quinidine sulphate The standard treatment for AF is quinidine sulphate, administered by stomach tube. Some clinicians recommend a test dose of 5 g per horse on the day before treatment is planned, to test for anaphylactic reactions. This is a rare problem and the author does not use a test dose. The dosage rate is 20 mg/kg (i.e. 10 g for a 500 kg horse), administered by stomach tube. The rate of absorption and half-life dictate the therapeutic regime. The aim of treatment is to titrate the drug to a plasma concentration within the therapeutic range (approximately 2.5–5.0 mg/l). Peak plasma levels are usually reached approximately 2 hours after administration. The dose is therefore repeated every 2 hours until the horse converts to normal sinus rhythm, or until toxic side-effects are recognised (see below). Increased dosage resulting in plasma levels above 5.0 mg/l is likely to result in side-effects and will not increase the chances of reversion to sinus rhythm because conversion normally only occurs with plasma concentrations in the therapeutic range. Ideally, on site quinidine assays can be used for monitoring plasma levels, but this is seldom possible in practice.

If the therapeutic range is exceeded, animals may convert to sinus rhythm when the plasma level falls back into the therapeutic range, after treatment has been stopped. Many horses revert to sinus rhythm after a dose of approximately 30–60 g. Side-effects are much more common after total doses in the range of 50–80 g have been administered. Continued dosage beyond this point may be unwise unless the clinician is confident that the toxic range has not been reached. Very few 500 kg horses have drug levels below the therapeutic range after 60 g of quinidine given at two hourly intervals.

The approach to treating horses with AF is summarised in Table 7.4.

If initial treatment is unsuccessful A number of steps can be taken if initial treatment is unsuccessful. One approach is to take a blood sample for a quinidine assay to see if therapeutic levels have been reached. Treatment can be stopped while the results are obtained. If absorption has been poor, the plasma levels may be below the therapeutic range. The treatment can be repeated at a later date, with a higher total dose, if necessary.

Table 7.4 Summary: Treatment of atrial fibrillation

Selection of cases

Consider:
 Signs of underlying heart disease, e.g. murmurs, tachycardia
 Duration of arrhythmia
 Type of work required from horse
 Cost
 Side-effects

Good prognosis:
 No pathological cardiac murmurs
 Normal heart rate
 Duration of AF < 4 months

Moderate prognosis:
 Murmur of Al, TR and MR but no volume overload on echocardiography
 Duration unknown or suspected to be > 4 months

Poor prognosis:
 Pathological murmur (especially MR) with volume overload
 Previous unsuccessful treatment
 Heart rate > 55 bpm

Treatment

Dose with 20 mg/kg every 2 hours up to total dose of 60–80 g per 500 kg horse
Monitor heart rate, ECG if possible
Monitor for side-effects
Monitor plasma levels if possible, to titrate drug level into therapeutic range of 2.5–5.0 mg/l
Do not move horse during course of treatment
If fail to convert after 60–80 g, or reaches upper end of therapeutic range, switch to 20 mg/kg
 every 6 hours. If uncertain, take a blood sample 2 hours after last dose and assay to see if
 therapeutic levels were reached
If still in AF after 24 hours, consider addition of digoxin at dose of 0.002 mg/kg I/V
If sufficiently severe side-effects develop, stop treatment and consider administration of
 balanced electrolyte solution, bicarbonate (1 mEq/kg IV), or if life threatening
 phenylephrine (10 mg in 500 ml of normal saline to effect)
If unsuccessful, and levels were theraupeutic, consider repeating treatment a few days later
 after starting on a maintenance level of digoxin
If converts, can return to light work after 3–5 days, full training 7–10 days
If reverts to AF later, can repeat treatment
If unsuccessful, consider if animal is capable of a reduced level of athletic work

Traditionally, if treatment was unsuccessful after the initial titration, it was resumed the following day. However, evidence suggests that the longer plasma levels are kept in the therapeutic range, the greater the chances of successful treatment. Since the half-life of quinidine is around 6 hours, doses can be repeated every 6 hours to try to maintain the drug level in the therapeutic range until conversion is achieved. If on-site assays are possible, it is desirable to repeat the assay 2 hours after administration of a dose and, if necessary, just before treatment, to obtain precise drug levels. The 6-hourly treatment can be repeated until side-effects become a problem or until the patience of the clinician is exhausted. Six-hourly administration of quinidine has been successful in some animals as long as three days after the beginning of treatment.

Digoxin is routinely used in addition to quinidine by some clinicians; however, there does not appear to be any particular advantage in the use of digoxin and, in the author's view, the additional drug only complicates evaluation of the patient. Interactions between the two drugs mean that administration of digoxin may increase plasma levels of quinidine, which may not be desirable. Under some circumstances the use of digoxin may be indicated. If, after 24 hours, treatment is still unsuccessful, intravenous administration of digoxin at a dose of 0.0025 mg/kg, followed by oral administration at a dose of 0.015 mg/kg twice daily, may result in a return to sinus rhythm. If treatment with the standard regime is unsuccessful, using an oral maintenance dose of digoxin for three to five days prior to repeating the administration of quinidine may be worthwhile.

Horses which fail to convert with the traditional initial titration regime, but convert after 6-hourly treatments or treatment on another day, are more likely to revert to AF at a later date than animals which respond to the initial titration. The reversion rate in these animals is approximately 50%. Most horses which stay in sinus rhythm for more than a year after treatment are unlikely to revert to AF. Some horses can be treated repeatedly and turn in useful performances in the interim period. The suitability of a case for repeated treatment depends on the value of the horse's performance or sentimental factors. Owners should be warned of the increased risk of failure or later reversion in animals which need repeated treatment.

Management of side-effects and toxicity Many of the side-effects which have been reported to be associated with the use of quinidine are likely to have resulted from drug levels well into the toxic range and out of the therapeutic range. With the treatment regime recommended above, drug levels in the toxic range are less likely to be reached than with some regimes used previously. The use of on-site assays of plasma levels is the ideal method of making sure that animals stay in the therapeutic rather than the toxic range. However, even with this facility, side-effects do occur, and it is important to recognise those which are to be expected in the course of normal successful treatment, those which are a cause of concern and indicate that further treatment should be stopped, and those which are life-threatening and require intensive treatment.

Side-effects which are frequently seen during successful treatment include depression, mild colic and mild diarrhoea. More serious signs include marked tachycardia (heart rate > 100–120 bpm), weakness, severe colic and nasal oedema. If these signs are encountered, the drug levels are likely to be above the therapeutic range and treatment should be restricted to a six-hour dosage regime or stopped if they do not resolve. Colic may be sufficiently severe to require the use of analgesics and even cessation of treatment. Occasionally, ataxia, diarrhoea, laminitis, hypotension and collapse are reported. These situations indicate that no further treatment should be given. Monitoring the ECG is helpful because it allows significant arrhythmias to be detected in addition to identifying the return of sinus rhythm. It may also be useful to monitor heart rate, which can be difficult to measure by palpation or auscultation at fast heart rates. Radiotelemetric monitoring of an ECG allows significant arrhythmias to be detected early, and corrective treatment can be instituted as soon as possible. A number of arrhythmias may develop during the course of treatment. Once AF has been terminated, a rapid supraventricular tachycardia with a higher heart rate than was present with AF can develop, and may be associated with a deterioration of clinical signs. Prolongation of the QRS complex by more than 25% has been reported to be an indication of toxicity.

The most significant cardiovascular side-effect of quinidine is hypotension. Therefore, where side-effects are a cause for concern, fluid therapy with a balanced electrolyte solution should be instituted. Ideally, an intravenous catheter should already be in place so that emergency treatment can be given if necessary. If the side-effects are severe, intravenous sodium bicarbonate (1 mEq/kg) should be administered because it will increase the protein binding of quinidine. Phenylephrine has been used occasionally in cases where hypotension is severe (dose rate 5–10 mg in 500 ml saline per 500 kg horse to effect). Digoxin can be used if the heart rate becomes very high (>120) and should be administered if an atrial tachycardia develops. Digoxin reduces the rate of conduction through the AV node; however, it may not affect the heart rate as much as might be hoped because it will not reverse the effects of high sympathetic tone. It is important that animals which require intensive treatment can be treated without moving them to another box. Absolute rest is advisable because moving a hypotensive animal may cause it to collapse.

In a very limited number of cases a horse may appear particularly sensitive to the effects of the drug and sudden death during treatment is a potential hazard. Although this is very uncommon, it is wise to warn owners of the potential dangers of treatment.

Stomach tube problems Passage of a stomach tube may be difficult in some horses, particularly when repeated dosing is required, or if nasal oedema or haemorrhage develop. The stomach tube should always be cleaned thoroughly because the taste of quinidine will make the horse resent its use even more. Sedation should be avoided if at all possible. Phenothiazines (e.g. acepromazine) will reduce blood pressure and may make side-effects more severe. Alpha$_2$ agonists (e.g. detomidine) will increase vagal tone, reduce myocardial contractility and may also decrease cardiac output in an animal in which it is already compromised. If necessary, the animal can be sedated to allow a tube to be passed and the tube left in place for treatment to commence once the effects of the sedative have worn off. The tube should be plugged to avoid aerophagia resulting in bloat; however, where possible the use of an indwelling tube should be avoided. It may be possible to administer a mixture of quinidine and molasses as a paste in unco-operative animals, but oral ulceration can occur because of the direct effect of the drug on the mucous membranes.

Contraindications for treatment It should be remembered that quinidine treatment is *contraindicated in cases of CHF*. The hypotensive and negatively inotropic effects of quinidine can be fatal to horses with CHF. Where there is a resting heart rate above 60 bpm, it is imperative to lower the heart rate with digoxin before quinidine is used. Few animals with a resting heart rate of >60 bpm are likely to be suitable for treatment even if the rate can be reduced. Because the long-term outlook for these animals is almost invariably poor, treatment is unlikely to be worthwhile. The exception to this rule would be animals with myocardial disease which may resolve. Even in this situation, a wiser course of action would be to control signs with the judicious dosage of digoxin and frusemide rather than risk the use of quinidine.

Intravenous use of quinidine gluconate for treatment of AF Where quinidine gluconate is available, it can be used to convert animals with AF to sinus rhythm. It appears to be most successful in horses which have been in AF for only a few days. The ease and speed of administration mean that it has some practical advantages compared to the use of quinidine sulphate. Side-effects are reported to be uncommon, provided that appropriate cases are selected.

Intravenous boluses of quinidine gluconate (0.5–1.0 mg/kg) are given at ten-minute intervals until conversion, or until a total dose of 10 mg/kg is reached.

Prevention of reversion to atrial fibrillation Most horses that have no underlying heart disease and which return to sinus rhythm during the initial titration period are unlikely to relapse into AF. However, there are steps which can be taken to determine which animals are in danger of reversion and which may need further managemental or therapeutic procedures.

It is important to consider conditions which might predispose to the development of AF at the time of treatment. The most common predisposing abnormality is thought to be the presence of an irritant focus in the atrial myocardium which results in APCs. APCs may trigger AF if they occur at a critical time during repolarisation. They may be more common in animals that have a recent history of respiratory disease, possibly due to a myocarditis. APCs may be detected by auscultation or standard ECG analysis after successful treatment of AF; however, they are more likely to be found by monitoring cardiac rhythm using a Holter monitor at rest and by radiotelemetry during exercise. Animals with APCs should be rested for at least a month and may need treatment with digoxin and/or corticosteroids (see above). After this period the ECGs should be repeated to see if the frequency of the APCs has decreased to a level where a return to work is advisable. If Holter monitoring is not available, a history of recent respiratory disease may be sufficient indication to rest the horse for 1–2 months after treatment in order to decrease the risk of reversion to AF. Animals without evidence of APCs may be returned to light work approximately 3 days after treatment and to full training after 7–10 days.

Electrolyte imbalance, particularly hypokalaemia, may also predispose animals to the development of AF. In animals in which AF recurs, electrolytes levels should be measured prior to repeat treatment and if necessary at intervals following treatment. Electrolyte analysis is also worthwhile in animals known or suspected to suffer from paroxysmal AF. Plasma or serum levels can be measured; however, there is some controversy about their value. Measurement of urinary fractional excretion of potassium can also be used to detect underlying potassium depletion (see section 2.2.6). Deficiencies can be treated by supplementation of the diet with potassium.

7.8.6 Paroxysmal atrial fibrillation

In some horses, AF occurs for a short period of time before sinus rhythm returns without treatment. This usually occurs during exercise. When sinus rhythm is reestablished within 24 hours this is termed paroxysmal atrial fibrillation. Paroxysmal AF can result in a significant reduction in performance during exercise. In racehorses, the usual pattern is for a sudden tailing-off from the rest of the field. In some cases, epistaxis and ataxia are seen. It can be difficult to establish the diagnosis in these cases because the paroxysm has often resolved by the time that a veterinary examination is performed. Horses with this history need a thorough examination for all potential causes of poor athletic performance (see section 8.2). Radiotelemetry is a very useful aid to detecting paroxysmal AF itself, or APCs which may predispose to AF. However, it not always possible to reproduce the clinical signs seen on the track and a presumptive diagnosis may have to be made. In horses in which repeated paroxysmal AF is suspected, trainers should be encouraged to seek a veterinary examination directly after the end of the race if the horse unexpectedly tails-off.

It is unclear how many horses have repeated bouts of paroxysmal AF. Many animals which have an episode of paroxysmal AF do not have repeated episodes even without treatment or rest. In most cases in which paroxysmal AF is suspected, no specific treatment can be given because of the restrictions on the use of drugs in animals in competition. Even if treatment of horses during competition was permitted, it would be difficult to ensure that paroxysmal AF did not occur. Therefore, in animals in which it occurs repeatedly, possible predisposing factors should be assessed. Valvular heart disease is a significant factor and, if present, carries a poor prognosis because there is no treatment. The most common predisposing factors are atrial myocardial disease (usually a myocarditis) and electrolyte imbalance. These should be evaluated in the same way as for persistent AF. Other conditions which reduce performance and may put extra pressure on the horse at exercise may also be important. For example, if respiratory disease has been present but is managed appropriately, paroxysmal AF may not recur. Upper airway obstruction may be a complicating factor in some cases and if corrected may make paroxysmal AF less likely to recur.

7.8.7 Pre-excitation syndromes

Pre-excitation syndromes, including the electrocardiographic equivalent of Wolff–Parkinson–White syndrome, (a well-recognised condition in humans), have been reported in a number of horses. These syndromes are associated with an abnormal conduction pathway which bypasses the AV node. This is recognised electrocardiographically by a short PR interval and a wide QRS complex, with a small notch at the initial portion of the complex (a delta wave). The clinical significance of the condition is unclear. In some animals it may not be associated with any clinical signs and is only detected if an ECG is recorded. In other animals, the aberrant conduction pathway may allow re-entrant supraventricular tachydysrhythmias to develop.

7.8.8 Ventricular premature complexes

Clinical examination and electrocardiography

VPCs are caused by abnormal impulses originating in the ventricular myocardium. Because they are premature they disturb the R–R interval, resulting in an irregular rhythm. Auscultation will reveal an early beat, usually followed by a longer than normal (compensatory) diastolic pause. The intensity of S1 may be greater than normal, and S2 may be relatively quiet, depending on the duration of diastole. Often a pulse deficit will be palpated.

VPCs are ectopic and do not follow the normal conduction pathways; therefore, the resultant QRS complex differs from normal. However, the normal range of QRS complex duration is quite variable in horses (0.08–0.14 sec) and the duration of a VPC may not exceed this value. VPCs may therefore have to be distinguished from sinus beats on the grounds that they have an abnormal configuration QRS complex (Figure 7.10). If the ventricular origin QRS morphology varies, the condition is described as multiform. This may mean that there are multiple ectopic foci (multifocal VPCs) or that conduction from one ectopic focus is variable. Two other features can also be useful to identify VPCs. The T wave is widened, larger and of opposite polarity to the QRS complex. In addition, a VPC is almost always followed by a full compensatory pause. The sinus beat which occurs fractionally after the VPC is not conducted because the ventricles are refractory, but the following sinus beat is conducted in the usual way. This means that the short diastolic interval which indicates a premature beat is followed by a longer diastolic interval, with an R′–R interval which is greater than the normal R–R interval. This can be a useful guide when a premature beat is auscultated because APCs are seldom followed by a compensatory pause. However, an ECG is always required to make a definitive diagnosis. Occasionally a VPC occurs between two normal QRS complexes without disrupting the R–R interval, in which case it is called an interpolated beat.

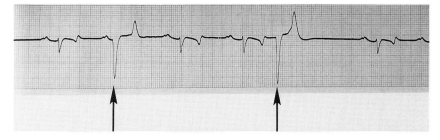

Fig. 7.10 Ventricular premature complexes.
Two VPCs are present (*arrowed*). These have a greater amplitude and duration than the normal sinus beats (recorded at 0.5 cm/mV). The first is preceded by a P wave, but the P–R duration is too short for it to have been responsible for the ventricular depolarisation. The second VPC is followed by a full compensatory pause.

The significance of VPCs

VPCs are relatively uncommon in horses in comparison with other species. However, the presence of an occasional, isolated VPC is not necessarily abnormal and is found in a few apparently normal individuals during a 24-hour ECG recording. If no other abnormalities are detected, the abnormal beat may be of no significance. However, detection of even a single VPC should alert the clinician to the possibility of myocardial disease and a thorough investigation should be performed. In some animals, the frequency of the VPCs may increase during exercise. This may be associated with poor athletic performance or even collapse. However, in a few cases, a normal increase in the sinus rate during exercise will result in abolition of the VPCs, if they have a slow intrinsic rate which is overridden by a raised sinus rate. In this instance, the VPCs are unlikely to limit performance. Radiotelemetry and 24-hour ECG recording may be useful to assess the significance of the arrhythmia.

Ectopic foci which cause VPCs can result from primary myocardial disease or from the effects of systemic disease on a normal myocardium. Investigation should be aimed at detecting underlying cardiac or systemic disease. If myocardial disease is the cause this may involve just a small focal lesion or the whole of the myocardium may be involved. Echocardiography may be required in order to identify underlying heart disease. Systemic disease may be evident on clinical examination. Routine biochemistry and haematology may also be helpful.

Management and treatment of horses with VPCs

Treatment is aimed at reversing the underlying condition in the first instance; only if clinical signs at rest are severe should antidysrhythmic drugs be used. However, specific treatment is seldom possible; the principal treatment is rest. A period of 1–2 months may be sufficient. The horse should then be re-evaluated and, if VPCs are still present, a further period of rest or treatment may be required. If a moderate number of VPCs are occurring (e.g. 1–6 per minute), and an inflammatory myocarditis is suspected, then corticosteroid treatment (as described for treatment of APCs) may be helpful (see Appendix). On some occasions corticosteroids have helped when the VPCs are more frequent or even if they dominate the rhythm.

If VPCs are frequent and constitute a ventricular tachycardia (see below), antidysrhythmic treatment may be required in some cases. Treatment may also be required if there are multiform VPCs, or if R-on-T phenomenon is observed (when the QRS complex of the VPC coincides with the T wave of the previous complex). The judgement of whether to treat or not is primarily dependent on the clinical condition of the horse. If the animal is weak then treatment is more likely to be required.

The drug of choice is quinidine gluconate given intravenously. Quinidine sulphate can be given by stomach tube if this is not available. Lignocaine can also be used to treat ventricular tachycardias, although it has the potential to cause neurological side-effects including seizures. In fact, this problem is seldom encountered and, if quinidine gluconate is not available, lignocaine (without adrenaline) can be used, particularly if the arrhythmia occurs during general anaesthesia. Monitoring of the ECG is advisable during the course of treatment of ventricular tachydysrhythmias.

In the majority of horses with VPCs, antidysrhythmic drugs are not required. If treatment is needed, great caution should be used because these drugs are negative inotropes. If widespread cardiac disease with poor myocardial contractility is detected, lignocaine may be preferable to quinidine because it is less likely to precipitate a profound fall in blood pressure. If the condition can be managed by box rest and reversal of underlying disease, this is preferable.

7.8.9 Ventricular tachycardia

Ventricular tachycardia is defined as four or more VPCs in succession. It may be paroxysmal or sustained (Figures 7.11 and 7.12). Ventricular tachycardia nearly always indicates the presence of serious underlying disease. Non-conducted P waves may be seen or may be hidden by the abnormal QRS complexes. Fusion beats (when the depolarisation starts from both the AV node and an ectopic focus simultaneously) or capture beats (when a sinus beat is conducted) may be seen. If no normal QRS complexes are seen it may be difficult to be sure that the QRS complexes are abnormally wide, because there is considerable overlap between the normal range of QRS duration and the QRS duration of ectopic ventricular beats in horses.

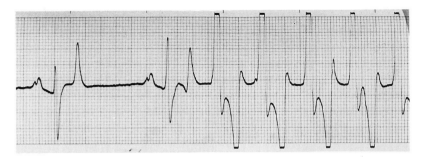

Fig. 7.11 Paroxysmal ventricular tachycardia.
The first two QRS complexes are normal complexes caused by sinus depolarisation (the slight difference in shape is within normal limits). The last five complexes are ventricular in origin (wide and bizarre compared with normal). Abberant conduction of a supra-ventricular tachycardia is unlikely to produce such bizarre complexes in the horse.

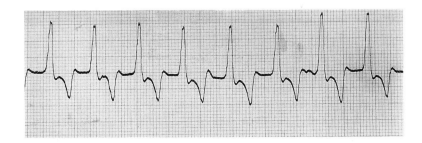

Fig. 7.12 Sutained ventricular tachycardia.
The fact that this recording was made with a conventional base-apex lead and yet has positive QRS complexes is helpful in identifying the rhythm as ventricular in origin. There are no normal QRS complexes with which to compare the width of these complexes; QRS complexes of ventricular origin can be within normal limits for duration in horses. Occasional P waves may be present but have no relation to the QRS complexes.

Auscultation will reveal a rapid rhythm (> ~60 bpm) which is regular in sustained ventricular tachycardia and periodically irregular if paroxysms occur. A weak, variable pulse is palpated. Signs of underlying cardiac or systemic disease may be seen. CHF may be present. Treatment is aimed at reversing underlying disease. Antidysrhythmic drugs may be required in some cases (see above). The prognosis is likely to be unfavourable unless the underlying disease can be resolved. When ventricular tachycardia develops as a result of a primary cardiac condition, it usually indicates severe disease. In this case, the prognosis is likely to be poor. Identification of the primary cause may indicate that euthanasia is the only humane course of action.

7.8.10   Junctional escape beats

A junctional escape beat is a protective mechanism that occurs when there has been no supraventricular stimulus to the ventricles to initiate systole. It is associated with failure of stimulus formation in the SA node (SA arrest) or conduction through the AV node, although the delay must be very marked for an escape beat to occur unless the junctional rate is raised (see below). On auscultation, a long diastolic pause is followed by a loud S1. An arrhythmia will be appreciated. When a junctional escape beat is present, the ECG shows a slow heart rate with a long pause followed by a normal or nearly normal QRS complex. Retrograde P waves may be seen just before, or coincident with the QRS complex.

7.8.11   Junctional escape rhythm

A junctional escape rhythm occurs when the junctional escape beats become regular and persistent because of the lack of SA stimulus or AV block. The rhythm is regular and usually slow. No A sound will be heard if SA arrest is present. The ECG shows a slow heart rate with regular R–R intervals and a normal or nearly normal QRS complexes. Retrograde P waves may be seen. This is a protective mechanism that does not require treatment.

7.8.12   Ventricular escape beats

Ventricular escape beats are similar to junctional escape beats except that the impulse starts within the ventricular myocardium. Because depolarisation does not follow normal pathways, it results in a QRS complex which differs from normal and may be wide and bizarre. A ventricular escape beat is indicative of a failure of the sinoatrial node, atria or junctional tissue to adopt the pacemaker role or of the AV node to conduct a sinus impulse. The escape beat itself is a normal response to the failure of activation and does not require treatment. However, investigation of underlying causes of atrial or junctional disease is advisable. Ventricular escape rhythms have a slow, regular rhythm. The ECG will show an absence of P waves, or non-conducted P waves which have no relationship to the regularly spaced, abnormal QRS complexes.

7.8.13   Accelerated idiojunctional and idioventricular rhythms

Idiojunctional and idioventricular rhythms occur when there is a slow sinoatrial rate but an abnormally high (accelerated) junctional or ventricular rate. The term idioventricular implies that the complexes are ventricular in origin, i.e. they have an abnormal configuration. A similar mechanism can result in an idionodal or idiojunctional rhythm when the complexes arise for the AV node or junctional tissue; this is defined as a supraventricular rhythm and the QRS complexes are normal in configuration. An idioventricular rhythm is a ventricular rhythm with a slow rate (usually of approximately 50 bpm). If the same pattern was seen with a higher rate (> ~60 bpm) the rhythm would be defined as a ventricular tachycardia. P waves occur less frequently than the QRS complexes, are unconducted, and therefore do not bear any relationship to the QRS complex (Figure 7.13). The separation of atrial and ventricular rhythms is called AV dissociation. Occasionally, a P wave is conducted and a normal QRS complex follows at a normal P–R interval (a capture beat). Fusion beats can also be seen when sinus beats are conducted and coincide with depolarisation from the ectopic focus. These are abnormal configuration QRS complexes which occur with a short P–R interval.

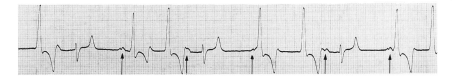

Fig. 7.13 An idioventricular rhythm.
This ECG was recorded from a horse with renal failure. There are pairs of abnormal QRS complexes which bear no relationship to the P waves (*arrowed*) which are also seen. The ventricular rate is 60 bpm so the idio-ventricular rhythm can be described as accelerated, while the sinus rate is 40 bpm. The small QRS complexes are capture beats with a P wave buried in the previous T wave. (Courtesy of Mark Hillyer)

Accelerated junctional or ventricular rhythms are most commonly seen in association with severe systemic disease, for example in horses after colic surgery where there is high vagal tone (and hence a low sinus rate, or AV block), but increased levels of catecholamines which raise the intrinsic junctional or ventricular rate from their normal level of approximately 8–20 bpm. Occasionally, idioventricular or idiojunctional rhythms occur during anaesthesia. The rate of the arrhythmia is usually normal or just greater than normal (40–50 bpm), so it has relatively little direct effect on cardiac function. Once the systemic disease has resolved, the rhythm usually returns to normal sinus rhythm. There is therefore usually no requirement to treat these rhythms, but the ECG and cardiovascular status should be closely monitored. However the systemic disease should be reversed if possible and this may require aggressive treatment.

7.8.14 *Ventricular fibrillation (VF)*

Ventricular fibrillation (VF) is usually a terminal event in which there are no organised ventricular depolarisations or contractions. It is associated with increased myocardial irritability, usually caused by severe systemic or cardiac disease. Auscultation reveals no clear heart sounds. There is no palpable pulse. The ECG shows baseline undulations with no QRS complexes, or P or T waves (Figure 7.14).

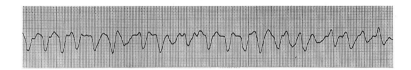

Fig. 7.14 Ventricular fibrillation.
This ECG was recorded from a foal with a ruptured bladder before the electrolyte imbalance
could be corrected. There is random movement of the baseline with no identifiable QRS
complexes. (Courtesy of Dr Celia Marr)

Intravenous lignocaine and support is needed immediately, but is seldom
successful in the horse. Administration of adrenaline is not sufficient to reverse
the arrhythmia. Electrical defibrillation is not practicable usually in the adult
horse, although it has been used successfully in small ponies. VF is almost
invariably fatal despite treatment.

7.8.15 Bradydysrhythmias

Bradydysrhythmias due to cardiac disease are very uncommon in horses. Syncope or weakness are the principal signs associated with these arrhythmias if
they are sufficiently severe.

Profound second degree heart block
In rare situations, prolonged periods of 2°AV block which are not abolished by
increasing sympathetic tone may occur and these may cause clinical signs. It may
be helpful to use radiotelemetry, or a 24-hour Holter monitor and timed
observations, to see if syncopal attacks coincide with periods of severe AV block.
Unfortunately, the intervals between these attacks are often very long and it may
not be possible to monitor the horse for prolonged periods. Occasionally the
arrhythmia may be related to an abnormally high vagal tone caused by extracardiac disease, in which case atropine may abolish the block. If AV node disease
is present, atropine will have little effect on heart rate or the AV block.

If 2°AVB is accompanied by syncope or weakness, an artificial pacemaker
may be required. If it occurs in an anaesthetised animal and leads to a marked
drop in blood pressure, anticholinergic drugs can be administered, and dopamine or dobutamine can be used to raise cardiac output and increase vascular
tone. However, sometimes the use of these catecholamines can in itself induce
AV block because of the baroreceptor mechanism.

Third degree AV block
Third degree AV block (complete heart block) is a condition in which the AV
node does not conduct any sinus impulses. The ventricles are 'rescued' by a
regular slow rate resulting from a junctional or ventricular escape rhythm.
Auscultation reveals regular ventricular contraction with A sounds heard during
the diastolic intervals. Jugular venous pulses may be seen at the atrial rate, with
cannon A waves occurring when atrial and ventricular contraction coincide. The
heart rate may be as low as 12–20 bpm. The ECG will show normal P waves
which do not bear any relationship to the escape complexes (Figure 7.15). There

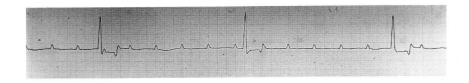

Fig. 7.15 Third degree atrioventricular block.
Regular P waves (rate 100/min) are seen with three ventricular escape complexes (rate 18/min). There is no relationship between the P waves and R waves, the P waves being completely blocked at the AV node. (Courtesy of Ian Crowe)

is usually a regular R–R interval between these escape complexes. The escape complexes are most likely to be junctional (and therefore appear normal or nearly normal) but may be ventricular (and therefore appear different from junctional beats, although they may not be particularly wide or bizarre). In a few cases ventricular tachydysrhythmias are thought to develop and further compromise cardiac output.

The condition is invariably pathological and carries a grave prognosis. Occasionally it is reversible, but this is probably the exception. It is exceptionally rare. Investigation should centre on identifying underlying disease. However, a specific cause is seldom found. Treatment consists of box rest and reversal of any underlying systemic or heart disease if possible. If no underlying disease is found or treatment is unsuccessful, an artificial pacemaker is required. Pacemakers have been successfully used in horses, but this requires specialist equipment and expertise. Reports are limited because severe bradyarrhythmias are very rare. With so little experience of their use in horses, it would be unwise to comment on their long-term value and possible complications.

Chapter 8

Problems in Equine Cardiology

8.1 The pre-purchase examination

8.1.1 General considerations

Cardiac murmurs and arrhythmias are frequently detected at a pre-purchase examination and may be a cause of concern for the examining veterinary surgeon. Most often, normal functional murmurs and physiological arrhythmias, which have no bearing on the suitability of the animal for any athletic use, will be present. On other occasions, the findings may indicate the presence of underlying pathology which may or may not have a significant effect on the horse's future use.

At a pre-purchase examination, a veterinary surgeon is asked for an opinion regarding the suitability of an animal for a specified intended purpose. This is a matter of judgement; there are no hard and fast rules. Ideally, the judgement can be given in terms of the degree of risk that prospective purchasers would be taking if they bought the horse. However, the existing system means that the animal has to be recommended as suitable or unsuitable for whatever purpose, taking the specific findings into consideration. Obviously, veterinarians are concerned about the possibility of litigation if a problem ensues and someone else does not agree with their opinion.

The principal concerns at a pre-purchase examination are the future athletic performance of the animal and its safety as a riding animal. The veterinarian should make a reasoned judgement about the significance of cardiac disease depending on individual circumstances. One is not asked to give 100% guarantees, and this should be made clear. To regard all animals with cardiac murmurs or arrhythmias as unsuitable for purchase would not be in the interests of prospective purchasers. If the clinical approach is sound, the findings are accurately recorded and the situation fully explained, then the best interests of all are served. The ground rules for the pre-purchase examination are therefore similar to those in the clinical evaluation of an animal which is presented for poor performance or other clinical signs which may relate to heart disease; the essential step is to establish a *specific diagnosis*. This can normally be based on careful examination and auscultation (Chapter 3). Sometimes, further diagnostic aids such as echocardiography and electrocardiography may be required to confirm a diagnosis and aid judgement of the severity of the condition. Unfortunately, less emphasis can reliably be placed on the clinical history at pre-purchase than during a conventional examination.

Once it has been established that a pathological process is present, the next step is to determine the significance of the problem. This primarily depends on the extent to which cardiovascular function is affected. However, at a pre-purchase examination it also depends on the level of athletic activity which the horse is likely to perform and the specific requirements of the potential purchaser. Seldom do two owners have exactly the same requirements.

8.1.2 Questions regarding the intended use of the animal

There are a number of questions regarding the intended use of the horse which are particularly important. These are summarised in Table 8.1. The horse's recent performance history may be a helpful guide if it is given on reliable authority, particularly if it is documented through the results of competition. It is also important to establish whether, in the future, the horse will be required to perform similar work to its present use or whether future athletic demands will be more arduous. Early tiring is much the most likely presenting sign in animals with valvular heart disease. Cardiac abnormalities present a hazard to safety when animals tire and then fall or take a bad step. If a valvular abnormality is present, the greatest risk is taken in expecting the horse to do more arduous work than it already performs.

Table 8.1 Summary: Evaluation of the cardiovascular system at pre-purchase examination

- Establish a specific diagnosis
  General clinical examination
  Auscultation
  Diagnostic aids such as electrocardiography
- Is the finding an abnormality resulting from pathological change or a physiological variant?
- What effect if any is the abnormality having on the horse at the present time? (The horse's recent performance history may be a helpful guide if it is given on reliable authority)
- Was there any evidence of lack of physical fitness during the exercise stage of the examination? Did the heart rate return to normal within a suitable period of time? Bear in mind the likely fitness of the animal depending on the circumstances of training and expected level of fitness
- Is the horse required to perform similar work in the future or will future athletic demands be more arduous?
- How long will the animal be used by the prospective purchaser?
- Does the prospective purchaser wish to insure the horse?
- Is the prospective purchaser likely to want to sell the horse in the near future?
- How experienced a rider is expected to ride the animal?

It is pertinent to consider how long the animal will be used by the prospective purchaser. This is an important consideration because if the animal is likely to be sold on, the same finding may be made at a subsequent purchase examination resulting in difficulty in making a sale, or a reduction in value.

Another important question is whether the prospective purchaser intends to insure the horse. If significant clinical findings are made, exclusion clauses may be placed on future insurance or the owners may be unable to obtain cover. It is worthwhile pointing this out to prospective purchasers.

A final and difficult question concerns the experience of the prospective rider. If a horse with a recognised cardiac problem which may result in poor exercise tolerance is ridden by an inexperienced rider, they may fail to recognise that the horse is getting unacceptably tired and continue riding when it would be wise to stop. Animals with conditions such as mitral regurgitation may be unsuitable for these riders.

8.1.3 Findings at the pre-purchase examination

Resting phase

If a murmur or an arrhythmia which is classified as functional is detected during the initial examination, no further steps need be taken. However, if a murmur is pan or holosystolic or holodiastolic, it is likely to result from a pathological process and needs further, careful evaluation. The vital part of the examination is therefore to decide whether a murmur is associated with a pathological process or is functional in origin (Table 3.4).

If the resting heart rate is elevated (> 45 per minute), cardiac disease should be suspected unless another cause is detected. It is therefore very important that a true resting heart rate is recorded. Animals with a loud heart murmur (grade 4 or greater) and a tachycardia, are unlikely to be suitable for purchase under any circumstances. However, assessment of the severity of pathological murmurs often requires further investigation such as echocardiography.

The period of time that a murmur has been known to be present can be a useful guide to the rate of progression and may be helpful during a pre-purchase examination if such information is reliable. A condition which has been present for some months or years with no deterioration is less likely to deteriorate rapidly after purchase. This is, however, only a guideline.

The exercise phase

The exercise section of the pre-purchase examination is often fraught with difficulty. Ideally the animal should be put through arduous work in surroundings which allow this to be performed safely. Often circumstances are far from ideal. In particular, lunging animals as an alternative to ridden exercise is to be avoided if possible because it is seldom possible to raise the heart rate to maximal levels. Some arrhythmias occur during the post-exercise period and may be confused with pathological arrhythmias. These are particularly common following submaximal exercise (see below).

The effect of exercise on cardiac murmurs is often taken as a useful guide to significance. This rule of thumb should be avoided if possible, as it is often used as an alternative to making a specific diagnosis of the source of a murmur. Murmurs which are functional in origin are variable at different heart rates and may become less apparent after exercise. However, mild or moderate intensity murmurs of valvular regurgitation, which may have an important bearing on future use, cannot always be heard easily under the conditions of a post-exercise examination. In addition, some functional murmurs become louder after exercise (see section 3.8.2).

During the exercise phase of the examination, it is very difficult to judge whether the level of physical fitness is affected by underlying heart disease or by the amount of training which the horse has been given. Guidelines for the expected heart rates at different gaits and expected rate of recovery to resting heart rates are given in section 3.8.3. However, a standardised exercise test cannot be performed during a pre-purchase examination, so the onus is on interpretation of the level of fitness, taking all factors into consideration, before any inference is drawn regarding the effects of cardiac disease.

8.1.4 Conditions resulting in a cardiac murmur

Mitral regurgitation

Murmurs thought to indicate the presence of mitral regurgitation (MR) are potentially the greatest cause for concern because they are often associated with poor athletic performance and even congestive heart failure. The significance of mitral regurgitation was described in detail in section 6.2.5. As a general rule, if a murmur of MR is quiet (grade 1 or 2) and localised, it is seldom a significant problem at the time of examination (even in high performance horses). However, the progression of the condition is difficult to predict and therefore there is some degree of risk involved in purchasing the animal, although it may be relatively small in some circumstances. The best way to predict the likely course of the disease is to examine the animal again in a few months time, and if possible to perform serial echocardiographic examinations. However, this is not always possible. The owner's intended use of the horse is also relevant because the longer the period over which they expect good performance, the greater the possibility of deterioration.

If a murmur of MR is grade 3/6 or greater, is widespread, or if there is any suggestion of poor exercise tolerance, echocardiography offers the best prospect of evaluating the severity of the condition. Whether this is performed will depend on the particular owner and prospective purchaser, but unless the animal is of little financial value it is well worthwhile even if this requires referral. Any signs of volume overload indicate that the condition is haemodynamically significant. Some purchasers may be able to take a risk with horses in the early stages of volume overload, because they may perform satisfactorily, particularly for activities such as dressage, show-jumping and hacking, while having moderate degrees of MR. If MR is associated with significant volume overload, pathological arrhythmias, or a resting tachycardia, purchase should not usually be recommended.

Mitral valve prolapse may have a better prognosis than degenerative mitral valve disease. If a murmur is thought to be due to prolapse, and preferably this assumption is backed up by echocardiographic evidence, a better prognosis for future athletic use is usually warranted.

Tricuspid regurgitation

Tricuspid regurgitation (TR) is a common finding in fit National Hunt racehorses, when it is seldom the cause of poor athletic performance. It may also be relatively common in other large fit horses. However, in some horses TR may affect performance and, in extreme cases, may even result in congestive heart failure.

When TR is detected at a pre-purchase examination it should be recorded on the examination form. In large, fit horses, if there is no suggestion of limited performance or other problems, it is probably acceptable to state that localised murmurs of TR are unlikely to be associated with sufficient regurgitation to prevent the animal's use for athletic activity. Judgement should be circumspect in other types of animal. The best method of estimating the significance of the finding is to perform an echocardiographic examination. Echocardiography is recommended if TR is detected in animals which are seldom affected such as horses under the age of 4, pleasure horses and ponies and, ideally, for accurate evaluation in racehorses.

Aortic regurgitation

Aortic regurgitation (AR) is a common finding in the older horse, although it may be found in animals as young as 4 years of age, or even in association with congenital heart disease. The intensity of a murmur of AR is a very poor guide to its significance. However, the resting heart rate and arterial pulse quality are useful guides in advanced disease. The best method of estimating the significance of AR is to perform an echocardiographic examination. Unless there are signs of volume overload, the animal may be suitable for athletic use (see section 6.5.3). Since loud heart murmurs are an obvious cause for concern, an echocardiographic evaluation is often of benefit for the vendor and prospective purchaser. Without this examination, perfectly useful horses will be turned down at pre-purchase examinations. The guidelines for monitoring the progression of AR are the same as for MR. If AR is associated with MR, or significant pathological arrhythmias are present, purchase should not usually be recommended.

Congenital disease

Animals with complex congenital heart disease are unsuitable for riding or breeding. However, animals with small ventricular septal defects (VSDs) may perform normally and may be suitable for sale for all but the most arduous activities. Unless signs of heart failure are present, the severity of a VSD is difficult to judge from clinical examination alone; they are nearly always associated with a murmur of grade 5 or 6/6 irrespective of the size of the defect (see section 5.5.3). The best method of estimating the significance of a VSD is to perform an echocardiographic examination. Two-dimensional echocardiography and Doppler echocardiography are very useful for assessing severity and guiding prognostication. Prospective purchasers of animals with a VSD should be informed that these animals are not suitable for breeding and that congenital lesions are often excluded from the conditions of insurance policies.

Summary

A guiding rule is that on the few occasions when a murmur is detected but a specific diagnosis cannot be made from accurate auscultation, a specialist opinion should be sought if the prospective purchasers wish to proceed. If the regurgitant murmur is relatively quiet it may not be relevant at the time of examination, but it may be important at some point in the future. If a murmur is relatively loud and the client is still interested in purchase, then an echocardiographic examination is worthwhile in order to quantify the degree of volume overload if any, and to give as accurate a prognosis as possible.

8.1.5 *Arrhythmias*

The same principles apply to arrhythmias detected at a pre-purchase examination as to murmurs, namely that a specific diagnosis of the type of arrhythmia should be made. Physiological arrhythmias include second-degree atrioventricular block (2°AVB) and sinus block. 2°AVB is the most common vagally mediated arrhythmia and is usually characteristic at rest with predictable periods of sinus beats followed by a blocked beat, during which an atrial contraction sound can usually be heard in the absence of S1 and S2. The arrhythmia disappears when the heart rate is raised by exercise or excitement (see section 7.7.2). Sinus block may also be identified at rest and is abolished by increased sympathetic tone. These vagally mediated arrhythmias are of no significance for the purposes of purchase.

If abnormal arrhythmias are noted, the most significant considerations are their rate and any evidence of underlying cardiac disease.

Atrial fibrillation

Atrial fibrillation (AF) is a relatively common cause of poor athletic performance. Animals with AF are not suitable for sale as performance animals. Some animals can perform less arduous work normally while in AF, particularly if there is no underlying heart disease. These animals may be suitable for some forms of activity. The resting heart rate, heart rate during exercise, and the significance of any underlying valvular and myocardial disease should all be investigated if animals with atrial fibrillation are to be ridden (see section 7.8.5). However, purchase of any animal with AF is a risk, even though they may perform normally in the short-term for relatively undemanding events such as dressage, show-jumping and hacking.

Atrial premature complexes

Occasional premature beats are a relatively common clinical finding and present a difficult problem at a pre-purchase examination because occasional atrial premature beats (APCs) can occur in normal horses. APCs result in the first heart sound (S1) being detected earlier than expected. It may also be louder than with sinus beats. APC are not usually followed by a compensatory pause (see section 7.8.3).

APCs are usually more frequent after exercise and if they are numerous during this period horses may not be suitable for athletic use until the arrhythmia has resolved. An ECG may be required to distinguish APCs from vagally mediated arrhythmias during the period of autonomic imbalance as it may not be possible to distinguish them on auscultation alone. Runs of APCs are more likely to be clinically significant than those which occur intermittently or cyclically. As a rough guide, 1–3 APCs per minute would prompt further investigation, without which purchase should not be recommended. If more than 3–10 APCs per minute are detected, the horse should not be recommended for purchase until the arrhythmia has resolved. This may need to be supported by radiotelemetric and 24-hour Holter recordings in order to ensure that the arrhythmia is not occurring intermittently (see section 7.8.3).

Premature ventricular complexes

Premature ventricular complexes (VPCs) are most commonly found in animals with myocardial disease, severe systemic disease or marked electrolyte imbalances. Animals in the second of these categories are unlikely to be subject to a pre-purchase examination. Occasional VPCs may be detected in normal animals. However, since the period of auscultation during a pre-purchase examination is relatively short, if a premature beat is detected, purchase should not be recommended without further investigation.

VPCs are recognised by auscultation of an early beat, in which S1 is often relatively loud, and are usually followed by a full compensatory pause (see section 7.8.8). An ECG, echocardiogram and laboratory investigations may be justified if more than the occasional beat is detected, should the prospective purchasers wish to pursue the case. If these tests show that there is no evidence of underlying heart disease or systemic disease, re-examination in a few months time might be worthwhile. Otherwise, purchase should not be recommended until the condition has resolved, if it does so. If VPCs are frequent or multiform, the animal is unlikely to be suitable for purchase. If exercise results in an increased frequency athletic use should be curtailed and purchase should not be recommended. Some VPCs will be absent once the sinus node rate increases above a certain level. These are less likely to be significant, although they may be sufficient cause for concern to prevent purchase because the arrhythmia could deteriorate. Exercise ECGs and 24-hour recordings are useful for assessing the significance of VPCs if further investigations are considered (see section 7.8.8).

Post-exercise arrhythmias

Arrhythmias commonly occur in the immediate post-exercise period, while the heart rate slows, and can be a cause for concern. If exercise has been submaximal, there may still be sufficient vagal tone present for vagally mediated arrhythmias to be detected. The period is therefore known as a phase of 'autonomic imbalance'. Post-exercise transient sinus arrhythmia is a well-recognised rhythm; sometimes 2°AVB also is present during this period (see section 7.7.2). A wandering pacemaker may be detected during the sinus arrhythmia and it may be difficult to determine whether this indicates the presence of an APC, or is due to a change in the position of origin of the impulse within the sinus node. If these APCs/wandering sinus beats occur periodically, in a cyclical manner, they are unlikely to be clinically significant. Occasionally, blocked APCs will be seen. Runs of atrial tachycardia, or frequent APCs would be a cause for concern, and these animals may not be suitable for athletic use until the arrhythmia has resolved (see above).

If arrhythmias are heard during the period of autonomic imbalance during heart rate slowing, they may be abolished by an increased level of exercise. Therefore, if an arrhythmia is detected and an ECG or radiotelemetry cannot be performed, it is sensible to exercise the animal further to see if the arrhythmia resolves. Exercise ECGs and 24-hour recordings may be useful for assessing the significance of arrhythmias detected during the post-exercise section of a pre-purchase examination if further investigation is considered necessary (see sections 4.1.6 and 4.1.8).

8.1.6 Suitability of animals for breeding

Animals with congenital heart disease should not be passed as suitable for breeding purposes because it is possible that these conditions have a hereditary element. At present, there is no evidence that acquired valvular or myocardial disease has a hereditary basis in the horse, although this is sometimes true in other species.

Horses with congestive heart failure may be maintained on suitable treatment to allow them to be used for breeding. Some stallions with severe cardiac disease only show clinical signs when covering mares. However, it would be difficult to recommend a stallion with moderate or severe valvular heart disease for use as a breeding animal. Mares with moderate or severe heart disease may be clinically unaffected in early pregnancy, but often show clinical signs towards the end of pregnancy. These signs may be controllable, with drug treatment if necessary, but further pregnancies cannot be recommended. It would therefore be unwise to recommend the purchase of a mare with moderate to severe volume overload for breeding purposes. Horses with AF but no underlying heart disease may remain useful for breeding for many years.

An echocardiographic examination is advisable before the purchase of breeding animals with valvular heart disease or AF because there is a risk that the breeding life of the animal would be curtailed compared with a normal animal. A full evaluation may show that there is little volume overload and that myocardial function is normal. Under these circumstances, an animal may be a suitable purchase for some owners. Insurance may be problematic for the purchasers of valuable breeding animals with cardiac disease. Specialist examination and an echocardiographic examination may be required before an underwriter will take on such cases, and it is worthwhile investigating this problem before the purchase of a valuable animal.

The significance of cardiac disease detected at a pre-purchase is summarised in Table 8.2.

8.2 Poor athletic performance

There are many causes of poor athletic performance. Many owners expect great results from their horse, particularly if they have made a substantial financial investment, and often animals are presented for examination because they have failed to achieve the owner's hopes. Therefore, one of the first requirements, when examining a horse presented for disappointing performance, is to establish whether there has been a recent loss of proven form, or whether the animal has never performed as the owners hoped. Only one animal will win a race and the others usually do not do so because they are not good enough on the day! It may be that the horse has not been trained appropriately, or that it has been entered for the wrong event. It may be very difficult to explain to owners that their horses lack ability.

Table 8.2 Summary: Interpretation of findings at pre-purchase examinations

Murmur detected

Functional heart murmur
(Early–mid systolic ejection-type with PMI over the left base, early diastolic high-pitched murmurs and pre-systolic murmurs, variable intensity at different heart rates.) No bearing on future use

MR, quiet and localised
Unlikely to be relevant in the near future but may deteriorate over future months or years. Consider follow-up examination or purchase on approval, if vendors/purchasers allow

MR, grade 3 or greater or widespread
Advise against purchase for athletic use unless echocardiogram shows no volume overload. If echocardiogram satisfactory consider potential rate of deterioration

AR any grade, normal pulse quality
Echocardiogram is helpful before an accurate prognosis can be given

AR, bounding pulse quality
Advise against purchase

TR, fit National Hunt horse
Echocardiography advisable, but many perform well

TR, other types of horse
Best evaluated echocardiographically if intended for athletic use

VSD
Not suitable for breeding, not suitable for athletic use unless restrictive size, normal RV volume, and normal IVS motion detected on echocardiography. Unlikely to be suitable for top flight performance

Arrhythmia detected

Arrhythmia diagnosed as 2°AVB or other vagally mediated arrhythmia
No bearing on future use

Post-exercise arrhythmia, identified as vagally mediated or cyclical
Increase level of exercise and re-examine, or perform ECG if possible
No bearing on future use

Occasional APCs or VPCs
Exercise ECG and 24-hour recording and echocardiography recommended if intended for athletic use

Frequent APCs or VPCs
Not suitable until problem identified and corrected

AF, no evidence of underlying heart disease
Not suitable for athletic use, may be suitable for low intensity work

AF, evidence of underlying heart disease
Not suitable for ridden exercise, unlikely to be suitable for breeding

These difficulties have placed a great deal of pressure on veterinarians to come up with a diagnosis in the poor performance case. Fortunately, this pressure has resulted in an improvement in diagnostic ability due to a greater understanding of equine disease and exercise physiology and to the development of new investigative techniques. No doubt the availability of these specialist investigative techniques will increase. The more widespread availability of high-speed treadmills will undoubtedly improve the proportion of cases in which a definitive diagnosis is reached.

Frequently, the problem in pinpointing the cause of poor athletic performance is that there is not one single condition which is responsible, but that it is due to a combination of minor abnormalities. The investigation of a horse with poor performance therefore requires a thorough examination of all body systems. In a referral centre, a number of different specialists may be involved in the examination. Even when a problem is identified, other systems should be investigated so that other problems are not missed. One of the difficulties in interpreting statistical analysis performed on case records by specialist centres is that the numbers are biased by the referral case load, the facilities available and the fields of interest of the clinicians involved.

Cardiovascular disease is often suspected as a cause of poor athletic performance in horses. Because so many horses have arrhythmias and murmurs which are physiological it is very important that these are not mistaken for signs of significant heart disease and used to explain poor performance. In the UK, musculo–skeletal disease, upper airway obstruction and lower airway disease are more common causes of poor athletic performance than cardiac disease. These diseases will be discussed briefly so that they can be considered when evaluating animals in which cardiac disease is suspected to be the cause of poor performance. More detailed descriptions are found in articles listed in the reading list.

8.2.1 Musculo–skeletal disease

Musculo–skeletal disease is probably an under-diagnosed cause of poor performance. Although lameness is usually recognised, some animals will win races or be placed when, under close examination, they are slightly lame. This is not to say that they would not do better if they were sound.

Horses with a unilateral lameness are unlikely to be presented as a poor performance case because this is usually apparent to the trainer or jockey. However, in some cases it will have been overlooked, or will have been dismissed as unimportant. Some animals may only be lame at high speeds and this may be difficult to detect without examination on a treadmill. Bilateral lameness is a common cause of poor athletic performance and it is frequently overlooked. This may be particularly true in young racehorses which have bilateral injury due to poor adaptation to stresses placed on bone. Careful clinical examination may detect changes suggestive of stress fracture of the dorsal metacarpus, but is less likely to detect remodelling changes in the proximal sesamoid bones or third carpal bone. Scintigraphy is particularly useful in demonstrating areas of high bone turnover in these cases. However, there is no clear demarcating margin between extremes of normal bone remodelling and a skeletal abnormality which is a cause of pain. The more widespread use of scintigraphy will no doubt increase the rate at which musculo–skeletal causes of poor performance are detected.

Myopathies

Myopathies are recognised to be a cause of lameness, stiffness, and poor performance. However, they are perhaps under-diagnosed in the latter category. Measurement of plasma CK before exercise and 6 hours later is usually sufficient to make a diagnosis. AST and LDH assays may help to identify the duration of the injury, or detect previous injury, because their levels decline more slowly than CK, which peaks after six hours. AST levels peak around 24 hours and may remain high for 7 days; LDH peaks within 12 hours and remains high for around 7 days. LDH is much less specific for muscle damage than CK or AST.

Aorto–iliac thrombosis

Aorto–iliac thrombosis is an uncommon cause of poor athletic performance, but should be considered in those animals which show hindlimb gait abnormalities after exercise (see section 6.10.5).

8.2.2 Upper respiratory disease

A large, clear airway is an essential requirement for athletic function. Static or dynamic obstructions of the upper airway are a common cause of poor athletic performance. Static obstructions are easily observed endoscopically at rest. To visualise a dynamic obstruction, endoscopy is best performed with the horse exercising on a treadmill.

History

Upper airway obstructions result in abnormal respiratory sounds at exercise. It is therefore important that the rider is carefully questioned about respiratory noise even in a horse which is presented for poor athletic performance which is suspected to be due to a cardiac problem. The way in which animals perform during a race can also be important in reaching a diagnosis. Most horses with heart disease start the race well and then fade. Occasionally they will stop suddenly, but this history should also suggest the possibility of a dorsal displacement of the soft palate (DDSP).

Clinical examination

Clinical examination of the poor performance horse should include careful palpation of the larynx. Evidence of atrophy of the dorsal cricoarytenoideus muscle is suggestive of a significant degree of recurrent laryngeal neuropathy (RLN). Exercise may be required to reproduce an abnormal respiratory noise which has been noted by the owners, for the benefit of the veterinarian.

A roaring or whistling sound is characteristic of RLN. A 'gurgling' noise is characteristic of DDSP, colloquially described as 'choking-up'. Occasionally, other forms of obstruction such as epiglottal entrapment, laryngeal chondritis, fourth brachial arch defects, sub-epiglottic cysts and abnormalities of the alar folds can occur and may produce an abnormal sound.

Endoscopy

The most important aid to the diagnosis of upper airway disease is endoscopy. Endoscopy in the resting horse is usually sufficient for a diagnosis to be made in the majority of cases. Animals with dynamic obstructions require endoscopy on a treadmill or a presumptive diagnosis from the history, clinical signs and description of upper respiratory noise from the jockey. Laryngeal hemiplegia resulting from RLN, nasal chamber obstruction, epiglottic entrapment, laryngeal chondritis and pharyngeal masses such as sub-epiglottic cysts can usually be observed by resting endoscopy. DDSP is often seen during resting endoscopy, but may not be a significant finding unless it is persistent. It is best demonstrated during exercise. If it is found, careful consideration should be given to underlying predisposing factors. Collapse of the pharynx is sometimes observed during exercise. Intermittent epiglottic entrapment has also been observed during treadmill endoscopy.

8.2.3 Lower respiratory tract disease

Lower respiratory tract disease (LRTD) is a common cause of poor athletic performance. While it is well-recognised that respiratory tract infections result in poor performance, lower respiratory tract disease is still under-diagnosed. Reactive small airway disease, which commonly affects animals following respiratory infections, but which is exacerbated by poor air hygiene, is being recognised with increasing frequency.

History

When investigating any case presented for poor athletic performance, careful questioning about incidents of infectious respiratory disease in the individual animal and in other in-contact horses is important. It is also important to ask detailed questions about the stable management and, if necessary, to conduct a review of the stable environment. The type of bedding, feed and ventilation are key factors in the likelihood of allergic small airway disease (COPD) affecting an animal. Even details of the surrounding stables and air hygiene during transportation are important.

Details of how horses perform at exercise are also an important clue to the diagnosis of LRTD. Usually, animals gradually fade, although if the condition results in abnormal pressures within the upper airways it may induce dynamic obstruction with the result that horses suddenly stop. Exercise induced pulmonary haemorrhage (EIPH) is also a common cause of poor performance. This may be evident from the history, although many more horses bleed during a race without blood being seen at the nostrils.

Clinical examination

Few animals are presented for investigation of potential cardiac disease when there is evidence of active respiratory infection. However, many are examined for this reason when they have clinical evidence of allergic small airway disease. Auscultation of lung sounds is an important part of the examination of horses which perform poorly and is greatly aided by the use of a re-breathing bag. A plastic bag such as a large dustbin liner is placed over the nostrils and held tight to produce an airtight seal. The bag should be prevented from occluding the nostrils. This makes the animal breath more deeply and consequently auscultation of abnormal respiratory sounds is easier. Fluid is often heard most clearly over the trachea at the level of the thoracic inlet. Deep breaths are often taken just as the bag is removed and may provide the clearest sounds. Some horses with marked COPD will cough during re-breathing. However, occasionally animals with significant LRTD have no abnormal respiratory sounds.

Diagnostic aids

Clinical pathology   Viral and bacterial respiratory infection may be suspected on the grounds of haematological findings. Paired viral titres and virus isolation are sometimes useful. Readers are referred to the reading list for further details. Culture of bacteria from lower airways is best performed by trans-tracheal lavage or using guarded endoscopic techniques.

Endoscopy Endoscopy is a very helpful diagnostic aid in cases of COPD. Long endoscopes (> 1.5 m) are particularly useful as they can be advanced to the carina. Exudate may be most easily seen after exercise, transportation, or the use of a re-breathing bag. Cytology can be performed from tracheal washes taken via an endoscope, but if bacterial culture is performed, the results should be interpreted in the light of likely contamination by upper airway tract commensals.

Cytology Cytology is best performed on samples obtained by broncho-alveolar lavage, although tracheal wash samples may be sufficient for a diagnosis to be made. The cells should be examined as soon as possible; if this cannot be performed within a few hours the sample should be spun down and a smear made. COPD results in an inflammatory response. Haemosiderin filled macrophages are suggestive of a recent episode of EIPH. Detailed descriptions of cytological findings are found in relevant articles in the reading list.

Bacteriology Bacteriological culture of a tracheal wash should be performed as soon as possible after sampling. BAL samples are unsuitable. The significance of bacterial isolates from wash samples is a matter of some debate at the present time. It appears that, in some horses, LRT bacterial infection may be a more important cause of poor athletic performance than was previously thought. The preferred method of storage and preparation of cytological specimens depends on the laboratory and their advice should be sought prior to submitting samples.

Radiology The utility of radiology for detection of changes associated with COPD is a matter of some debate. Good quality radiographs are essential for meaningful interpretation. A bronchial and interstitial pattern has been regarded as a sign of small airway disease by some clinicians; however, a wide range of radiographic changes are seen in normal animals. If COPD is severe, it may result in small pulmonary vessels due to the raised intra-pulmonary pressure and an increase in interstitial and bronchial markings. Evaluation of these changes is extremely subjective except in severe cases. Exercise induced pulmonary haemorrhage may be evident as an area of increased density in the dorso-caudal extremity of the lung fields.

Nuclear scintigraphy Perfusion and ventilation scans are a useful method of evaluating the distribution of blood and air within the lungs. Both techniques require the use of a large-field gamma camera and a computer. Ventilation scans need additional specialised equipment in order that radionuclides can be delivered to the lung and cleared without contamination of the environment. Aerosols of Technetium 99m are suitable. The technique is primarily a research tool.

Perfusion scans are more easily performed. They may be particularly useful in demonstrating the changes in perfusion of the dorso-caudal lung fields associated with EIPH. However, the technique is probably insufficiently sensitive to be used as a screening technique to detect cases of mild COPD.

Lung function tests   Pulmonary function tests require expensive equipment and an expertise in exercise physiology. They have been used for many years as a research tool, primarily to attempt to quantify the level of fitness of a horse. More recently they have become a useful clinical aid.

The tests are performed on a treadmill. Most horses are able to gallop on a treadmill after two to three days of training. Pulmonary function tests and blood lactate measurement may be helpful in cases in which a diagnosis has not been reached using other diagnostic methods. They seldom provide a definitive diagnosis, but can be helpful to guide the diagnosis and to quantify the approximate level of athletic performance which an animal is capable of producing.

8.2.4 Cardiovascular disease

The effects of different cardiovascular diseases on athletic performance were discussed in the appropriate chapter describing each condition. It is difficult to quantify the cardiovascular effects of heart disease exactly; evaluation of each case is a matter of judgement. As a rule, valvular heart disease is not as common a cause of poor athletic performance as is widely thought. However, arrhythmias which occur during exercise, and which may affect performance, may not be detected without the aid of exercise ECGs and may be under-diagnosed. Echocardiography allows an accurate estimate of the significance of valvular regurgitation in horses which are presented with a history of poor performance.

Mitral regurgitation
MR is the most common valvular condition resulting in poor athletic performance. Localised grade 2/6 murmurs are unlikely to be associated with poor athletic performance, but more widespread and louder murmurs should be regarded with suspicion. Animals with a grade 5/6 murmur of MR are unlikely to perform athletic work normally. Tachycardia and pathological arrhythmias, particularly AF, may be present if marked volume overload results from the valvular incompetence. Animals with moderate or severe MR are likely to start a race normally but tire quickly. Epistaxis is observed in some cases during exercise. After pulling up there is likely to be marked tachycardia and tachypnoea. The recovery period is usually prolonged. Echocardiography is the best method of assessing the severity of grade 3 and 4 murmurs (see section 6.2.6).

Aortic regurgitation
Many horses with AR perform normally. This may be partly accounted for by the fact that it usually affects older horses which often perform lower intensity work than young animals. However, in some circumstances, it may be responsible for poor athletic function. Where a tachycardia or abnormal pulse quality is detected, or when the condition is found in association with significant arrhythmias or MR, it is more likely that performance will be restricted. The murmur associated with AR can be extremely loud (even grade 5 or 6) in horses with normal exercise tolerance. When AR appears to be sudden in onset it is more likely to affect race times. Other causes of poor performance should also be investigated. However,

where other causes do not appear to account for the signs seen, echocardiography and possibly blood pressure measurement are useful guides to severity (see section 6.5.3).

Tricuspid regurgitation

TR is a common finding in National Hunt racehorses which have a normal performance history, or even an excellent racing record. It may therefore be an incidental finding when it is detected in a horse which is presented for poor athletic performance. Other causes of poor performance should be investigated, but when no other significant findings are made, an echocardiographic assessment examination should be performed (see section 6.3.3).

Congenital heart disease

Complex congenital heart disease is incompatible with athletic performance. Small restrictive ventricular septal defects (VSDs) are found in some animals which are able to record useful racing performances, but seldom in the very best athletes. Affected animals may be able to perform less demanding work satisfactorily. Normal right ventricular size, normal interventricular septal motion and a defect of less than 2.0–2.5 cm are good prognostic signs. Doppler echocardiography is very useful; a velocity of greater than 4.0–4.5 m/sec indicates that the defect is likely to be restrictive (see section 5.5.5).

Atrial fibrillation

AF is the most common arrhythmia to cause poor athletic performance. Few horses will perform well in competitive events while in AF. AF should therefore be considered as the likely cause of poor performance in animals presented for this reason. Treatment is usually required for them to recover normal performance levels. If treatment is successful and there is no significant underlying heart disease, it is likely that the horse will return to previous levels of performance. Animals which need repeated treatment may perform normally between bouts of AF. Some horses with AF have significant underlying heart disease and may not respond to treatment or recover normal performance even if they can be treated successfully.

Although animals have been reported to win races while in paroxysmal AF, it usually results in poor performance. It can be very difficult to diagnose. Paroxysmal AF usually only occurs during the stress of a race rather than at home on the gallops or on a treadmill, although there are exceptions. Unless the horse is examined before normal sinus rhythm returns it may be difficult to prove that paroxysmal AF is the cause of fading. It may be worthwhile visiting the racecourse to record an ECG if the episode of poor performance is repeated. Exercising and 24-hour ECGs may be helpful in establishing that an arrhythmia is the cause of the problem. Although the recordings may not show AF, an increased number of APCs may be detected and this would make a horse more likely to develop paroxysmal AF during a race. Fractional excretion tests may be useful because electrolyte disturbances predispose the horse to AF (see section 2.3.6). Echocardiography may be worthwhile to ensure that there is no evidence of underlying heart disease.

Atrial premature complexes, atrial tachycardia and ventricular arrhythmias
APCs and/or VPCs may be detected during a routine clinical examination or during heart rate slowing after exercise. It is frequently difficult to determine the significance of these abnormalities with regard to athletic performance. Exercising ECGs are invaluable in determining whether APCs occur more frequently or less frequently during exercise and therefore whether they are likely to affect performance. Similar tests to those described above for paroxysmal AF should be performed to determine whether there is any predisposing factors. Treatment and management of these conditions were discussed in sections 7.8.3 and 7.8.8.

Myocarditis
Myocarditis may be suspected if arrhythmias are detected. Investigation should include echocardiography to assess myocardial function and identification of any other conditions which predispose to arrhythmias. 'Heart strain' has been a popular concept in some areas of the world; however, there is little evidence that training can have any deleterious effects on the heart, except in exacerbating the effects of a virally mediated myocarditis. T wave abnormalities have been said to indicate the presence of heart strain, but there is no clear evidence that they are reliable indicators of cardiac disease. They may be found in animals with poor athletic performance, however, they are also found in horses with good racing records (see section 4.1.4).

A summary of causes of poor athletic performance is shown in Table 8.3. Useful diagnostic aids are summarised in Tables 8.4 and 8.5.

8.3   Episodic collapse

A horse which collapses is obviously a potential danger to the rider and handlers. Often owners of these animals assign diagnoses such as a 'heart attack' or a 'fit'. At the outset, it is worth informing owners that coronary artery disease is exceptionally rare in the horse. A thorough investigation is required to ensure that any abnormalities are detected and to reassure the rider so that their confidence is restored if the animal is safe to ride again. As in all clinical evaluations, the first aim when examining a horse which collapses is to reach a specific diagnosis. Cardiovascular and neurological diseases are the most commonly identified causes of episodic collapse; however, a specific diagnosis is seldom made. In these cases the role of the veterinarian is to offer sensible advice on the management of the horse.

Episodic collapse can be defined as a loss of consciousness or ataxia leading to recumbency and should be distinguished from a fall, stumbling or slipping. This distinction is not always easy. Ideally, it is helpful to examine animals during a collapsing episode, but this is seldom possible, such events can very rarely be reproduced for the benefit of an examining veterinary surgeon. The first requirement in investigation of these cases is therefore to acquire an accurate history.

Table 8.3 Summary: Causes of poor athletic performance

Intrinsic problems
Lack of ability
Inappropriate or inadequate training
Behaviour

Cardiovascular disease
Mitral regurgitation
Atrial fibrillation
Other supraventricular arrhythmias
Ventricular arrhythmias
Myocarditis
Aortic regurgitation, tricuspid regurgitation, congenital heart disease
Aorto–iliac thromboembolism

Musculo-skeletal
Unilateral lameness
Bilateral lameness
Multiple lameness
Myopathies

Upper airway disease
Recurrent laryngeal neuropathy (static or dynamic)
Dorsal displacement of the soft palate (dynamic)
Epiglottic entrapment (static or dynamic)
Dynamic collapse of the pharynx
Mass in pharynx
Laryngeal chondritis
Alar fold obstruction
Nasal chamber obstruction

Lower airway disease
Respiratory infections
Allergic small airway disease
Exercise induced pulmonary haemorrhage

Table 8.4 Summary: Evaluation of the poor performance case suspected of having cardiovascular disease. Baseline information

Thorough clinical examination, including palpation of larynx, use of a re-breathing bag, examination of horse at exercise and basic lameness examination.

Endoscopy of the upper and lower respiratory tract
Tracheal wash cytology
Echocardiography
Resting and exercising ECG
Chest radiograph of dorso-caudal lung fields
Pre- and post-exercise CK assay
Haematology

8.3.1 History

In addition to the general health and management of the animal, the exact circumstances surrounding the incident should be ascertained. Inciting causes should be pinpointed if possible, particularly in animals in which the collapsing episode has occurred on more than one occasion. Important points are

Table 8.5 Summary: Diagnostic aids in evaluation of the poor performance case

Musculo-skeletal
Lameness examination
Radiology
Regional anaesthesia
Ultrasonography
Scintigraphy
Gait analysis
High-speed video analysis
Treadmill studies
Muscle enzyme assay

Upper airway disease
Resting endoscopy
Radiography
Dynamic endoscopy on a treadmill

Lower airway disease
Haematology
Endoscopy
Cytology of broncho-alveolar lavage
Cytology of tracheal lavage
Radiography
Bacterial culture from trans-tracheal lavage or guarded endoscopic tracheal lavage
Viral titres
Virus isolation
Scintigraphy
Ultrasonography
Respiratory function tests

Cardiovascular disease
Echocardiography
Resting ECG
Exercising ECG
24-hour ECG
Laboratory tests

summarised in Table 8.6. It is very important to establish whether the episode of collapse occurred during exercise or at rest. Cardiovascular conditions may cause collapse either at rest or during exercise. If an episode of collapse occurs during exercise it is helpful to know whether the horse tired and then collapsed or collapsed without warning. If the animal collapsed at rest, it may be helpful to know whether it was being attended or was alone in its box or field. If the owners were in attendance, it is helpful to establish exactly what were they doing, what had they just done and what were they about to do. Any possible inciting events should be noted. It may be useful to know whether the possible inciting event was part of a regular routine (such as grooming or tacking-up) or was unexpected (such as being scared by a car or another animal).

The details of the episode of collapse itself may also be important. It is helpful to establish how long the animal was on the ground, whether it made any movements when on the ground and whether it was aware of its surroundings. It can be useful to know whether there was any eye movement because these will be absent if the horse was actually unconscious. Owners should be asked what

Table 8.6 Summary: Important historical information in a collapsing horse

Events surrounding the collapsing episode
- Did the animal collapse at exercise or at rest?
- If at exercise, how tired was it at the time?
- If the animal collapsed at rest, was it being attended or was it alone in its box or field?
- If the owners were in attendance, what exactly were they doing, what had they just done and what were they about to do?
- Was the inciting event part of a regular routine such as grooming or tacking-up or was the inciting cause an unusual occurrence?

The collapse itself
- How long was the animal on the ground?
- Did it make any movement when on the ground?
- Was it aware of its surroundings when it was collapsed?
- Was any eye movement noted?
- What did it do when it recovered?

the horse did when it recovered, particularly whether it was apparently normal or remained dazed for some time. Animals which collapse as a result of a cardiac problem are usually normal immediately they stand up, although they may be stunned or scared by the event.

Almost invariably a veterinarian arrives to examine the animal after it has recovered. Under these circumstances a complete clinical examination should be carried out, but points which are particularly worthy of note are summarised in Table 8.7.

8.3.2 Cardiovascular causes of collapse

Severe cardiac disease may result in collapse of an animal at rest, but more frequently it occurs during exercise. Animals which collapse due to a sudden fall in cardiac output may show no signs of motion when on the ground and in effect show flaccid paralysis. This often lasts only a few seconds.

Collapse during exercise
Poor athletic performance is usually the first clinical sign associated with cardiac disease and is therefore seen before any condition is sufficiently severe to result in collapse. Intermittent arrhythmias, or myocardial or valvular disease of recent onset may result in collapse because the animal may be worked hard without knowledge of the presence of disease. Severe valvular heart disease can cause collapse during exercise, but this is remarkably uncommon. In addition, it would be a mistake to assume in every case in which a cardiac murmur associated with pathological change is detected, that cardiac disease is the cause of collapse. Severe myocardial disease or pericardial disease may also cause collapse at exercise, but these conditions are uncommon. Echocardiographic examination should be performed to assess their severity.

By far the most important cardiovascular causes of collapse during exercise are dysrhythmias. The development of AF during exercise may result in an animal suddenly tiring and collapsing or falling. Atrial or ventricular tachycardias may produce similar sudden reductions in cardiac output resulting in unexpected

Table 8.7 Summary: Examination of the collapsing horse

At the time of the event
First aid
A: Airway
B: Breathing
C: Cardiac
Do not endanger people by examining the animal during the episode unless experienced handlers are available and can approach the horse safely.

Examination
What is the mental stage of the animal? Is the animal conscious?
Are there any rapid eye movements?
What is the heart rate?
What is the heart rhythm?
Examine the capillary refill time, mucous membrane colour and arterial pulse quality.

After the event
General inspection
Has the animal recovered a normal mental state?
Is there evidence of traumatic damage caused by the event?

Cardiovascular system
Check the mucous membrane colour and refill time, pulse rate, rhythm and quality, check for signs of congestive heart failure. Auscultation

Neurological examination
Conscious or unconscious
Ocular motion
Pupillary light reflex
Peripheral reflexes

tiring or collapse. Usually there will be some evidence of these conditions when the animal is examined at rest. However, a diagnosis is often difficult in horses which develop paroxysmal AF because sinus rhythm may be present by the time that a veterinary examination is performed.

Some respiratory conditions can result in collapse during exercise. Exercise induced pulmonary haemorrhage can cause collapse and even death in horses, usually just after the end of exercise. This only occurs if the condition is very severe, in which case epistaxis will be evident. Only rarely do exercise-induced upper respiratory tract obstructions result in collapse, although they frequently result in a sudden tiring of the animal, which may predispose it to falling.

Occasionally acute musculo-skeletal problems such as bilateral fractures or rhambdomyolysis result in collapse during exercise. Stumbling or falling, with subsequent winding must also be considered.

Collapse may also occur during the immediate post-exercise period. This may be due to exhaustion, dehydration, heat stress, haemorrhage, or musculo–skeletal problems, but is unlikely to be primarily due to cardiac disease. Unfortunately, an ECG is seldom recorded at these times so it is difficult to exclude the possibility of an arrhythmia. It is also unlikely that this diagnostic dilemma will ever be resolved. Similar problems occur in man and are frequently undiagnosed.

Collapse at rest

The majority of horses which are presented for investigation of a collapsing episode have collapsed while at rest. Reaching a definitive diagnosis in these cases is often extremely difficult because the intermittent nature of the problem means that the animal will be normal when it is examined.

Animals with severe valvular heart disease may collapse, but usually they will have been showing clinical signs of severe heart disease for some time and congestive heart failure will be present. Some of these horses collapse because of the sudden development of a dysrhythmia, or because of rupture of a major vessel such as the pulmonary artery. Tachydysrhythmias may develop as a result of systemic disease, and these may cause a sudden reduction in cardiac output and resultant collapse. Pericardial disease will result in a severe limitation of the preload and therefore limit cardiac output so that collapse may ensue if there is an increased demand, for example on excitement. Severe myocardial disease may have a similar effect.

Bradycardias

Bradydysrhythmias, including extreme forms of vagally mediated arrhythmias such as 2°AVB and sinus arrest/block, are very seldom responsible for collapse. Usually, light exercise will result in the abolition of these arrhythmias. Sinus bradycardia is more commonly a pathological situation and may result in collapse. However, it is common for animals with this arrhythmia to show signs of systemic disease of which the arrhythmia is a secondary feature.

Collapse is likely to be one of the prominent presenting signs in horses with third degree atrioventricular block (3°AVB or complete heart block). This condition is usually persistent and results in collapse when the animal is first exercised because of an inability to increase heart rate to meet the demands for increased cardiac output. 3°AVB is very rare in horses. Treatment is with a pacemaker (see section 7.8.15).

If an intermittent bradycardia or tachycardia is suspected to be the cause of a collapsing episode, 24-hour and/or radiotelemetric ECG recording may be worthwhile. However, if the collapsing episodes are infrequent, it may not be possible to identify the cause of collapse even with this technique.

Vaso–vagal syncope

Vaso–vagal syncope is a cause of episodic collapse which is well-recognised in humans, but is poorly documented in animals. In people it is associated with fear, i.e. a classic 'fainting attack' and is most commonly found in very highly strung individuals. Although horses are not entirely analogous, it seems likely that a similar mechanism may occur in this species. Usually the animals affected are at rest and are then suddenly excited by a precipitating event. Recognised causes are grooming of the head or tightening of the girth, although other events may be responsible and should be identified if possible. In some cases the inciting cause will be a sudden, unexpected event. The mechanism of vaso–vagal syncope is thought to involve an inappropriate combination of sympathetic and para-sympathetic responses. In the 'flight-fight' mechanism, animals which are excited have an increased heart rate, myocardial contractility and central arterial tone, resulting in an increase in blood pressure. This is required to counteract a marked vasodilation in the skeletal musculature. These changes allow muscular perfusion to increase dramatically, enabling the animal to respond rapidly. In vaso–vagal syncope, baroreceptors in the left ventricle, carotid sinuses and aorta may be over-sensitive and, when stroke volume is increased, a reflex may cause a vagally mediated bradycardia, or prevent the heart rate rising in an appropriate manner. The imbalance due to the lack of increased cardiac output and peripheral vasodilation results in a precipitous drop in blood pressure to the brain and collapse ensues. The drop in blood pressure is only momentary and corrective mechanisms result in the animal rapidly regaining consciousness and standing, unless serious trauma has occurred.

It should be emphasised that the existence of this mechanism in horses is conjecture. There is no specific treatment; however, it is very unlikely that the episode will occur once the heart rate has risen while the horse is being ridden. If there is a specific inciting cause, it is wise to take steps to avoid it being repeated, if possible. In preparation for exercise it may be worthwhile lunging these animals, or trotting them in hand, so that a mild tachycardia is present before the horse is ridden.

8.3.3 Neurological causes of collapse

There are a number of different neurological conditions which result in collapse. Those which produce flaccid paralysis should be distinguished from those which produce recumbency as a result of ataxia or due to seizure activity. Spinal injuries, such as cervical malformation and fractures resulting in spinal cord trauma, may also cause flaccid collapse. Ataxia is not usually associated with cardiovascular causes of collapse except when the animal tires during arduous exercise. Cardiovascular disease seldom results in seizures.

Seizures
Seizures are characterised by involuntary motion, including paddling of the limbs. Urination and defecation may occur. Behavioural abnormalities may be noted in the form of pre-ictal aura and post-ictal bewilderment. Neurological causes of seizures include epilepsy, toxins, viral conditions and trauma.

Narcolepsy
An important differential diagnosis in cases of flaccid collapse is narcolepsy. This is a sleep disorder which results in cataplectic collapse and may appear very similar to vaso–vagal syncope. An inciting cause may or may not be identified. Inciting causes have been described which are similar to those listed for vaso–vagal syncope. Narcoleptic attacks may also occur during light exercise. The condition has been recorded in a variety of breeds including related Shetland ponies and Suffolk horses. Any age or sex of animal can be affected. Animals may fall, or may catch themselves in the process of falling. Narcoleptic, areflexic collapse may result in trauma to the carpi and head.

Diagnosis in cases of narcolepsy can be made in some cases on the basis of a physostigmine stimulation test. The test is best performed on a deep straw bed or in an induction/recovery box. Around 0.08 mg/kg is injected slowly intravenously; collapse may follow in 5–20 minutes. Administration of physostigmine can result in colic. The drug can be difficult to obtain and is highly toxic. Failure to respond to administration of physostigmine does not exclude a diagnosis of narcolepsy.

Prevention of narcolepsy has been recorded following administration of 20–60 mg atropine intravenously or imipramine at a dose of 250 mg intravenously or 750 mg orally. However, collapse is seldom sufficiently frequent for this to be used diagnostically, and it is not practical to continue treatment in the long-term. Some animals recover from the condition for unknown reasons.

Psychological/behavioural causes of collapse

It has been suggested that some horses may collapse for behavioural reasons. This may be because the animal does not want to be groomed, saddled or ridden. Back pain might be responsible for these behavioural abnormalities in some horses, but back problems are notoriously difficult to diagnose with certainty. Ponies have been known to collapse by rearing and falling backwards when attended in these ways. It is difficult to prove that behavioural abnormalities are responsible. Vaso–vagal syncope occurs in similar situations and may be related. It may be difficult to distinguish some of these episodes from narcolepsy. It is possible that collapse can become a patterned behaviour and it is worthwhile changing the management of the animal so that the inciting associations are broken.

8.3.4 Other potential causes of collapse

Other causes of collapse at rest include colic, rhabdomyolysis, laminitis and a number of rare metabolic disorders such as hypoglycaemia. If these conditions have been severe enough to cause an animal to collapse, the animal is usually still recumbent when examined. Biochemical and radiographic examination may be required in some cases.

Possible causes of collapse are summarised in Table 8.8.

8.3.5 Management of horses which collapse

Specific treatment of the conditions which result in collapse is seldom possible. Because these animals are potentially dangerous, it is incumbent on the veterinarian to advise against riding horses which repeatedly collapse, unless a management regime which significantly reduces the chance of further episodes occurring can be suggested. It is more difficult to give advice to the owner of a horse which has collapsed only once. In these circumstances a thorough discussion with the owner is required and each case should be judged according to individual circumstance. Sometimes the episodes are one-off events. It may be best to ride the horse in a fairly controlled area such as a sand school for a time rather than returning to competition or road work. If vaso–vagal syncope is likely, raising the heart rate by exercising the horse before it is ridden is advisable. Unfortunately, it is very difficult to be sure that the condition will not recur and the owner should be advised accordingly. Any degree of risk may be unacceptable in some cases such as children's ponies. However, in the author's opinion, conditions which result in collapse of an animal at rest are very unlikely to occur during exercise unless significant findings are made on a thorough clinical examination.

Table 8.8   Summary: Causes of episodic collapse

Cardiovascular
At rest
Vaso-vagal syncope
Severe valvular heart disease, usually in association with CHF
Tachydysrhythmias
Bradydysrhythmias, e.g. extreme 2°AVB, 3°AVB, sinus arrest, sinus bradycardia
Pericardial disease
Severe myocardial disease

At exercise
Severe valvular heart disease
Tachydysrhythmias
Pericardial disease
Severe myocardial disease

Neurological
Narcolepsy
Seizures:
  Epilepsy
  Toxins
  Viral
  Trauma
Cervical fractures and spinal cord trauma
Cervical malformation and spinal cord trauma

Musculo-skeletal
Rhabdomyolysis
Acute laminitis
Back pain
Bilateral fractures

Psychological
Does not want to be groomed
Does not want to be saddled
Does not want to be ridden

When investigating the cause of an episode of collapse, it should be explained to the owner at the outset that a diagnosis is seldom obtained. Furthermore, even if a diagnosis is reached, this may not alter the advice regarding riding the animal in future. The situation regarding loss of use insurance claims in these cases can be problematic. The role of the first opinion veterinarian in this instance is to make a thorough report of the clinical findings and any further diagnostic investigations undertaken and to reach a reasoned conclusion regarding further use of the animal. If this includes actual observation of the episodes the claim is easier to handle. The situation is further complicated because some animals appear to recover. A period of rest or change of environment may apparently resolve the problem, however, it is difficult to predict whether or not the animal may collapse again in the future.

8.4   Sudden death

Sudden death in horses is frequently attributed to cardiac disease. However, surveys have shown that in many cases there is no identifiable cause of death. It can be postulated that malignant arrhythmias may result in sudden death with no abnormal findings at PM; however, it may never be possible to prove or disprove this theory.

Usually animals are found dead in a box or in a field. Occasionally, animals collapse and die while at exercise or immediately after exercise. The most commonly identified causes of sudden death may not have been detectable prior to death even with a thorough examination; however, owners are usually concerned to identify a reason. Post-mortem examination (PM) should be carried out with great care because significant cardiac lesions may be difficult to find without careful observation (see section 2.4.1). Frequently PMs are unrewarding and, if conducted thoroughly, are likely to be expensive. In particular, toxicological tests are extremely expensive. Owners should be warned of these facts before a PM is performed, particularly if they are suspicious of malicious causes because these are very difficult to diagnose conclusively and owners are likely to be frustrated.

8.4.1 Causes of sudden death

Cardiac disease

There is no evidence that animals with mild-moderate valvular insufficiency are any more likely to drop dead than any other horse. Sudden death in animals with previously diagnosed valvular disease is only likely to result from rupture of a major chorda tendinea, rupture of the pulmonary artery, or a severe arrhythmia. Coronary artery disease is exceptionally rare in horses. Certainly they do not develop atheromatous plaques in the coronary arteries which result in occlusion and cause a 'heart attack'. This term is commonly used to account for sudden death in horses because it seems a plausible and understandable explanation to owners, but it is entirely inaccurate.

Acute onset tachydysrhythmias and bradydysrhythmias may be the cause of sudden death in animals in which no abnormalities are detected at routine examination. Unfortunately there is no way of proving this diagnosis without an ECG recorded at the time of death. Arrhythmias which are sufficiently severe to account for sudden death are very seldom encountered on clinical examination, even in sick animals. However, despite limited documentary evidence in animals or man, arrhythmias are still thought to cause sudden death in some cases.

Horses with congestive heart failure (CHF) may die suddenly. In animals with left-sided heart disease this is may be as a result of rupture of the pulmonary artery following pulmonary hypertension. Clinical signs usually develop from the point of poor athletic performance to CHF over a period of weeks to years. Horses with severe mitral regurgitation are particularly at risk and should be monitored echocardiographically if possible. For this reason animals with CHF should not be ridden under any circumstances. However, very few horses with valvular heart disease are in CHF.

Rupture of a major chorda tendinea may result in sudden left-sided cardiac failure. The clinical signs usually develop over a few hours to days, but occasionally result in sudden death. If this cause is suspected, PM should be carried out with great care so that the chordae are not damaged in the course of opening the left ventricle.

Peripheral cardiovascular disease

Peripheral cardiovascular disease, in the broadest sense of the term, is a relatively common cause of sudden death. The most common cause of sudden death recognised at PM is rupture of a major artery. This may be traumatic or result from pre-existing disease. Conditions include rupture of the pulmonary artery, aortic root, a major pulmonary vessel, a carotid artery (due to mycotic infection of the guttural pouch), a major abdominal artery (likely to be associated with parasitic damage), and rupture of a uterine artery (usually in the near-term mare). Major arteries may also be damaged as a result of fractures, particularly pelvic fractures.

A summary of the potential causes of sudden death, including non-cardiovascular disease is shown in Table 8.9. Readers are advised to refer to papers in the list of further reading for more detailed discussions.

Table 8.9 Summary: Causes of sudden death

Cardiovascular
Rupture of the pulmonary artery
Rupture of the aortic root
Rupture of a major pulmonary vessel (+/– severe EIPH)
Rupture of a carotid artery due to mycotic infection of the guttural pouch
Rupture of a major abdominal artery, likely to be associated with parasitic damage
Rupture of a uterine artery
Severed arteries associated with skeletal trauma
Tachydysrhythmia
Bradydysrhythmia (very rare)
Rupture of a major chorda tendinea
Congestive heart failure of any cause

Other causes
Abdominal catastrophe
Acute colitis
Trauma
Poisoning, e.g. yew
Gunshot wound
Hypomagnesemia

232

Appendix

Drugs Used in Equine Cardiology

(Approximate doses)

Antidysrhythmic drugs

(none licensed for use in horses)

Quinidine gluconate: Soluble preparation different from quinidine sulphate, not available in the UK at present. If available can be used to treat supraventricular and ventricular arrhythmias at 0.5–1.0 mg/kg IV every 10 minutes, or as an infusion to a maximum dose of 4 mg/kg.

Quinidine sulphate:
For AF: 10 g/500 kg every 2 hours by stomach tube up to total dose of 60–80 g (guideline). Then every 6 hours until conversion. Aim to keep in therapeutic range of 2.0–4.5 mg/l.
For VPCs: may have to be used for protracted treatment at 10 mg/kg by stomach tube every 6 hours if quinidine gluconate is not available

Lignocaine: IV 0.5 mg/kg boluses every 5 minutes, or as an infusion. Do not exceed total dose of 2.0–4.0 mg/kg. Ataxia/convulsions can occur (uncommon). These can be treated with diazepam at a dose of 0.1–0.2 mg/kg IV if necessary.

Propanalol: 0.05–0.15 mg/kg twice daily IV or 0.3–0.7 mg/kg PO. Little experience with this drug is reported.

Digoxin: (See positive inotropes.)

Atropine: Use for bradycardias which are sufficiently severe to result in prolonged clinical signs. Dose 0.01–0.015 mg/kg IV.

Glycopyrolate: 0.005–0.01 mg/kg IV used as an alternative to atropine.

Diuretics

Frusemide: 0.5–2 mg/kg IV, IM, PO twice or three times daily, or as needed.

Positive inotropes

(none licensed for use in horses)

Digoxin: Slows heart rate. May act as a positive inotrope. Use to control CHF when frusemide alone is not sufficient. Also to reduce ventricular response to supraventricular tachycardias.

IV dose 0.002–0.003 mg/kg twice daily.
Use oral dose if possible 0.01–0.015 mg/kg twice daily (or double this dose once daily).
Try to maintain within therapeutic range of 1.0– 2.0 μg/kg/min IV).

Dopamine: Used as an infusion at 1–5 μg/kg/min IV.

Dobutamine: Used as an infusion at 1–5 μg/kg/min IV.

Vasodilators

(estimated, untested doses)

Hydralazine: 0.5 mg/kg twice daily.

Acepromazine: 0.04–0.1 mg/kg twice daily.

Enalapril: 0.25–0.5 mg/kg once daily
Nitroglycerine ointment, nitroprusside and ACE antagonists (very expensive) have unknown dosages and side-effects in horses.

Antibiotics

Trimethoprim sulphur: 15 mg/kg once or twice daily PO.

Penicillin sodium: 20 000–40 000 iu/kg four times daily IV, and
Gentamycin: 2.2 mg/kg four times daily IV.

Ceftiofur: 1.0–2.0 mg/kg once daily IM.

Anti-inflammatory drugs

Corticosteroids:

Dexamethasone: Used to reduce inflammatory component of myocarditis. Controversial. Do not use during an active viral infection. Use only if rest is not successful or a rapid return to work is imperative after treatment. IV or PO 0.02–0.15 mg/kg in decreasing doses over the course of 2–4 weeks.

Prednisolone: An alternative to dexamethasone which may have fewer side-effects. PO or IM 0.02–1.0 mg/kg twice daily initially, gradually reducing the dose over the course of 2–4 weeks.

NSAIDs:

Flunixine meglamine: IV, IM or PO 0.25–1.0 mg/kg once/twice/three times daily depending on dose (for a limited period).

Phenylbutazone: IV or PO 2.0–4.0 mg/kg once/twice daily depending on dose (for a limited period).

Further Reading

Anatomy and physiology

General

Black, L.S., Monroe, W.E., Lee, J.C. and Robertson, J.L. (1994) Atrial natriuretic peptide. *Compendium of Continuing Education*, **16**, 717–729.

Braunwald, E. (1988) *Heart Disease. A textbook of cardiovascular medicine.* Saunders, Philadelphia, USA.

Brown, C.M. and Holmes, J.R. (1978) Haemodynamics in the horse: 1. Pressure pulse contours. *Equine Veterinary Journal*, **10**, 188–193.

Brown, C.M. and Holmes, J.R. (1978) Haemodynamics in the horse: 2. Intracardiac, pulmonary arterial and aortic pressures. *Equine Veterinary Journal*, **10**, 207–215.

Brown, C.M. and Holmes, J.R. (1978) Haemodynamics in the horse: 3. Duration of the phases of the cardiac cycle. *Equine Veterinary Journal*, **10**, 216–223.

Brown, C.M. and Holmes, J.R. (1979) Assessment of myocardial function in the horse: 1. Theoretical and technical considerations. *Equine Veterinary Journal*, **11**, 244–247.

Brown, C.M. and Holmes, J.R. (1979) Assessment of myocardial function in the horse: 2. Experimental findings in resting horses. *Equine Veterinary Journal*, **11**, 248–255.

Brown, C.M. and Holmes, J.R. (1979) Phonocardiography in the horse: 1. The intracardiac phonocardiogram. *Equine Veterinary Journal*, **11**, 11–18.

Brown, C.M. and Holmes, J.R. (1979) Phonocardiography in the horse: 2. The relationship of the external phonocardiogram to intracardiac pressure and sound. *Equine Veterinary Journal*, **11**, 183–186.

Hamlin, R.L. (1988) Normal physiology of the cardiovascular system. In: *Canine and feline cardiology* (Ed. P.R. Fox), Churchill Livingstone, New York, USA, pp. 15–25.

Hamlin, R.L., Klepinger, W.L., Gilpin, K.W and Smith, C.R. (1972) Autonomic control of heart rate in the horse. *American Journal of Physiology*, **222**, 976–978.

Holmes, J.R. (1986) *Equine Cardiology*. Vol. 1, part 1. Applied anatomy and physiology. Published by the author, Langford, England, pp. 1–49.

Itkin, R.J. (1994) Effects of the renin-angiotensin system on the kidneys. *Compendium of Continuing Education*, **16**, 753–763.

Kittleson, M.D. (1994) Left ventricular function and failure – Part I. *Compendium of Continuing Education*, **16**, 287–308.

Kittleson, M.D. (1994) Left ventricular function and failure – Part II. *Compendium of Continuing Education*, **16**, 1001–1017.

Miller, P.J. and Holmes, J.R. (1984) Observations on structure and function of the equine mitral valve. *Equine Veterinary Journal*, **16**, 457–460.

Shepherd, J.T. and Vanhoutte, P.M. (1979) *The human cardiovascular system.* Raven Press, New York, USA.

Sisson, D. (1989) The clinical evaluation of cardiac function. In: *Textbook of Veterinary Internal Medicine*, 3rd ed. (Ed. S.J. Ettinger), Saunders, Philadelphia, USA, pp. 923–939.

Vanselow, B., McCarthy, M. and Gay, C.C. (1978) A phonocardiographic study of equine heart sounds. *Australian Veterinary Journal*, **54**, 161–170.

Welker, F. and Muir, W.W. (1990) An investigation of the second heart sound in the normal horse. *Equine Veterinary Journal*, **22**, 403–407.

Electrophysiology

Darke, P.G.G. and Holmes, J.R. (1969) Studies on the equine cardiac electric field. 1. Body surface potentials. *Journal of Electrocardiology*, **2**, 229–234.

Darke, P.G.G. and Holmes, J.R. (1969) Studies on the equine cardiac electric field. 2. The integration of body surface potentials to derive resultant cardiac dipole moments. *Journal of Electrocardiology*, **2**, 235–244.

Glazier, D.B., Littledike, E.T. and Cook, H.M. (1983) The electrocardiographic changes in experimentally induced bundle branch block in the equine heart. *Irish Veterinary Journal*, **37**, 71–76.

Hamlin, R.L. and Smith, C.R. (1965) Categorisation of domestic mammals based upon their ventricular activation process. *Annals of the New York Academy of Sciences*, **127**, 195–203.

Hamlin, R.L., Himes, J.A., Guttridge, H. and Kirkham, W. (1970) P wave in the electrocardiogram of the horse. *American Journal of Veterinary Research*, **31**, 1027–1031.

Hamlin, R.L., Smetzer, D.L., Senta, T. and Smith, C.R. (1970) Atrial activation paths and P waves in horses. *American Journal of Physiology*, **219**, 306–313.

Meyling, H.A. and TerBorg, H. (1957) The conducting system of the heart in hoofed animals. *Cornell Veterinarian*, **47**, 419–447.

Muylle, E. and Oyaert, W. (1977) Equine electrocardiography. The genesis of the different configurations of the QRS complex. *Zentralblatt für Veterinarmedizin*, **24**, 762–771.

Exercise physiology

Bayly, W.M., Gabel, A.A. and Barr, S.A. (1983) Cardiovascular effects of submaximal aerobic training on a treadmill in Standardbred horses, using a standardized exercise test. *American Journal of Veterinary Research*, **44**, 544–553.

Kubo, K., Senta, T. and Sugimoto, O. (1974) Relationship between training and heart in the Thoroughbred racehorse. *Experimental Reports of the Equine Health Laboratory*, **11**, 87–93.

Milne, D.W., Gabel, A.A., Muir, W.W. and Skarda, R.T. (1977) Effects of training on heart rate, cardiac output and lactic acid in Standardbred horses, using a standardised exercise test. *Journal of Equine Medicine and Surgery*, **1**, 131–135.

Physick-Sheard, P.W. (1985) Cardiovascular response to exercise and training in the horse. *Veterinary Clinics of North America (Equine Practice)*, **1**, 383–417.

Rodiek, A.V., Lawrence, L.M. and Russell, M.A. (1987) Cardiovascular effects of intermittent or continuous treadmill conditioning in horses. *Equine Veterinary Science*, **7**, 14–19.

Rose, R.J. and Evans, D.L. (1991) Cardiovascular and respiratory function in the athletic horse. Proceedings of the Third International Conference on Equine Exercise Physiology. In: *Equine Exercise Physiology*, **3**, 1–23.

Sexton, W.L., Erickson, H.H. and Coffman, J.R. (1987) Cardiopulmonary and metabolic responses to exercise in the Quarter horse: effects of training. Proceedings of the Second International Conference in Equine Exercise Physiology. In: *Equine Exercise Physiology*, **2**, 77–91.

Thomas, D.P., Fregin, G.F., Gerber, N.H. and Ailes, N.B. (1983) Effects of training on cardiorespiratory function in the horse. *American Journal of Physiology*, **245**, R160–165.

Weber, J-M., Dobson, G.P., Parkhouse, W.S., Wheeldon, D., Harman, J.C., Snow, D.H. and Hochachka, P.W. (1987) Cardiac output and oxygen consumption in exercising horses. *American Journal of Physiology*, **253**, R890–895.

Pathology

Pathophysiology

Hamlin, R.L. (1988) Pathophysiology of heart failure. In: *Canine and feline cardiology* (Ed. P.R. Fox), Churchill Livingstone, New York, USA, pp. 159–171.

Kittleson, M.D. (1994) Left ventricular function and failure – Part I. *Compendium of Continuing Education*, **16**, 287–308.

Kittleson, M.D. (1994) Left ventricular function and failure – Part II. *Compendium of Continuing Education*, **16**, 1001–1017.

Knight, D.H. (1989) Pathophysiology of heart failure. In: *Textbook of Veterinary Internal Medicine*, 3rd ed. (Ed. S.J. Ettinger). Saunders, Philadelphia, pp. 899–922.

Clinical pathology

Harris, P. and Gray, J. (1992) The use of the fractional electrolyte excretion test to assess electrolyte status in the horse. *Equine Veterinary Education*, **4**, 162–166.

Leadon, D.P. (1992) Clinical pathology data. In: *Current Therapy in Equine Medicine*, 3rd ed. (Ed. N.E. Robinson). W.B. Saunders, Philadelphia, pp. 822–828.

Gross pathology

Bishop, S.F., Cole, C.R. and Smetzer, D.L. (1966) Functional and morphological pathology of equine aortic insufficiency. *Path. Vet.*, **3**, 137–158.

Dixon, P.M., Nicholls, J.R., McPherson, E.A., Lawson, G.H.K., Thomson, J.R., Pirie, H.W. and Breeze, R.G. (1982) Chronic obstructive pulmonary disease anatomical studies. *Equine Veterinary Journal*, **14**, 80–82.

Else, R.W. and Holmes, J.R. (1971) Pathological changes in atrial fibrillation in the horse. *Equine Veterinary Journal*, **3**, 56–62.

Else, R.W. and Holmes, J.R. (1972) Cardiac pathology in the horse (1) Gross pathology. *Equine Veterinary Journal*, **4**, 1–8.

Else, R.W. and Holmes, J.R. (1972) Cardiac pathology in the horse (2) Microscopic pathology. *Equine Veterinary Journal*, **4**, 57–62.

Holmes, J.R. and Else, R.W. (1972) Cardiac pathology in the horse (3) Clinical correlations. *Equine Veterinary Journal*, **4**, 195–203.

Holmes, J.R., Rezakhani, A. and Else, R.W. (1973) Rupture of a dissecting aortic aneurysm into the left pulmonary artery in a horse. *Equine Veterinary Journal*, **5**, 65–70.

Mahaffey, L.W. (1958) Fenestration of the aortic and pulmonary semilunar valves in the horse. *Veterinary Record*, **70**, 415–420.

Clinical examination

Bonagura, J.D. (1985) Equine heart disease: an overview. *Veterinary Clinics of North America (Equine Practice)*, **1**, 267–274.

Bonagura, J.D. (1990) Clinical examination and management of heart disease. *Equine Veterinary Education*, **2**, 31–37.

Glendenning, S.A. (1964) A distinctive diastolic murmur observed in healthy young horses. *Veterinary Record*, **76**, 341–342.

Glendenning, S.A. (1977) The clinician's approach to equine cardiology. *Equine Veterinary Journal*, **9**, 176–177.

Littlewort, M.C.G. (1962) The clinical auscultation of the equine heart. *Veterinary Record*, **74**, 1247–1260.

Littlewort, M.C.G. (1977) Cardiological problems in equine medicine. *Equine Veterinary Journal*, **9**, 173–175.

Machida, N., Yasuda, J. and Too, K. (1987) Auscultatory and phonocardiographic studies on the cardiovascular system of the newborn Thoroughbred foal. *Japanese Journal of Veterinary Research*, **35**, 235–250.

Paterson, D.F., Detweiler, D.K. and Glendenning, S.A. (1965) Heart sounds and murmurs of the normal horse. *Annals of the New York Academy of Sciences*, **127**, 242–305.

Patteson, M.W. and Cripps, P.J. (1993) A survey of cardiac auscultatory findings in horses. *Equine Veterinary Journal*, **25**, 409–415.

Reef, V.B. (1985) Evaluation of the equine cardiovascular system. *Veterinary Clinics of North America (Equine Practice)*, **1**, 275–288.

Rossdale, P.D. (1967) Clinical studies on the newborn Thoroughbred foal. II. Heart rate, auscultation and electrocardiogram. *British Veterinary Journal*, **123**, 521–523.

Smetzer, D.L. and Smith, C.R. (1965) Diastolic sounds of horses. *Journal of the American Veterinary Medical Association*, **146**, 937–944.

Smetzer, D.L., Bishop, S. and Smith, C.R. (1966) Diastolic murmur of equine aortic insufficiency. *American Heart Journal*, **72**, 489–497.

Smetzer, D.L., Smith, C.R. and Hamlin, R.L. (1965) The fourth heart sounds of horses. *Annals of the New York Academy of Sciences*, **127**, 305–321.

Stockman, S. (1894) Contribution to the study of heart disease in the horse. *Journal of Comparative Pathology*, **7**, 138–160.

Diagnostic techniques

Echocardiography

Adams-Brendemuehl, C. and Pipers, F.S. (1987) Antepartum evaluations of the equine fetus. *Journal of Reproduction and Fertility* (Suppl), **35**, 565–575.

Bertone, J.J., Paull, K.S., Wingfield, W.E. and Boon, J.A. (1987) M-mode echocardiograms of endurance horses in the recovery phase of long-distance competition. *American Journal of Veterinary Research*, **48**, 1708–1712.

Bonagura, J.D. (1983) M-mode echocardiography: basic principles. *Veterinary Clinics of North America (Small Animal Practice)*, **13**, 299–319.

Bonagura, J.D. and Herring, D.S. (1985) Echocardiography: congenital heart disease. *Veterinary Clinics of North America (Small Animal Practice)*, **15**, 1195–1208.

Bonagura, J.D. and Herring, D.S. (1985) Echocardiography: acquired heart disease. *Veterinary Clinics of North America (Small Animal Practice)*, **15**, 1209–1224.

Bonagura, J.D. and Pipers, F.S. (1981) Echocardiographic features of pericardial effusion in dogs. *Journal of the American Veterinary Medical Association*, **179**, 49–56.

Bonagura, J.D. and Pipers, F.S. (1983) Diagnosis of cardiac lesions by contrast echocardiography. *Journal of the American Veterinary Medical Association*, **182**, 396–402.

Bonagura, J.D. and Pipers, F.S. (1983) Echocardiographic features of aortic valve endocarditis in a dog, a cow, and a horse. *Journal of the American Veterinary Medical Association*, **182**, 595–599.

Bonagura, J.D., Herrings, D.S. and Welker, F. (1985) Echocardiography. *Veterinary Clinics of North America (Equine Practice)*, **1**, 311–333.

Bonagura, J.D., O'Grady, M.R. and Herring, D.S. (1985) Echocardiography: principles of interpretation. *Veterinary Clinics of North America (Small Animal Practice)*, **15**, 1177–1194.

Carlsten, J.C. (1987) Two-dimensional echocardiography in the horse. *Veterinary Radiology*, **28**, 76–87.

Carlsten, J.C. (1986) Imaging of the equine heart. An angiocardiographic and echocardiographic investigation. Thesis. Uppsala, Sweden.

DeMadron, E., Bonagura, J.D. and O'Grady, M.R. (1985) Normal and paradoxical ventricular septal motion in the dog. *American Journal of Veterinary Research*, **46**, 2546–2552.

Feigenbaum, H. (1986) *Echocardiography*, 4th ed. Lea and Ferbinger, Philadelphia, USA.

Goldberg, S.J., Allen, H.D., Marx, G.R. and Donnerstein, R.L. (1988) Doppler echocardiography, 2nd ed. Lea and Febinger, Philadelphia, USA.

Henry, W.L., DeMaria, A., Gramiak, R., King, D.L., Kisslo, J.A., Popp, R.L., Sahn, D.J., Schiller, N.B., Tajik, A., Teichholz, L.E. and Weyman, A.E. (1980) Report of the American Society of Echocardiography Committee on Nomenclature and Standards in two-dimensional echocardiography. *Circulation*, **62**, 212–217.

Herring, D.S. and Bjornton, G. (1985) Physics, facts and artefacts of diagnostic ultrasound. *Veterinary Clinics of North America (Small Animal Practice)*, **15**, 1107–1122.

Kuramoto, K., Shiraishi, A., Nakanishi, Y., Kau, M., Ueno, Y. and Ueda, Y. (1989) Application of echocardiography for assessing left ventricular function of Thoroughbred horses at a resting stage. *Bulletin of the Japanese Equine Research Institute*, **26**, 23–30.

Kvart, C., Carlsten, J.C., Jeffcott, L.B. and Nilsfors, L. (1985) Diagnostic value of contrast echocardiography in the horse. *Equine Veterinary Journal*, **17**, 357–360.

Leadon, D., McAllister, H., Mullins, E. and Osbourne, M. (1991) Electrocardiographic and echocardiographic measurements and their relationships in Thoroughbred yearlings to subsequent performance. Proceedings of the Third International Conference on Equine Exercise Physiology. *Equine Exercise Physiology*, **3**, 22–29.

Lescure, F. and Olivier, J.L. (1980) L'echocardiographie chez le cheval. *Practique Vétérinaire Equine*, **12**, 207–212.

Lescure, F. and Tamzali, Y. (1983) L'echocardiographie TM chez le cheval. 1 ieme partie: la technique. Le Point Veterinaire, **15**, 215–223.

Lescure, F. and Tamzali, Y. (1983) L'echocardiographie TM chez le cheval. 2 ieme partie: les cardiopathies orificielles acquises. *Le Point Vétérinaire*, **15**, 267–275.

Lescure, F. and Tamzali, Y. (1983) L'echocardiographie TM chez le cheval. 3 ieme partie: cardiopathies congenitale et trouble du rhythme. *Le Point Vétérinaire*, **15**, 373–380.

Lescure, F. and Tamzali, Y. (1984) Valeurs de reference en echocardiographie TM chez le cheval de sport. *Revue Medicine Vétérinaire*, **135**, 405–418.

Lombard, C.W., Evans, M., Martin, L. and Tehrani, J. (1984) Blood pressure, electrocardiographic and echocardiographic measurements in the growing pony foal. *Equine Veterinary Journal*, **16**, 342–347.

Long, K.J. (1990) Doppler echocardiography in the horse. *Equine Veterinary Education*, **2**, 15–17.

Long, K.J. (1992) Two-dimensional and M-mode echocardiography. *Equine Veterinary Education*, **4**, 303–310.

Long, K.J., Bonagura, J.D. and Darke, P.G.G. (1992) Standardised imaging technique for guided M-mode and Doppler echocardiography in the horse. *Equine Veterinary Journal*, **24**, 226–235.

Mahony, C., Rantanen, N.W., DeMichael, J.A. and Kincaid, B. (1992) Spontaneous echocardiographic contrast in the Thoroughbred: high prevalence in racehorses and a characteristic abnormality in bleeders. *Equine Veterinary Journal*, **24**, 129–133.

Miller, M.W., Knauer, K.W. and Herring, D.S. (1989) Echocardiography: principles of interpretation. *Seminars in Veterinary Surgery and Medicine*, **4**, 58–76.

Moise, N.S. (1989) Doppler echocardiographic evaluation of congenital cardiac disease. *Journal of Veterinary Internal Medicine*, **3**, 195–207.

O'Callaghan, M.W. (1985) Comparison of echocardiographic and autopsy measurements of cardiac dimensions in the horse. *Equine Veterinary Journal*, **17**, 361–368.

Patteson, M.W. (1994) Echocardiographic evaluation of horses with aortic regurgitation. *Equine Veterinary Education*, **6**, 159–166.

Paull, K.S., Wingfield, W.E., Bertone, J.J. and Boon, J.W. (1987) Echocardiographic changes with endurance training. Proceedings of the Second International Conference on Equine Exercise Physiology. In: *Equine Exercise Physiology*, **2**, 34–40.

Pipers, F.S. and Hamlin, R.L. (1977) Echocardiography in the horse. *Journal of the American Veterinary Medical Association*, **170**, 815–819.

Pipers, F.S., Hamlin, R.L. and Reef, V.B. (1979) Echocardiographic detection of cardiovascular lesions in the horse. *Journal of Equine Medicine and Surgery*, **3**, 68–77.

Rantanen, N.W. (1986) Diseases of the heart. *Veterinary Clinics of North America (Equine Practice)*, **2**, 33–47.

Rantanen, N.W., Byars, T.D., Hauser, M.L. and Gaines, R.D. (1984) Spontaneous contrast and mass lesions in the hearts of racehorses: ultrasound diagnosis – preliminary data. *Journal of Equine Veterinary Science*, **4**, 220–223.

Reef, V.B. (1990) Color flow Doppler mapping of horses with valvular insufficiency. Proceedings of the Eighth Annual Veterinary Medical Forum of the American College of Veterinary Internal Medicine, pp. 483–485.

Reef, V.B. (1990) Echocardiographic examination in the horse: the basics. *Compendium of Continuing Education for the Practicing Veterinarian*, **12**, 1312–1319.

Reef, V.B. (1991) Advances in echocardiography. *Veterinary Clinics of North America (Equine Practice)*, **7**, 435–450.

Reef, V.B. (1991) Echocardiographic findings in horses with congenital heart disease. *Compendium of Continuing Education for the Practicing Veterinarian*, **13**, 109–117.

Reef, V.B., Lalezari, K., DeBoo, J., Van Der Belt, A.J., Spencer, P.A. and Dik, K.J. (1989) Pulsed-wave Doppler evaluation of intracardiac blood flow in 30 normal Standardbred horses. *American Journal of Veterinary Research*, **50**, 75–83.

Reef, V.B., Maxson, A.D. and Lewis, M. (1994) Echocardiographic and ECG changes in horses following exercise. Proceedings of the Twelfth Annual Veterinary Medical Forum of the American College of Veterinary Internal Medicine, pp. 256–258.

Reef, V.B. and Spencer, P.A. (1987) Echocardiographic evaluation of equine aortic insufficiency. *American Journal of Veterinary Research*, **48**, 904–909.

Sisson, D.D. (1989) Quantitative echocardiography. Proceedings of the Seventh Annual Veterinary Medical Forum of the American College of Veterinary Internal Medicine, pp. 291–294.

Stadler, P., D'Agostino, U. and Deegen, E. (1988) Methodik der Schnittbildechokardiographie beim Pferd. *Pferdeheilkunde*, **4**, 161–174.

Stewart, J.H., Rose, R.J. and Barko, A.M. (1984) Echocardiography in foals from birth to three months old. *Equine Veterinary Journal*, **16**, 332–341.

Voros, K., Felkai, C., Szilagyi, Z. and Papp, A. (1991) Two-dimensional echocardiographically guided pericardiocentesis in a horse with traumatic pericarditis. *Journal of the American Veterinary Medical Association*, **198**, 1953–1956.

Voros, K., Holmes, J.R. and Gibbs, C. (1991) Measurement of cardiac dimensions with two-dimensional echocardiography in the living horse. *Equine Veterinary Journal*, **23**, 461–465.

Wilde, P. (1989) *Doppler echocardiography*. Churchill Livingstone, Edinburgh and London.

Wingfield, W.E., Miller, C.W., Voss, J.L., Bennett, D.G. and Breukels, J. (1980) Echocardiography in assessing mitral valve motion in three horses with atrial fibrillation. *Equine Veterinary Journal*, **12**, 181–184.

Electrocardiography

Buss, D.D., Rawling, C.A. and Bisgard, G.E. (1975) The normal electrocardiogram of the domestic pony. *Journal of Electrocardiography*, **8**, 167–172.

Evans, D.L. (1991) T-waves in the equine electrocardiogram: effects of training and implications for race performance. *Equine Exercise Physiology*, **3**, 475–481.

Fregin, G.F. (1982) The equine electrocardiogram with standardized body and limb positions. *Cornell Veterinarian*, **72**, 324.

Gatti, L. and Holmes, J.R. (1990) ECG recording at rest and during exercise in the horse. *Equine Veterinary Education*, **2**, 28–30.

Grauerholz, H. and Jaeschke, G. (1986) Problems in measuring and evaluating QRS duration in the ECG of the horse. *Berliner und Munchener Tierarztliche Wochenschrift*, **99**, 365–369.

Gross, D.R., Muir, W.W., Pipers, F.S. and Hamlin, R.L. (1974) Re-evaluation of the equine heart score. *South-West Veterinarian*, **27**, 231–233.

Hamlin, R.L., Smetzer, D.L. and Smith, C.R. (1964) Analysis of ARS complex recorded through a semi-orthogonal system in the horse. *American Journal of Physiology*, **207**, 325–333.

Holmes, J.R. (1976) Spatial vector changes during ventricular depolarisation using a semi-orthogonal lead system. *Equine Veterinary Journal*, **8**, 1–16.

Holmes, J.R. (1984) Equine electrocardiography: some practical hints on technique. *Equine Veterinary Journal*, **16**, 477–479.

Holmes, J.R. (1990) Electrocardiography in the diagnosis of common cardiac arrhythmias in the horse. *Equine Veterinary Education*, **2**, 24–27.

Holmes, J.R. and Alps, B.J. (1967) Studies into the equine electrocardiograph and vectorcardiography. 1. Cardiac electric forces and the dipole vector theory. *Canadian Journal of Comparative Medicine and Veterinary Science*, **31**, 92–102.

Holmes, J.R. and Alps, B.J. (1967) Studies into the equine electrocardiograph and vectorcardiography. 2. Cardiac vector distribution in apparently healthy horses. *Canadian Journal of Comparative Medicine and Veterinary Science*, **31**, 150–155.

Holmes, J.R. and Darke, P.G.G. (1968) Foetal electrocardiography in the mare. *Veterinary Record*, **79**, 651–655.

Holmes, J.R. and Darke, P.G.G. (1970) Studies on the development of a new lead system for equine electrocardiography. *Equine Veterinary Journal*, **2**, 12–21.

Holmes, J.R. and Else, R.W. (1972) Further studies on a new lead for equine electrocardiography. *Equine Veterinary Journal*, **4**, 81–87.

Holmes, J.R. and Rezakhani, A. (1975) Observations on the T wave of the equine electrocardiogram. *Equine Veterinary Journal*, **7**, 55–62.

Holmes, J.R., Alps, B.J. and Darke, P.G.G. (1966) A method of radiotelemetry in equine electrocardiography. *Veterinary Record*, **79**, 90–94.

Irvine, C.H.G. (1964) Electrocardiography in the horse – a review of J.D. Steel's monograph. *Australian Veterinary Journal*, **40**, 272–273.

Lannek, N. and Rutqvist, L. (1951) Normal area of variation for the electrocardiogram of horses. A statistical examination of extremity leads and unipolar leads. *Norsk Veterinaertidsskrift Medicin*, **3**, 1094–1117.

Leadon, D.P., Cunningham, E.P., Mahon, G.A. and Todd, A.J. (1982) Heart score and performance ability in the United Kingdom. *Equine Veterinary Journal*, **14**, 89–90.

Matsui, K., Amada, A., Sawasaki, T. and Kano, Y. (1983) Changes in electrocardiographic parameters with growth in Thoroughbred horses and Shetland ponies. *Bulletin of the Equine Research Institute*, **20**, 77–86.

Miller, P.J. and Holmes, J.R. (1984) Beat-to-beat variability in QRS potentials recorded with an orthogonal lead system in horses with second degree partial atrio-ventricular block. *Research in Veterinary Science*, **36**, 334–338.

Miller, P.J. and Holmes, J.R. (1984) Interrelationship of some electrocardiogram amplitudes, time intervals and respiration in the horse. *Research in Veterinary Science*, **36**, 370–374.

Moodie, E.W. and Sheard, R.P. (1980) The use of electrocardiography to estimate heart weight and predict performance in the racehorse. *Australian Veterinary Journal*, **56**, 557–558.

Muylle, E. and Oyaert, W. (1971) Clinical evaluation of cardiac vectors in the horse. *Equine Veterinary Journal*, **3**, 129–136.

Neilsen, K. and Vibe-Petersen, G. (1980) Relationship between QRS duration (heart score) and racing performance in trotters. *Equine Veterinary Journal*, **12**, 81–84.

Physick-Sheard, P.W. and Hendren, C.M. (1987) Heart score: physiological basis and confounding variables. *Equine Exercise Physiology*, **2**, 781–785.

Robertson, S.A. (1990) Practical use of ECG in the horse. *In Practice*, **12**, 59–67.

Senta, T., Smetzer, D.L. and Smith, C.R. (1970) Effects of exercise on certain electrocardiographic parameters and cardiac arrhythmias in the horse. A radiotelemetric study. *Cornell Veterinarian*, **60**, 552–569.

Steel, J.D. (1963) *Studies on the electrocardiogram of the racehorse.* Australian Medical Publishing Co., Sydney.

Steel, J.D. and Stewart, G.A. (1974) Electrocardiography of the horse and potential performance ability. *Journal of the South African Veterinary Association*, **45**, 263–268.

Steel, J.D., Stewart, G.A. and Toyne, A.H. (1970) Application of the heart score concept to the ECG of Olympic athletes. *Medical Journal of Australia*, **2**, 728–730.

Steel, J.D., Taylor, R.I., Davis, P.E., Stewart, G.A. and Salmon, P.W. (1976) Relationship between heart score, heart weight and body weight in greyhound dogs. *Australian Veterinary Journal*, **52**, 561–564.

Stewart, G.A. (1980) The use of electrocardiography to estimate heart weight and predict performance in the racehorse. *Australian Veterinary Journal*, **56**, 558–559.

Stewart, G.A. (1981) The heart score theory in the racehorse. *Australian Veterinary Journal*, **57**, 422–428.

Stewart, G.A. and Steel, J.D. (1970) Electrocardiography and the heart score concept in the racehorse. Proceedings of the American Association of Equine Practitioners Annual Convention, **16**, 363–381.

White, N.A. and Rhode, E.A. (1974) Correlation of electrocardiographic findings to clinical disease in the horse. *Journal of the American Veterinary Medical Association*, **164**, 46–56.

Other imaging techniques

Carlsten, J., Kvart, C. and Jeffcott, L.B. (1984) Method of selective and non-selective angiography for the horse. *Equine Veterinary Journal*, **161**, 47–52.

Koblick, P.D. and Hornof, W.J. (1985) Diagnostic radiology and nuclear cardiology: their use in the investigation of equine cardiovascular disease. *Veterinary Clinics of North America (Equine Practice)*, **1**, 289–309.

Koblick, P.D., Hornof, W.J., Rhode, E.A. and Kelly, A.B. (1985) Left ventricular ejection fraction in the normal horse determined by first-pass nuclear angiocardiography. *Veterinary Radiology*, **26**, 53–62.

Marr, C.M. (1990) Ancillary aids in equine cardiology. *Equine Veterinary Education*, **2**, 18–21.

Blood pressure measurement and catheterisation data

Bonagura, J.D. and Muir, W.W. The cardiovascular system. In: Equine Anaesthesia: Monitoring and Emergency Therapy, (Eds W.W. Muir and J.A.E. Hubble) Mosby Year Book, St Louis, USA, pp. 39–104.

Brown, C.M. and Holmes, J.R. (1978) Haemodynamics in the horse: 2. Intracardiac, pulmonary arterial and aortic pressures. *Equine Veterinary Journal*, **10**, 207–215.

Eberly, V.E., Gillespie, J.R. and Typler, W.S. (1964) Cardiovascular parameters in the Thoroughbred horse. *American Journal of Veterinary Research*, **25**, 1712–1716.

Johnson, J.H., Garner, H.E. and Hutcheson, D.P. (1976) Ultrasonic measurement of arterial blood pressure in conditioned Thoroughbreds. *Equine Veterinary Journal*, **8**, 55–57.

Milne, D.W., Muir, W.W. and Skarda, R.T. (1975) Pulmonary arterial wedge pressure, blood gas tensions and pH in the resting horse. *American Journal of Veterinary Research*, **36**, 1431–1434.

Muir, W.W., Skarda, R.T. and Milne, D.W. (1976) Estimation of cardiac output in the horse by thermodilution techniques. *American Journal of Veterinary Research*, **37**, 697–700.

Taylor, P.M. (1981) Techniques and clinical application of arterial blood pressure measurement in the horse. *Equine Veterinary Journal*, **13**, 271–275.

Congenital heart disease

Bayly, W.M., Reed, S.M., Leathers, C.W., Brown, C.M., Traub, J.L., Paradis, M.R. and Palmer, G.H. (1982) Multiple congenital heart anomalies in five Arabian foals. *Journal of the American Veterinary Medical Association*, **181**, 684–689.

Buergelt, C.D., Carmichael, J.A., Tashijan, R.J. and Das, K.M. (1970) Spontaneous rupture of the left pulmonary artery in a horse with a patent ductus arteriosus. *Journal of the American Veterinary Medical Association*, **157**, 313–320.

Button, C., Gross, D.R., Allert, J.A. and Kitxman, J.V. (1978) Tricuspid atresia in a foal. *Journal of the American Veterinary Medical Association*, **172**, 825–830.

Chaffin, M.K., Miller, M.W. and Morris, E.L. (1992) Double outlet right ventricle and other associated congenital cardiac anomalies in an American Minature horse foal. *Equine Veterinary Journal*, **24**, 402–406.

Critchley, K.L. (1976) An interventricular septal defect, pulmonary stenosis and bicuspid pulmonary valve in a Welsh pony foal. *Equine Veterinary Journal*, **8**, 176–178.

Derksen, F.S., Reed, S.M. and Hall, C.C. (1981) Aneurysm of the aortic arch and bicarotid trunk in a horse. *Journal of the American Veterinary Medical Association*, **179**, 692–694.

Hinchcliff, K.W. and Adams, W.M. (1991) Critical pulmonic stenosis in a newborn foal. *Equine Veterinary Journal*, **23**, 318–320.

Lombard, C.W., Scarratt, W.K. and Buergelt, C.D. (1983) Ventricular septal defects in the horse. *Journal of the American Veterinary Medical Association*, **183**, 562–565.

McClure, J.J., Gaber, C.E., Watters, J.W. and Qualls, C.W. (1983) Complete transposition of the great arteries with ventricular septal defect and pulmonary stenosis in a Thoroughbred foal. *Equine Veterinary Journal*, **15**, 377–380.

Mussleman, E.E. and LoGuidice, R.J. (1984) Hypoplastic left ventricular syndrome in a foal. *Journal of the American Veterinary Medical Association*, **185**, 542–543.

Orisini, J.A., Koch, C. and Stewart, B. (1981) Peritoneopericardial hernia in a horse. *Journal of the American Veterinary Medical Association*, **179**, 907–910.

Pipers, F.S., Reef, V.B. and Wilson, J. (1985) Echocardiographic detection of ventricular septal defects in large animals. *Journal of the American Veterinary Medical Association*, **187**, 810–816.

Pricket, M.E., Reeves, J.T. and Zent, W.W. (1973) Tetralogy of Fallot in a Thoroughbred foal. *Journal of the American Veterinary Medical Association*, **162**, 552–555.

Reef, V.B. (1985) Cardiovascular disease in the equine neonate. *Veterinary Clinics of North America (Equine Practice)*, **1**, 117–129.

Reef, V.B. (1988) Pulsed and continuous wave Doppler echocardiographic evaluation of congenital heart disease in large animals. Proceedings of the Sixth Annual Veterinary Medical Forum of the American College of Veterinary Internal Medicine, pp. 382–384.

Reef, V.B. (1991) Echocardiographic findings in horses with congenital heart disease. *Compendium of Continuing Education for the Practicing Veterinarian*, **13**, 109–117.

Reef, V.B., Mann, P.C. and Orsini, P.G. (1987) Echocardiographic detection of tricuspid atresia in two foals. *Journal of the American Veterinary Medical Association*, **191**, 225–228.

Rooney, J.R. and Franks, W.C. (1964) Congenital cardiac anomalies in horses. *Path Vet.*, **1**, 454– 464.

Scott, E.A., Chaffee, A., Eyster, G.E. and Kneller, S.K. (1978) Interruption of the aortic arch in two foals. *Journal of the American Veterinary Medical Association*, **172**, 347–350.

Scott, E.A., Kneller, S.K. and Witherspoon, D.M. (1975) Closure of ductus arteriosus determined by cardiac catheterisation and angiography in newborn foals. *American Journal of Veterinary Research*, **36**, 1021–1023.

Tadmore, A., Fischel, R. and Shem Tov, A. (1983) A condition resembling hypoplastic left heart syndrome in a foal. *Equine Veterinary Journal*, **15**, 175–177.

Taylor, F.G.R., Wotton, P.R., Hillyer, M.H., Barr, F.J. and Lucke, V.M. (1991) Atrial septal defect and atrial fibrillation in a foal. *Veterinary Record*, **128**, 80–81.

Zamora, C.S., Vitums, A., Foreman, J.H., Bayly, W.M. and Weidner, J.P. (1985) Common ventricle with separate pulmonary outflow chamber in a horse. *Journal of the American Veterinary Medical Association*, **186**, 1210–1213.

Acquired heart disease

Ball, M.A. and Weldon, A.D. (1992) Vegetative endocarditis in an Appaloosa gelding. *Cornell Veterinarian*, **82**, 301–309.

Baumbaugh, G.W., Thomas, W.P., Enos, L.R. and Kaneko, J.J. (1983) A pharmacokinetic study of digoxin in the horse. *Journal of Veterinary Pharmacology and Therapeutics*, **6**, 163–172.

Bernard, W., Reef, V.B., Clark, E.S., Vaala, W. and Ehnen, S.J. (1990) Pericarditis in horses: six cases (1982–1986). *Journal of the American Veterinary Medical Association*, **196**, 468–471.

Brown, C.M., Bell, T.G., Paradis, M-R. and Breeze, R.G. (1983) Rupture of mitral valve chordae tendineae in two horses. *Journal of the American Veterinary Medical Association*, **182**, 281–283.

Brumaugh, G.W., Thomas, W.P. and Hodge, T.G. (1982) Medical management of congestive heart failure in a horse. *Journal of the American Veterinary Medical Association*, **180**, 787–883.

Buergelt, C.D., Cooley, A.J., Hines, S.A. and Pipers, F.S. (1985) Endocarditis in six horses. *Veterinary Pathology*, **22**, 333–337.

Button, C., Gross, D.R., Johnston, J.T. and Yaketon, T.G. (1980) Digoxin pharmacokinetics, bioavailability, efficacy and dosage regimens in the horse. *American Journal of Veterinary Research*, **41**, 1388–1395.

Collatos, C., Clark, E.S. and Reef, V.B. (1990) Atrial fibrillation, cardiomegaly, left atrial mass and *Rhodococcus equi* septic osteoarthritis in a foal. *Journal of the American Veterinary Medical Association*, **197**, 1039–1042.

Cranley, J.J. and McCullagh, K.G. (1981) Ischaemic myocardial fibrosis and aortic strongylosis in the horse. *Equine Veterinary Journal*, **13**, 35–41.

Dedrick, P., Reef, V.B., Sweeney, R.W. and Morris, D.D. (1988) Treatment of bacterial endocarditis in a horse. *Journal of the American Veterinary Medical Association*, **193**, 339–342.

Dill, S.G., Sinoncini, B.S., Bolton, G.R., Rendanao, V.T., Crissman, L.W., King, J.M. and Tennant, B.M. (1980) Fibrinous pericarditis in the horse. *Journal of the American Veterinary Medical Association*, **180**, 266–271.

Edwards, G.B. and Allen, W.E. (1988) Aorto-iliac thrombosis in two horses: clinical course of the disease and use of real-time ultrasonography to confirm diagnosis. *Equine Veterinary Journal*, **20**, 384–387.

Ewart, S., Brown, C., Derksen, F. and Kufor-Mensa, E. (1992) *Serratia marcescens* endocarditis in a horse. *Journal of the American Veterinary Medical Association*, **200**, 961–963.

Freestone, J.F., Thomas, W.P., Carlson, G.P. and Brumbaugh, G.W. (1987) Idiopathic effusive pericarditis with tamponade in the horse. *Equine Veterinary Journal*, **19**, 38–42.

Hardy, J., Robertson, J.T. and Reed, S.M. (1992) Constrictive pericarditis in a mare: attempted treatment by partial pericardiectomy. *Equine Veterinary Journal*, **24**, 151–154.

Harrington, D.D. and Page, E.H. (1983) Acute vitamin D_3 toxicosis in horses: case reports and experimental studies of the comparative toxicity of vitamins D_2 and D_3. *Journal of the American Veterinary Medical Association*, **182**, 1358–1369.

Hillyer, M.H., Mair, T.S. and Holmes, J.R. (1990) Treatment of bacterial endocarditis in a shire mare. *Equine Veterinary Education*, **2**, 5–7.

Hines, M.T., Heidel, J.R. and Barbee, D.B. (1993) Bacterial endocarditis with thrombus formation and abscessation in a horse. *Veterinary Radiology and Ultrasound*, **34**, 47–51.

Hoskinson, J.J., Wooten, P. and Evans, R. (1991) Nonsurgical removal of a catheter embolus from the heart of a foal. *Journal of the American Veterinary Medical Association*, **199**, 233–235.

Kasari, T.R. and Roussel, A.J. (1989) Bacterial endocarditis. Part 1. Pathophysiologic, diagnostic and therapeutic considerations. *Compendium of Continuing Education for the Practicing Veterinarian*, **11**, 655–671.

Lees, M.J., Read, R.A., Klein, K.R., Chennel, K.R., Clark, W.T. and Weldon, A. (1989) Surgical retrieval of a broken jugular catheter from the right ventricle of a foal. *Equine Veterinary Journal*, **21**, 384–387.

Marr, C.M., Love, S., Pirie, H.M. and Northridge, D.B. (1990) Confirmation by Doppler echocardiography of valvular regurgitation in a horse with a ruptured chorda tendinea of the mitral valve. *Veterinary Record*, **127**, 376–379.

Miller, P.J. and Holmes, J.R. (1984) Three cases of ruptured mitral valve chordae in the horse. *Equine Veterinary Journal*, **16**, 125–135.

Miller, P.J. and Holmes, J.R. (1985) Observations on seven cases of mitral insufficiency in the horse. *Equine Veterinary Journal*, **17**, 181–190.

Muir, W.W. and McGuirk, S.M. (1985) Pharmacology and pharmacokinetics of drugs used to treat cardiac disease in horses. *Veterinary Clinics of North America* (Equine Practice), **1**, 335–352.

Nilsfors, L., Lombard, C.W., Weckner, D. and Kvart, C. (1991) Diagnosis of pulmonary valve endocarditis in a horse. *Equine Veterinary Journal*, **23**, 479–482.

Patteson, M.W. (1994) Echocardiographic evaluation of horses with aortic regurgitation. *Equine Veterinary Education*, **6**, 159–166.

Pearson, E.G., Ayres, J.W., Wood, G.L. and Watrous, B.J. (1987) Digoxin toxicity in a horse. *Compendium of Continuing Education for the Practicing Veterinarian*, **9**, 958–964.

Reef, V.B. (1987) Mitral insufficiency associated with ruptured chordae tendineae in three foals. *Journal of the American Veterinary Medical Association*, **191**, 329–331.

Reef, V.B. (1990) A monesin outbreak in horses in the Eastern United States: pathogenesis, clinical signs and epidemiology. Proceedings of the Eighth Annual Veterinary Medical Forum of the American College of Veterinary Internal Medicine, pp. 619–621.

Reef, V.B. and Spencer, P.A. (1987) Echocardiographic evaluation of equine aortic insufficiency. *American Journal of Veterinary Research*, **48**, 904–909.

Reef, V.B., Gentile, D.G. and Freeman, D.E. (1984) Successful treatment of pericarditis in a horse. *Journal of the American Veterinary Medical Association*, **185**, 94–98.

Reef, V.B., Klump, S., Maxson, A.D. and Sweeney, R.W. (1990) Echocardiographic demonstration of an intact aneurysm in a horse. *Journal of the American Veterinary Medical Association*, **197**, 752–755.

Reef, V.B., Roby, K.A.W., Richardson, D.W. and Johnston, J.K. (1987) Use of ultrasonography for the detection of aortic-iliac thrombosis in horses. *Journal of the American Veterinary Medical Association*, **190**, 286–288.

Reimer, J., Reef, V.B. and Sommer, M. (1991) Echocardiographic detection of pulmonic valve rupture in a horse with right-sided heart failure. *Journal of the American Veterinary Medical Association*, **198**, 880–882.

Roby, K.A.W., Reef, V.B., Shaw, D.P. and Sweeney, C.R. (1986) Rupture of an aortic sinus aneurysm in a 15-year-old brood mare. *Journal of the American Veterinary Medical Association*, **189**, 305–308.

Rouseel, A.J. and Kasari, T.R. (1989) Bacterial endocarditis. Part II. Incidence, causes, clinical signs and pathologic findings. *Compendium of Continuing Education for the Practicing Veterinarian*, **11**, 769–773.

Shaftoe, S. and McGuirk, S.M. (1987) Valvular insufficiency in a horse with atrial fibrillation – a case report. *Compendium of Continuing Education for the Practicing Veterinarian*, **9**, 203–208.

Trim, C.M. (1994) Inotropic agents and vasopressors in equine anesthesia. *Compendium of Continuing Education for the Practicing Veterinarian*, **16**, 118–121.

Wagner, P.C., Miller, R.A., Merrit, F., Pickering, L.A. and Grant, B.D. (1977) Constrictive pericarditis in the horse. *Journal of Equine Medicine and Surgery*, **1**, 242–247.

Arrhythmias

Bertone, J.J. and Wingfield, W.E. (1987). Atrial fibrillation in horses. *Compendium of Continuing Education for the Practicing Veterinarian*, **9**, 763–769.

Bertone, J.J., Traub-Dargatz, J.L. and Wingfield, W.E. (1987) Atrial fibrillation in a pregnant mare: treatment with quinidine sulfate. *Journal of the American Veterinary Medical Association*, **190**, 1565–1566.

Cooper, S.A. (1962) Ventricular pre-excitation (Wolff–Parkinson–White syndrome) in a horse. *Veterinary Record*, **74**, 527–530.

Cornick, J.L. and Seahorn, T.L. (1990) Cardiac arrhythmias in horses with duodenitis/proximal jejunitis: six cases (1985–1988). *Journal of the American Veterinary Medical Association*, **197**, 1054–1059.

Dangman, K.H. and Boyden, P.A. (1988) Cellular mechanisms of cardiac arrhythmias. In: *Canine and feline cardiology*. (ed. P.R. Fox) Churchill Livingstone, New York, USA, pp. 269–287.

Deem, D.A. and Fregin, G.F. (1982) Atrial fibrillation in horses: a review of 106 clinical cases with consideration of prevalence, clinical signs and prognosis. *Journal of the American Veterinary Medical Association*, **180**, 261–265.

Epstein, Y. (1984) Relationship between potassium administration, hyperkalaemia and the electrocardiogram: an experimental study. *Equine Veterinary Journal*, **16**, 453–456.

Gelberg, H.B., Smetzer, D.L. and Foreman, J.H. (1991) Pulmonary hypertension as a cause of atrial fibrillation in young horses: four cases (1980–1989). *Journal of the American Veterinary Medical Association*, **198**, 679–682.

Glazier, D.B., Littledike, E.T. and Evans, R.D. (1979) Electrocardiographic changes in inducated hypocalcaemia and hypercalcaemia in horses. *Journal of Equine Medicine and Surgery*, **3**, 489–494.

Glazier, D.B., Littledike, E.T. and Evans, R.D. (1982) Electrocardiographic changes in induced hyperkalaemia in ponies. *American Journal of Veterinary Research*, **43**, 1934–1937.

Glendenning, S.A. (1965) The use of quinidine sulphate for the treatment of atrial fibrillation in 12 horses. *Veterinary Record*, **77**, 951–960.

Hamir, A.N. and Reef, V.B. (1989) Complications of a transvenous pacing catheter in a horse. *Journal of Comparative Pathology*, **101**, 317–326.

Hilwig, R.W. (1977) Cardiac arrhythmias in the horse. *Journal of the American Veterinary Medical Association*, **170**, 153–163.

Holmes, J.R., Darke, P.G.G. and Else, R.W. (1969) Atrial fibrillation in the horse. *Equine Veterinary Journal*, **1**, 212–222.

Holmes, J.R. (1987) Cardiac arrhythmias on the racecourse. *Equine Exercise Physiology*, **2**, 781–785.

Holmes, J.R., Henigan, M., Williams, R.B. and Witherington, D.H. (1986) Paroxysmal atrial fibrillation in racehorses. *Equine Veterinary Journal*, **18**, 37–42.

Marr, C.M. (1991) An echocardiographic study of atrial fibrillation in horses before and after treatment with quinidine sulphate. Proceedings of the Ninth Annual Medical Forum of the American College of Veterinary Internal Medicine, p. 367.

McGuirk, S.M., Muir, W.W. and Sams, R.A. (1981) Pharmacokinetic analysis of intravenously and orally administered quinidine in horses. *American Journal of Veterinary Research*, **42**, 938–942.

McGuirk, S.M. and Muir, W.W. (1985) Diagnosis and treatment of cardiac arrhythmias. *Veterinary Clinics of North America* (Equine Practice), **1**, 353–370.

Miller, P.J. and Holmes, J.R. (1984) Relationships of left side systolic time intervals to beat-by-beat heart rate and blood pressure variables in some cardiac arrhythmias of the horse. *Research in Veterinary Science*, **37**, 18–25.

Morris, D.D. and Fregin, G.F. (1982) Atrial fibrillation in horses: factors associated with response to quinidine sulfate in 77 clinical cases. *Cornell Veterinarian*, **72**, 339–349.

Muir, W.W. and McGuirk, S.M. (1983) Ventricular pre-excitation in two horses. *Journal of the American Veterinary Medical Association*, **183**, 573–576.

Muir, W.W. and McGuirk, S.M. (1984) Haemodynamics before and after conversion of atrial fibrillation to normal sinus rhythm in horses. *Journal of the American Veterinary Medical Association*, **184**, 965–970.

Muir, W.W. and McGuirk, S.M. (1985) Pharmacology and pharmacokinetics of drugs used to treat cardiac disease in horses. *Veterinary Clinics of North America* (Equine Practice), **1**, 335–352.

Muir, W.W., Reed, S.M. and McGuirk, S.M. (1990) Treatment of atrial fibrillation in horses by intravenous administration of quinidine. *Journal of the American Veterinary Medical Association*, **197**, 1607–1610.

Pibarot, P., Vrins, A., Salmon, Y. and Difruscia, R. (1993) Implantation of a programmable atrioventricular pacemaker in a donkey with complete atrioventricular block and syncope. *Equine Veterinary Journal*, **25**, 248–251.

Reef, V.B. (1991) New perspective on the treatment of equine atrial fibrillation. Proceedings of the Ninth Annual Medical Forum of the American College of Veterinary Internal Medicine, pp. 363–365.

Reef, V.B., Clark, E.S., Oliver, J.A. and Donawick, W.J. (1986) Implantation of a permanent transvenous pacing catheter in a horse with complete heart block and syncope. *Journal of the American Veterinary Medical Association*, **189**, 449–452.

Reef, V.B., Levitan, C.W. and Spencer, P.A. (1989) Factors influencing prognosis and treatment in horses with atrial fibrillation. *Journal of Veterinary Internal Medicine*, **2**, 1–6.

Reimer, J.M., Reef, V.B. and Sweeney, R.W. (1992) Ventricular arrhythmias in horses: 21 cases (1984–1989). *Journal of the American Veterinary Medical Association*, **201**, 1237–1243.

Wagner, A.E., Muir, W.W. and Hinchcliffe, K.W. (1991) Cardiovascular effects of xylaxine and detomidine in horses. *American Journal of Veterinary Research*, **52**, 651–657.

Yamamoto, K., Yasuda, J. and Too, K. (1992) Arrhythmias in newborn Thoroughbred foals. *Equine Veterinary Journal*, **24**, 169–173.

Problem situations

Brown, C.M. (1989) Poor or reduced athletic performance. In: *Problems in Equine Medicine*, (ed. C.M. Brown). Lea & Febinger, Philadelphia, pp. 229–244.

Brown, C.M., Kaneene, J.B. and Taylor, R.F. (1988) Sudden and unexpected death in horses and ponies: and analysis of 200 cases. *Equine Veterinary Journal*, **20**, 99–103.

Brown, C.M., Taylor, R.F. and Slanker, M.R. (1987) Sudden and unexpected death in adult horses. *Compendium of Continuing Education for the Practicing Veterinarian*, **9**, 78–86.

Dixon, P.M. (1995) Collection of tracheal respiratory secretions in the horse. *In Practice*, **17**, 66–69.

Gelberg, H.B., Zachary, J.F., Everitt, J.I., Jensen, R.C. and Smetzer, D.L. (1985) Sudden death in training and racing Thoroughbred horses. *Journal of the American Veterinary Medical Association*, **187**, 1354–1356.

Lucke, V.M. (1987) Sudden death. *Equine Veterinary Journal*, **19**, 85–86.

Lunn, D.P., Cuddon, P.A., Shaftoe, S. and Archer, R.M. (1993) Familial occurrence of narcolepsy in Minature horses. *Equine Veterinary Journal*, **25**, 483–487.

Mair, T. (1992) Diagnostic techniques for lower respiratory tract diseases. In: *Current Therapy in Equine Medicine*, 3rd ed. (Ed. N.E. Robinson). W.B. Saunders, Philadelphia, pp. 299–303.

Mayhew, I.G. (1989) Coma and altered states of consciousness. In: *Large animal neurology: a handbook for veterinary clinicians*, Lea and Febinger, Philadelphia, USA, pp. 133–146.

Morris, E.A. (section Ed.) (1992) Assessment of performance problems. In: *Current Therapy in Equine Medicine*, 3rd ed. (Ed. N.E. Robinson). W.B. Saunders, Philadelphia, pp. 771–814.

Morris, E.A. and Seeherman, H.J. (1991) Clinical evaluation of poor performance in the racehorse: the results of 275 evaluations. *Equine Veterinary Journal*, **23**, 169–174.

Platt, H. (1982) Sudden and unexpected death in horses: a review of 69 cases. *British Veterinary Journal*, **138**, 417–429.

Reef, V.B. Clinical approach to poor performance in horses. Proceedings of the Seventh Annual Medical Forum of the American College of Veterinary Internal Medicine, pp. 566–569.

Sweeney, C.R., Hendricks, J.C., Beech, J. and Morison, A.R. (1983) Narcolepsy in a horse. *Journal of the American Veterinary Medical Association*, **183**, 126–128.

Index